Conduct Unbecoming a Woman

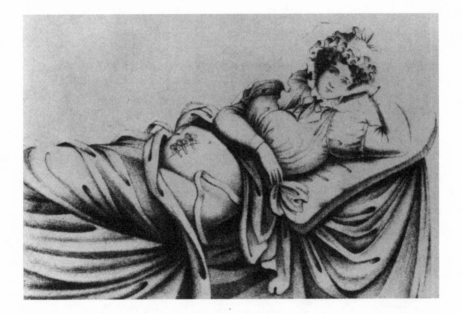

Conduct Unbecoming a Woman

Medicine on Trial in Turn-of-the-Century Brooklyn

Regina Morantz-Sanchez

New York Oxford
Oxford University Press
1999

Oxford University Press

Oxford   New York

Athens   Auckland   Bangkok   Bogotá   Buenos Aires   Calcutta
Cape Town   Chennai   Dar es Salaam   Delhi   Florence   Hong Kong   Istanbul
Karachi   Kuala Lumpur   Madrid   Melbourne   Mexico City   Mumbai
Nairobi   Paris   São Paulo   Singapore   Taipei   Tokyo   Toronto   Warsaw

and associated companies in
Berlin   Ibadan

Published by Oxford University Press, Inc.
198 Madison Avenue, New York, New York 10016

Oxford is a registered trademark of Oxford University Press

Library of Congress Cataloging-in-Publication Data
Morantz-Sanchez, Regina Markell.
Conduct unbecoming a woman : medicine on trial in turn-of-the-
century Brooklyn / Regina Morantz-Sanchez.
p.   cm.
Includes bibliographical references and index.
ISBN 0-19-512624-6
1. Gynecology—United States—History—19th century.   2. Dixon
Jones, Mary Amanda—Trials, litigation, etc.   3. Brooklyn daily
eagle—Trials, litigation, etc.   4. Gynecology—Law and legislation—
United States—History—19th century.   5. Gynecologists—Legal
status, laws, etc.—New York (State)—History—19th century.
6. Brooklyn (New York, N.Y.)   I. Title.
RG67.U6M67   1999
618.1'00973'09034—dc21   98-29764

Frontispiece: From J. P. Maygrier mit Eduard von Siebold, *Abbildungen aus dem
Gesammtgebiete der theoretischen-praktischen Geburtshülfe, nebst beschreibender
Erklärung derselben*, Taf LX. Reutlinger: Verlag von Jacob von Ensslin, 1836.
Courtesy of the University of Kentucky Library.

1 3 5 7 9 8 6 4 2

Printed in the United States of America
on acid-free paper

for ghe

Contents

Acknowledgments

Long projects accumulate a lot of debt. I owe thanks to many people. Skilled archivists facilitated my research at every juncture. Special thanks are due to a group of dedicated souls at the Archives on Women in Medicine at the Medical College of Pennsylvania, now Allegheny University of the Health Sciences, whose willingness to service this project always resulted in a cheerful and speedy response to my requests. I am grateful beyond measure to Sandra Chaff, Margaret Jerrido, Jill Gates Smith, Teresa R. Taylor, and, more recently, Barbara Williams. Equally helpful were the people in Special Collections at the New York Academy of Medicine, especially Caroline Melish. Barbara L. Krieger facilitated photograph reproduction at Dartmouth University Library. Susan Rishworth, head of the Archives of the American College of Obstetricians and Gynecologists, was the gracious and cheerful administrator of a research grant from that organization that gave me a month of unprecedented freedom to browse among a wonderful collection of gynecology textbooks and old medical journals in an extraordinarily comfortable and serviceable setting. The staff at King's County Medical Society cheerfully allowed me to poke through papers and manuscripts stored in their records room. Librarians at the Brooklyn Historical Society, the New-York Historical Society, the New York Municipal Archives, and the National Library of Medicine also extended aid. Librarian Gordon Mestler, Kathy Powderly of the Division of Humanities in Medicine, and archivist Jack E. Termine, all at the State University of New York Health

Science Center at Brooklyn, were enormously giving of their time. At the Lawson Tait Collection in Birmingham, England, Stan Jenkins, Mrs. Elaine Simpson, Mrs. Lilian Salt, and especially Dr. Brian Gough made my research there a memorable experience. Librarians at the Wellcome Institute and the Royal College of Physicians in London also deserve thanks. Other institutional staffs offering aid were at the Oregon Historical Society, Harvard University Special Collections, the Louise Darling Medical Library at UCLA, and the interlibrary loan departments of UCLA and the University of Michigan.

The painstaking detective work this book required could not have been accomplished without generous financial support from several sources. In addition to the ACOG fellowship mentioned above, I received a National Endowment for the Humanities summer fellowship, a grant from the National Library of Medicine, and two NEH Senior Fellowships. The NEH's Division of Science, Technology, and Medicine enabled me to complete the project, and Dan Jones at the helm of that division was a particularly supportive administrator. UCLA and the University of Michigan also offered generous help in the form of faculty research grants.

The department of history at the University of Michigan extended me a different kind of encouragement. Its administrative and support staff has proved to be among the most efficient and good-natured I have ever encountered. As for my colleagues, I cannot sing their praises too highly. From them I have been granted an abiding nourishment rare in many academic settings and have found myself welcomed into an intellectual community made up of scintillating scholars as well as compassionate human beings.

I have been blessed with a collection of graduate students, some of whom have already gone on to successful academic careers, whose research assistance has been invaluable. Sue Zschoche and Margaret Finnegan took this project as seriously as if it were their own. Both went above and beyond the call of duty repeatedly and without complaint and also provided a stimulating sounding board for my ideas and theories. At UCLA, Pat Moore, Joan Johnson, John Olmstead, and, especially, Sue Gonda and Charles Romney deserve thanks. Maureen Stewart, Becky Conekin, Ruth Hartman, John Mogul, and Leslie Paris at the University of Michigan also made important contributions toward moving the research along. Leslie offered ideas and interpretations as well. Michelle Seldin handled the frustrating task of tracking down photographs with efficiency and good cheer and helped prepare the index. Charles Romney and Maureen Henke, at Fourth Dimension Interactive, provided technical assistance in rendering the map of Brooklyn.

Early in this project, the encouragement and intellectual support of Barbara Bair, Jane Sewell, Dale C. Smith, Anita Clair Fellman, Gert Brieger, Gerald Grob, Ed Tenner, Burt Hansen, Sue Zschoche, Sue Gonda, Charles Romney, Ann Lombard, Margaret Finnegan, and George Sanchez was invaluable. Others read and critiqued parts or all of the manuscript. Joel Howell, Jane Sewall, Russ Maulitz, Tom Bonner, and Dale C. Smith monitored the accuracy of the medical history. Joel Howell read the entire manuscript at least twice. Other indefatigable critics were Ellen Chesler, Arleen Tuchman, Sara Blair, Bruce Shulman, Deborah Kuhn McGregor, Susan Douglass, Charlotte Borst, Leslie Paris, Robyn Muncy, Nancy Theriot, and members of the Center for the Study of Social Transformation at the University of Michigan. Finally, the unstinting intellectual input of Louise Newman and Geoff Eley cannot be measured. They read and reread drafts of chapters every step of the way and in the end became collaborators who pushed and pushed until I got it right.

I am also grateful for the bountiful sustenance of a number of extraordinary friends who helped move me through some rough spots. Geoff Eley, Anita Clair Fellman, John Efron, Barbara Bair, Louise Newman, Alice Blue and Marc Fitzerman, Karl and Diane Pohrt, Joan Meisel and Lee Hunt, Ellen Chesler and Matt Mallow, Susan Douglass and T. R. Durham, David Scobey and Denise Thal, Kathy Dalton and Tony Rotundo, Kate Schechter and Ari Roth, Jonathan Freedman and Sara Blair, Anita Norich, Peggy Somers, Kathleen Canning, Sonya Rose, Kali Israel, Bruce Shulman and Alice Killian, Julia Adams and Jeff Jordan, Robin Kelley and Dierdre Harris-Kelley, Bill and Lorna Chafe, Mitch and Phyllis Miller, John Chambers, Harvard Sitkoff, Valerie Matsumoto, and Brenda Stevenson deserve special mention.

Thomas LeBien of Oxford University Press is an old-fashioned, hands-on editor. His insights are impeccable, and it has been an utter pleasure working with him. I was very fortunate. His assistant, Susan Ferber, couldn't have been more efficient or encouraging. Joellyn Ausanka was a cheerful and skilled production editor, and I was particularly pleased to be able to renew her acquaintance.

My family is forever a source of personal growth: I thank my children, Adam Max Sanchez, Alison Morantz, and Jessica and Shaya Billowitz; my grandchildren, Sara Chana, Bracha, and Dovid Mordecai; my brother, Jon Markell, and his wife, Carrie; my mother, Rosalind Markell; and May and Ralph Ziskin.

Conduct Unbecoming a Woman

Introduction

Nothing that has ever happened should be regarded as lost for history.
  —*WALTER BENJAMIN, Theses of the Philosophy of History*

In February and March 1892, Brooklyn's one million citizens were riveted by the spectacle of an extraordinary libel trial pitting their largest newspaper, the Brooklyn *Daily Eagle*, against Dr. Mary Amanda Dixon Jones, a female gynecological surgeon of considerable national and international reputation. The newspaper had printed a series of lurid articles in the spring of 1889 that not only hinted at financial improprieties but portrayed the doctor as an ambitious and unscrupulous social climber, a knife-happy, over-eager, and irresponsible practitioner who forced unnecessary operations on unsuspecting women and used the specimens gleaned from their bodies to advance her reputation in diagnosis and treatment. These startling feature stories set off an avalanche of public criticism, eventually giving rise to two manslaughter indictments and eight malpractice suits. It took almost two years for Dixon Jones to clear her name of all criminal and civil charges. She then retaliated by suing the *Eagle*, seeking $150,000 in damages.[1]

  The two-month legal extravaganza of 1892 was the longest libel suit tried in the United States to date. It involved leading physicians in New York and Brooklyn, as well as an array of witnesses, including humble craftsmen and seamstresses, immigrants speaking only broken English, tradesmen and their industrious wives, former patients with babies in their arms, and prominent members of Brooklyn's professional and commercial elite. Roughly 300 people testified. For the first time, jars full of specimens and surgical mannequins became common sights in the courtroom, while the indications for radical gynecological surgery were discussed in obscure and technical language by leading pathologists and surgeons from New York, Brooklyn, New Jersey, and Philadelphia. According to the *Eagle*, the trial attracted a throng of curious onlookers, decidedly not the "idle loungers that form the divorce or murder trial audience," but professional men, "citizens of standing and reputation," and significant numbers of respectable women.[2] Lawyers estimated that the *Eagle*'s court costs were in the range of $30,000.[3]

In his charge to the jury, Judge Willard Bartlett, whose legal career had rendered him particularly experienced in libel cases, apologized for his inability to summarize the proceedings adequately, noting that "hundreds of witnesses have been examined, thousands of pages of testimony have been taken. My own notes," he admitted, pointing to the stack of four notebooks beside him, "amount merely to a skeleton of the proof." Indeed, what made the trial unique in legal history was the fact that the offending libelous passages encompassed an unprecedented 69,000 words, comprising reading material considerably longer than an ordinary novel.[4] Moreover, at the end of twenty-three hours of deliberation, a frustrated jury begged the judge to be discharged. Incensed, Bartlett refused. They debated an additional eighteen hours before reaching their verdict.[5]

The press covered the proceedings with interest. The New York *Tribune* dubbed the inquiry "by far the most important ever tried in this city." The Brooklyn *Citizen*, the Brooklyn *Times*, the New York *Times*, and the New York *World* highlighted the story. The *Brooklyn Medical Journal* claimed that the event involved the "honor and reputation" of its medical establishment, and even the *Journal of the American Medical Association* commented on the verdict. The *Eagle* reported from court almost daily, and printed much of the testimony verbatim, while the Philadelphia *Ledger* hailed the case as "the most important . . . since the Beecher" scandal, a reference to the salacious Beecher–Tilton adultery trial that had riveted citizens in the New York area in the early 1870s.[6]

A month after the decision was handed down, Charles Dixon Jones, Mary's son and surgical partner, broke into the home of Dr. Joseph H. Raymond, former Brooklyn Health Commissioner and the editor of the *Brooklyn Medical Journal*. Enraged, Charles dragged the older man from his bed and horsewhipped him when he refused to retract a negative editorial just published by the *Journal*. Though the affair was eventually settled with the offer of an apology, the incident seemed a graphic ending to an electrifying couple of months.[7]

Manifestly a remarkable event in 1892, the Dixon Jones imbroglio disappeared from the historical record only a few years later. The newspaper quickly turned to bigger and better campaigns, while Dixon Jones closed her surgical practice and moved to New York City. Using slides and specimens she had accumulated during her surgical career, she spent the next decade working in and publishing articles on the clinical pathology of the female reproductive system. Already advanced in years when the trial occurred, she died in 1908 at the age of eighty. By 1928, when the editors of the *Dictionary of American Medical Biography* alluded to the episode in their published biographical sketch of this admittedly singular woman, the incident had largely been forgotten.[8]

Yet the Dixon Jones affair compels our attention. A marvelous tale, it has all the components of an intricately crafted suspense novel. Innocent patients died. Others recovered from dangerous surgery only to discover that they could never bear children. Investigative reporters doggedly tracked rumors of malfeasance. A female physician went on trial for manslaughter. Brooklyn's leading newspaper conducted a protracted smear campaign, accusing Dixon Jones of displaying a "mania" for the knife. The libel trial that resulted brought the city's upper crust under scrutiny. The management of public and private structures of philanthropy was called into question.

What follows is unabashedly a work of historical reconstruction. Dixon Jones's story was obscured in the historical record. It intruded into my research now and then, much as tiny patches of desert vegetation appear when seen from an airplane—like blotches encroaching aimlessly on the uniform character of the landscape. Knowledge of the event accumulated just as serendipitously. Traces presented themselves in random fashion: an article of Dixon Jones's on ovariotomy with a footnote referring vaguely to the betrayal of jealous colleagues in Brooklyn, a letter to the dean from a female physician colleague inquiring about Dixon Jones's record at the Woman's Medical College of Pennsylvania, a negative report from another well-meaning woman doctor in Brooklyn describing an unnamed woman physician whose obvious talent could not compensate for her coarse manners and questionable reputation. These fragments hinted at an interesting tale waiting to be told. Using letters, trial proceedings published in the Brooklyn *Eagle*, summaries of events described elsewhere, newspaper accounts, maps, city archives, medical articles, biographical information, and medical school, hospital, and specialty society proceedings and archives, I offer the results of ten years of detective work.

The story is a resifting of the evidence pondered by Dixon Jones's two juries and a revisiting of their verdicts, guided by hindsight and a better grasp of context. Though the gaps in the record are real, and the motivations and private thoughts of leading participants unattainable, there is much that can be said to make this affair comprehensible. While my own perspective is every bit as partial as that of the eleven men who judged Dixon Jones,[9] I have also had access to evidence beyond their knowledge: private remarks voiced about the outcome, the opinions and responses of contemporaries after the trials, an historian's understanding of the social change that provided a formative, if default backdrop. This makes my perspective a very different one from theirs.

Of course, I believe there is more here than simply a good story. Adequately contextualized, this fascinating incident opens a window onto complex processes of social change, not just in Brooklyn, but in the nation at large. For example, the trial represents a chapter in the social history of medicine, marking in all its complexity the emergence of new models of professional identity and the birth of a challenging medical subspecialty—gynecological surgery—that catalyzed a rethinking of attitudes toward specialization and toward the female body. Because not all physicians saw these developments as positive, the event is also a study in professional rivalry and competition. Additionally, the affair speaks eloquently of public perceptions of medicine, offering insight into how ordinary men and women viewed some of the most dramatic technological and scientific advances in medical practice generated in the last third of the nineteenth century. It reveals much about the intimate relations between patients and their doctors as well. Nor can the complex implications of the trial be properly understood without considering the emerging culture of the urban middle class, or weighing the growing importance of Brooklyn as a metropolitan center. The specific habits and character of the city's respectable elites had much to do with the attention given the affair as a public event. Moreover, it is unlikely the libel suit would ever have occurred had it not been for the increasing importance of the press as an instrument of cultural production and social control in the city. Finally, because its leading actor was a woman accused of murder and mayhem, the episode compels us to ask how and in what specific ways gender tensions structured these other themes.

Work on this book has benefited in countless ways from recently expanded scholarly definitions of what counts as history. In particular, historians' experiments with what Robert Darnton has called "history in the ethnographic grain" had yielded exhilarating results. This approach to the study of the past has uncovered uniquely striking source material in popular trials and other public spectacles, which scholars have read revealingly as social theater.[10]

Given our own experience with sensational trials in the last decade, we cannot help but be impressed by the rhetorical significance of such events. Trials, for example, by using a variety of techniques of persuasion and dramatization, carefully construct arguments that can advance the causes of participants, both within and outside the courtroom. Each side hopes to appear narratively coherent and rational to the larger public, which will eventually ponder and judge. The Dixon Jones libel case was just such a contest—one that imbued ordinary social life with dramatic meaning. That the incident attracted considerable public notice suggests that it marked a moment of collective self-reflection, crisis resolution, and transformation.[11]

To explain how this occurred, this book draws heavily on recent work in feminist theory and the history of medicine, especially scholarship on professionalization, doctors and patients, and the female body.[12] By insisting that gender be separated from biological sex as a category of analysis, feminist scholars have been busy demonstrating how and in what specific ways modern gender roles were fashioned, as was modern science itself, through culture.

My past work on women physicians in the United States, for example, argued that in the colonial period women participated in healing as nurses, midwives, and practitioners of folk medicine. Professional medicine was closed to them because in Anglo-American tradition, a physician had to be a *gentleman.* Though reality in the United States fell far short of the ideal, the identification of formal medical knowledge with men continued until the mid-nineteenth century. By then, complicated social changes, including the development of the ideology of domesticity and a powerful popular critique of professional expertise in general, accompanied by holistic approaches to illness that required sympathy and intuitive medical judgment from all practitioners, opened up opportunities for women to study medicine. Based on the limitations of mid-nineteenth century physicians' power to cure, there were strong arguments for women's superior ability to care for ill patients and provide the emotional support many of them required. Eventually, new concepts of professionalism and a new ideology of science emerged in the second half of the nineteenth century that repositioned women in the profession in complicated ways but eventually worked to curtail their increasing numbers and marginalize their contributions within the twentieth-century professional world. At every juncture in this long process, had the historical circumstances been slightly altered, women might have developed a different relationship to medicine. The present study of Mary Dixon Jones's career reopens some of these questions about late nineteenth century professionalization, offering an in-depth perspective on some of the issues which only a case study can provide.[13]

Politics, male anxiety about shifts in power relations between the sexes, social and political upheaval, professional concerns, and changes in the family all had an impact on women's fate as professional practitioners. But these forces also produced new knowledge regarding the female body, including the "discovery," invention, and treatment of a wide range of female ailments, from anorexia nervosa to fibroid tumors. As gynecology emerged as a specialty, it targeted women's bodies as a case apart, elaborating on the theme of women's biological difference, a subject that, along with parallel theories about race, dominated the newer disciplines of biology, embryology, genetics, and the emerging social sciences of anthropology, psychology, and sociology.[14]

Mary Dixon Jones practiced gynecology and gynecological surgery at a time when many members of her specialty sought to fashion a coherent program for female health and a shared explanation for women's social role based on biological theory. Some invented a therapeutic regimen that ultimately entailed the invasion of the body through the surgical removal of the reproductive organs. How she managed to balance her sense of herself as a woman and as a professional who participated actively in these developments is a central theme in this study.

There is another reason that Mary Dixon Jones's story is important. Because in many respects she invented herself, her career reveals a great deal about the fashioning of a culture and life-style unique to the urbanizing middle class in the late nineteenth century. Scholars in the last decade have been particularly interested in how new notions of public space and public responsibility emerged in western Europe and the United States during and after the Age of Revolution.[15] American historians have used this work to describe the characteristics of an urbanized, class-stratified, mixed-sex public culture that began to appear in the nation's cities in the decades after the Civil War. They have argued that middle-class identity was constructed from the "physical milieux" and "social round of daily life" that gave rise to new styles and manners, new notions of proper behavior and social responsibility, new constructions of family life, gender roles, child nurturance and education, domestic space, and taste. Carpets, sofas, and pianos—artifacts of a new life-style—shaped social relations and taught etiquette in complex ways, even as they helped distinguish the living quarters of the respectable from those of the very rich, as well as the poor.[16]

The social values, styles, and networks that gave the emerging bourgeoisie coherence often did not seek expression directly through politics, but were based on a "canon of domestic privatism and intraclass sociability" that was powerfully catalyzed by women.[17] Indeed, the boundaries between public and private in the nineteenth century were constantly shifting, always permeable, and often intertwined.[18] Thus female reform and professional activity in this period has been understood as "quasi-political." Though produced on behalf of and flowing out of private domestic life, female charitable and benevolent enterprise, which expanded and diversified in complex ways after the Civil War, could be represented as one form of women's entry into the public sphere. For a time, Mary Dixon Jones and her Woman's Hospital in Brooklyn were lavish recipients of this uniquely female-organized social largesse.[19]

Indeed, the work of women doctors like Mary Dixon Jones represented the ways in which many middle-class women eroded the gulf between women's private life and the public domain. Women entered the medical profession as part of a determined effort to apply the civilizing effects of womanhood to the needs of an increasingly unstable and rapidly industrializing society. Like female teachers, they were comfortable touting their special skills at nurturance, and armed themselves with the conviction that the profession of medicine needed the "leaven of tender humanity that women represent."[20]

But once women entered the field, they were socialized as professionals, and they quickly learned that the ethos of professionalism was a profoundly gendered phenomenon. Increasingly, toward the end of the century, medical school curricula, residency programs, specialty societies, and teaching methods were structured around cultural conceptions of masculinity and geared toward the male life-cycle. Those who attempted to alter the direction of medical practice in significant ways were generally marginalized, while women who were willing to "blend in" had to work harder than their male colleagues for lesser public recognition and reward. Other female physicians developed their own version of female professionalism, one that combined a belief in women's special gifts at patient care with a willingness to defer to men by concentrating their attention on preventive medicine and the treatment of women and children.[21] Refracted through the narrative of the libel trial, Mary Dixon Jones's life speaks eloquently to these group dilemmas, demonstrating that there were limits to how, when, and in what manner women could enter the professional public sphere.

The Dixon Jones affair indirectly illuminates another source of women's entrance into the public realm, one that emerged most noticeably in the last third of the century. This was middle-class housewives' gradual appearance in specific commercialized spaces of the city, which were remade to accommodate their new responsibilities as consumers. Women's role as family purchasing agents became increasingly elaborate, as dynamic urban locales, with magnificent department stores, specialty shops, restaurants, and newly refurbished theaters, enticed women out of the home and competed with more traditional forms of leisure and benevolent activity for their attention and patronage. It was a world where style, fashion, display, opulence, materialism, and the buying and selling of goods melded together to demand a special kind of competence, helping to create new models of the "lady in public." It was also a world in which women became more responsible for their own health and the health of their families. Their role as consumers of health care is an essential part of Dixon Jones's rise to prominence as a gynecologist.

Scholars attracted to what has been called "the linguistic turn" in the social sciences have attempted to understand cultural formation by focusing on the interrelationship between language and the creation of individual consciousness, social organization, and structures of power. Their emphasis on the necessity of multiple perspectives has challenged traditional depictions of culture as unified and coherent, and they stress the instability of meanings and the numerous contradictions inherent in particular historical events.[22] These cautions have guided my interpretations of the Mary Dixon Jones trial. The nature of the evidence makes it impossible to reach immutable and consistent conclusions about the motives of each of the participants. Nor can one argue that one version of the story is more "true" than any of the others. I have a point of view, but, in the final analysis, it is the reader who must choose which narrative presented here makes the most sense.

The book consists of nine chapters. The first will describe and measure the ramified effects of the original twenty-four articles published by the *Eagle* from April 24 to June 16, 1889. Chapter 2 draws an in-depth portrait of Brooklyn as a burgeoning metropolis, seeking to explain at least in part what made this city such a logical site for an event of this kind. The middle four chapters turn to issues in medicine. Chapter 3 chronicles Mary Dixon Jones's route to becoming a surgeon, demonstrating that this woman kept company with some very talented male surgeons who shared her approach to patient care. Chapter 4 offers what I hope is a unique historical overview of the emergence of gynecology in the United States, arguing that surgery as a whole, and gynecological surgery in particular, was highly contested among practitioners, with some endorsing radical procedures and others calling them into question. Chapter 5 examines gynecologists' and gynecological surgeons' ideas about female health, seeking to consider how and in what ways the practitioner's gender shaped attitudes. Chapter 6 explores the complexities of the physician-patient encounter by reconstructing the patient's world and attempting to understand why many women might have actively sought operations. In Chapter 7 we return to the courtroom for a detailed examination of the manslaughter trial, and in Chapter 8 we examine the rhetorics and narratives of the libel trial itself. The final chapter speculates on the larger social and cultural meanings of the affair.

The surgeon Howard Kelly's curious sketch of Mary Dixon Jones in the 1920 edition of the *Dictionary of American Medical Biography* speaks to her complexity as an historical figure. Kelly was a younger contemporary, a brilliant surgeon who made his career as one of the shining stars of the faculty at Johns Hopkins Medical School, which opened its doors in 1893. His report of Dixon Jones's suit against the Brooklyn *Eagle* for allegations of malpractice is clearly reproachful in tone, not because he necessarily believed the accusations, but for Dixon Jones's willingness to risk making herself a public spectacle. Summing up her life, he observed:

> Dr. Jones was peculiar in person, flashy, and tawdry in appearance, but undoubtedly a student. Lack of judgment and of intimate contact with the better members of the profession may have been responsible for a certain mental obliquity with which she is accredited. The Nestor of surgery in Brooklyn declared that "she was quite a pachyderm."[23]

One takes note of Kelly's admiration for Dixon Jones's intellectual drive, but pauses at the use of the word "tawdry." As our story unfolds, we shall see that the Brooklyn *Eagle* took pains to paint Dixon Jones in a negative light, but though the newspaper often discussed her appearance, it never claimed that she looked cheap or gaudy. Moreover, in Victorian parlance, "pachyderm" referred to a person who was thick-skinned and insensitive, an individual who did not shrink from a fight. Her biographer's choice of words suggests that Victorian men had no appropriate language to describe the unconventionality of this singular woman. They resorted instead to familiar terms of female denigration. Dixon Jones may or may not have forced life-threatening operations on timid patients, botched surgery that ultimately led to death, and mismanaged funds at her small hospital. Of these matters we will learn a great deal more before we judge. Mary Dixon Jones deliberately avoided close connections with the female professional networks that proffered support and affiliation after she completed her medical education. She chose a more aggressive and individualistic path to professional success, one that prompted her to seek out male colleagues, rather than female ones. Whatever we conclude about her skills as a surgeon, it is also true that she was a woman who either deliberately or unknowingly ignored the gender scripts that dictated professional behavior for a female physician of her time. And for that, among other things, she was punished.

My attempt to read Mary Dixon Jones, the woman doctor, back into the historical record gives her something she deeply craved during her lifetime: a place in history. Ironically, she will not necessarily be remembered for the reasons she might have wished. How could she have known in 1892 that her angry libel suit against the Brooklyn *Eagle* would locate her at the center of an intense debate bringing together for public consideration important and weighty questions in medicine, professionalization, social relations, and gender roles? In the final analysis, it was not her remarkable surgical achievements, of which she was justly proud, but the transgressive nature of her professional career that rescues her from historical obscurity, making her, at long last, a worthy subject for history.

1

Saving the City from Corruption: The *Eagle* Launches a Campaign

On February 14, 1889, Ida Hunt, the twenty-six-year-old wife of a printer, checked herself into the Woman's Hospital of Brooklyn for the removal of a tumor. According to the account published in the Brooklyn *Eagle*, Ida was robust and physically fit. L. P. Grover, a physician who had treated her since childhood, found her "beautiful and healthy" when he had examined her six months before. Though he admitted to noting a sensitive and "slightly irritated" organ "on the left side," he assured her that she suffered a minor reflex irritation that would readily yield to bromides. When Ida asked whether she needed an operation, he "strongly advised against it."[1]

But Ida was dissatisfied with Grover's diagnosis. Plagued with headaches, she visited several local physicians and T. Gaillard Thomas, the world-renowned gynecologist at the Woman's Hospital in New York City, before settling on Mary Dixon Jones. Countering the advice of the male practitioners, Dixon Jones diagnosed the presence of a worrisome tissue mass and cautioned that the growth could burst without warning, killing her or driving her insane. Though her skeptical husband begged her to reconsider, Ida trusted Dixon Jones, insisting that the doctor was "a very nice lady and a good Christian and very pious, that she always prayed before she performed an operation, and that she had . . . saved the wife of an eminent banker from the same trouble." Ida seemed delighted to share a physician with the wife of a prominent businessman, and was much reassured by the doctor's claim to have performed eighty-five laparotomies without losing a patient.[2] After nine days' preparatory in the hospital, Ida Hunt submitted to surgery.

Participants disagree as to what happened next. The operation went badly, and peritonitis ensued. Several days later, Dixon Jones told James Hunt that the cancerous tumor had burst during "one of the most terrible operations I have ever performed." Hunt understood that his wife was dying and called Ida's father, a bricklayer and veteran fireman, to the hospital. Together they sat by her bedside for hours, leaving late in the evening. The next morning, according the *Eagle*, Hunt received a request by telephone to hurry to the hospital. When he arrived, Dixon Jones asked him to take Ida home. Her case was hopeless, the doctor explained, and she needed familiar surroundings. But a little later, when Hunt brought the carriage to fetch his wife, Dixon Jones announced that the patient had rallied, and refused to let her leave. Then, at eleven that evening, there was a knock at their door, waking both Hunt and Ida's parents, the DeVoes. On Dixon Jones's behalf, Mary, the hospital nurse, urged a rapid return to the hospital. Ida must be brought home immediately.

The anxious family complied. A storm was gathering. Bitter cold, it was already snowing hard, with accumulation so far of half an inch. At two o'clock in the morning, the *Eagle* reported, the dying Ida was gently laid into a carriage, sandwiched between Dixon Jones and her mother, and resting on blankets and pillows provided, not by the doctor, but by her father. Friction ensued between Dixon Jones and Ida's parents. When Mrs. DeVoe complained about taking her daughter out in the snow, Dixon Jones allegedly dismissed the idea, insisting that "the ride will do her good." The father told the *Eagle* that it later dawned on him that Dixon Jones wanted the girl moved so that death would occur "at some other place than the hospital." The doctor deliberately waited until nighttime, he asserted, "so that the neighbors would not see."

Once settled in her own bed, Ida denounced Dixon Jones and Jones's son Charles, her surgical assistant, calling them "murderers and hypocrites." She claimed that at the very last moment she had changed her mind about having the procedure. "I fought as hard as I could and screamed," an expiring Ida told her mother. But Mrs. Jones administered the ether by force, insisting, "You've gone this far and now you've got to go through with it." When Ida regained consciousness after the surgery, she heard someone admit that "something had gone wrong." Distraught until the very end, Ida Hunt expired in her mother's arms at 11:30 the next morning.[3]

Only days later, Mr. DeVoe visited Dixon Jones, seeking certification of the cause of death on Ida's insurance papers. The doctor responded by presenting a bill for her medical services, promising to sign the insurance forms as soon as it was paid. DeVoe asked to see the tumor Dixon Jones had removed from his daughter's body. "Oh, why didn't you come before?" she answered. "We've just shipped it to Paris." "I told a doctor that," DeVoe informed the *Eagle*'s reporter, "and he laughed and said they had tumors enough of their own in Paris without importing any. I don't believe Ida ever had a tumor," he added. Even more curious, the undertaker and embalmer judged Ida's body to be in a suspicious state. Apparently, the stitches from the abdominal incision had ripped open and the body cavity was stuffed with ether-soaked rags "covered with loose flaps of skin left by the operation."[4]

The high drama of Ida's last ride, accomplished stealthily in the darkest of night in near blizzard conditions, became for the Brooklyn *Eagle* a central marker in a larger narrative crafted with great care and sensitivity, particularly to readers hungry for good copy. Ida is portrayed as an innocent young victim in the prime of life, beloved by a loyal and caring family, whose unhappy fate was sealed by a sadistic and knife-happy woman surgeon. Later in this chapter, we will meet Ida Hunt again in a very different scenario from the one described by the *Eagle* in 1889. We will learn that she had been chronically ill since early in her marriage, and that the real cause of her poor health may well have been the venereal disease she contracted from her significantly older husband. Later still in this book, we will entertain the idea that Hunt was not simply the victim of an overly ambitious female physician, but a decisive patient who could speak casually and without embarrassment about her illness, while actively seeking aid from referral networks of laywomen and a variety of physicians. For the *Eagle*, however, she symbolized the innocent young woman betrayed, abandoned, and forced to die under the cruelest and most shocking conditions.

Appearing on May 3, the tale of "Ida's Last Ride" marked a crucial moment of escalation in the series featuring Dr. Mary Dixon Jones and the Woman's Hospital of Brooklyn launched by the newspaper on April 24, 1889. Composed of twenty-four pieces, some of them quite lengthy, the exposé ran almost daily, tantalizing readers from the last week in April through the middle of June. Beginning innocently enough, with a promise to investigate the hospital, the articles rose gradually to a resounding crescendo, displaying all the trappings of a sensationalist campaign.

It was a campaign, however, that was contoured to fit the newspaper's specific image and needs. Though originally a Democratic party organ, the Brooklyn *Eagle* had emerged by the 1880s as an independent newspaper, projecting the stable values of the business-oriented, Protestant bourgeoisie. Staid and respectable compared with its counterparts across the river like the New York *World*, a shining exemplar of the new "yellow journalism," the paper identified strongly with the city of Brooklyn. The *Eagle*'s editors, sensitive to the high profits New York rivals earned from melodrama, were not above initiating an occasional assault of their own, particularly when it served to convince readers of the *Eagle*'s vaunted role as a "public service." The paper chose its targets carefully, however, wary of offending its "sacred cows"—primarily the city's businessmen and the professionally prominent. In the case of Dixon Jones, the newspaper's accusations contained a variety of interesting motifs, including charges of the misuse of public funds to finance what was allegedly a private hospital. Posing as a pious woman with an unblemished record of medical service, Dixon Jones was shown to have misrepresented the institution to key members of the philanthropic elite. Adding insult to injury, the *Eagle* also intimated that the doctor operated indiscriminately on patients, endangering countless lives and deliberately misinforming clients of their true physical condition. The newspaper cited numerous examples of unprofessional conduct, implying that the respectable medical community suspected her of charlatanism. Our story begins, then, with an examination of each of these arrogations in detail.[5]

DUPING THE ARISTOCRACY AND BILKING PUBLIC COFFERS

Accusations of deception and fraud were launched in the *Eagle*'s very long first feature, which began by describing a lavish benefit parlor concert attended by the wealthy inhabitants of Brooklyn's "Heights and Hill" districts. The affair was held at the home of Joseph Knapp, one of the city's several millionaires.[6] The *Eagle* pictured in detail the "rare and costly" flowers, "the finest singers and instrumentalists that money could buy," and a banquet of such culinary perfection that "Lucullus" himself would have been forced to "acknowledge that he was a barbarian." It was, the *Eagle* opined, "as highly satisfactory a gathering as ever was collected in the name of charity." Yet a closer examination of the festivities revealed that few of the guests knew much about the institution they had been brought together to support. Even the hostess could not offer adequate details, and was obliged to summon to her side Mary Dixon Jones, described by the *Eagle* as a "stout, voluble, middle aged lady, with a captivating smile and a very plausible and insinuating way of talking" to elaborate to the curious about the Woman's Hospital of Brooklyn. With great gusto she entered into an explanation, calling the hospital "the most wonderful . . . in the world," citing its "extraordinary record of results in treatment" and its "grand work" in the cause of charity. But though the rich and well born of Brooklyn were content, the *Eagle* clearly was not. Its reporter observed caustically that guests went away "as wise in regard to the institution they were helping as the host himself," who, he added pointedly, "did not know where it was situated."[7] As more of the Woman's Hospital's story was unfolded, many of Brooklyn's first men and women faced increasing embarrassment. Though the newspaper would eventually let Brooklyn's rich and well born off the hook, its first article highlighted the gullibility of Brooklyn's elite.

Chronicling the newspaper's efforts to sort through layers of misconception in preparation for this opening salvo, the article's next paragraph turned to reporter Sidney Reid's interview with Mary Dixon Jones and her son Charles at their home a few weeks after the Knapp concert. Hoping to glean an accurate history of the institution in an unrehearsed conversation with the Joneses, Reid found himself obligated instead to listen to a prepared statement detailing their charity, self-sacrifice, courage, and perseverance.

Her hospital, Dixon Jones explained, was founded in 1881, when she was unable to secure a bed for an ailing patient in the renowned Women's Hospital in New York City. Believing that Brooklyn's good women also needed "such a refuge," she took the lead in establishing it. A number of prominent individuals joined in supporting the work, but she took pains to point out that the institution's first report featured *her* "earnest and self-sacrificing labor in the cause." There were, of course, other staunch advocates, including the institution's corresponding secretary, Mrs. E. E. Baldwin, the wife of Dr. S. L. Baldwin, recording secretary of the Methodist Episcopal Foreign Missionary Society. Indeed, several of the "best" men and women of Brooklyn were forthcoming with financial aid. Judge George G. Reynolds, a city judge and former state supreme court justice, drew up the papers of incorporation. Thomas Pearsall, another well-known lawyer, secured the deed for the institution's first dispensary on Tillary Street, and donated money from time to time. Additional contributors were John Gibb, a successful businessman active in club circles, philanthropist C. N. Hoaglund, whose special interest in medical research led him to endow Brooklyn's first pathology laboratory, future mayor David M. Boody, and Wall Street stockbrokers S. V. White and Arthur B. Claflin. Also interested were Mrs. Seth Low, whose husband had become Brooklyn's first reform mayor in 1881, her wealthy father-in-law, A. A. Low, and philanthropists George I. Seney, P. C. Cornell, A. S. Barnes, and D. W. McWilliams. Like Mrs. Low, several prominent wives were also active in the cause. Indeed, the list of Board of Trustees and the Advisory Board members first presented to Reid, which, according to the *Eagle*, even included the president of the Eagle Association, Colonel Hester, and the *Eagle*'s publisher, St. Clair McKelway, read like a *Who's Who* of Brooklyn's socially prominent. Skeptics had to agree that the assemblage was impressive.[8]

But Reid was not yet prepared to let the matter drop, partly because the *Eagle* had received some curious mail after the Knapp concert. Dixon Jones herself had written the newspaper a note, asking for a feature highlighting the hospital's charitable activities. "Pardon this tresspass," it began:

Some two years ago you told me you would gladly allow something in the *Eagle* for the Woman's Hospital of Brooklyn. The faculty and Board of Trustees want to report some of the good work of the hospital, as it is right that it should, as many good people and the city help support the hospital. Of course, the Woman's Hospital of Brooklyn, like all special hospitals, is not large, but has done some most successful surgical work. No hospital has better statistics. If you will kindly send a reporter to my house tomorrow at any hour I will give him some facts from the records of the hospital. Will you please drop me a line stating the hour.

Dr. Mary A. Dixon Jones

Initially inclined to comply, the *Eagle* became troubled when a second, anonymous communication arrived the same day, accusing the hospital and Dixon Jones of fraud. Addressed to the editor and signed only with the title "M.D.," this letter-writer called for an investigation. "I have reason to believe that it is a private institution obtaining public money," it read. "It gets $2000 from the city this year and I think that if you looked the thing up you would find it was not entitled to a cent."[9]

Thus, already on his guard when the interview with the Joneses began, Reid was further put off by the prepared statement, which was accompanied by disparaging remarks about the competition, the Women's Homeopathic Hospital of Brooklyn. In addition, mother and son denigrated the Hospital Saturday and Sunday Association, a charitable clearinghouse that had recently refused to grant money to their institution. Reid also puzzled over an odd slip of Charles's, who had playfully voiced relief that *his* hospital had "no unmanageable lady managers" with which to contend.[10]

After his interview with the Joneses, the reporter visited the office of Paul C. Grening, a real estate developer and hotelier who was listed as the Woman's Hospital president. Reid noted that, while waiting for Grening to accede to the interview, Dixon Jones appeared, visibly shaken, and met with Grening for at least ten minutes before reemerging into the outer office. There she questioned Reid about what he intended to print. Explaining that he couldn't reveal such information in advance, she left with a plea to "be sure you say something nice."[11]

Reid pursued a hard line of questioning with Grening, who acknowledged his connection with the institution since its establishment and confirmed the list of incorporators and trustees that the Joneses had already supplied. Grening compared his interest in the cause to that of "many other good people," adding that he thought it to be "a good thing." When Grening asked why the *Eagle* was pursuing an inquiry, Reid mentioned the allegation that the institution was a private one accepting public money. Vigorously denying the charge, Grening reminded Reid that the hospital functioned like all other institutions of its kind, and was "entirely open and above board."[12] When pressed, however, he was compelled to add that only he, Charles, and Mary Dixon Jones were in attendance at most trustees' meetings. He admitted further that Howard A. Smith, vice president of the Bedford Bank and cited as treasurer of the Woman's Hospital, had actually resigned some time ago. "But," he added, "I wouldn't say anything about that if I were you. Leave him in as treasurer." Further questioning revealed that it was Grening himself who transacted the hospital's business, signing the checks, paying the bills, and handling "all funds." Conceding to the reporter that he was dependent on the Joneses for information regarding the amounts of contributions, reports of the number of patients, and accounts of operations, he added, "I have the utmost confidence in them."[13]

So ended the narrative portion of the *Eagle*'s first article. Summarizing its conclusions and throwing down the gauntlet to the Doctors Jones and their supporters, the newspaper offered readers fifteen troubling "facts" it would elaborate on in the next several weeks. The *Eagle* would prove that hospital trustees did not authorize Dixon Jones to make any statement on their behalf, although Dixon Jones claimed that her prepared remarks gave the history of the hospital as "the trustees understand it." Moreover, the newspaper alleged, other members of the board did not even know that they were trustees *until the reporter informed them of the use of their names*. Most did not recall ever being summoned to a meeting and had never seen the hospital. What they did remember was that Dixon Jones had visited them from time to time, asking for money. Grening, in contrast, knew only what the Joneses told him. In addition, the *Eagle* would show that in actuality there was not *one* Woman's Hospital of Brooklyn, but *two*. The first was indeed incorporated in 1881, as Dixon Jones attested. The second's incorporation had not been legally recorded until May 7, 1885! Though Dixon Jones was connected with both institutions, conflict with the first hospital's Board of Lady Managers in February 1883 led to its dispanding soon afterward and the sale of the institution's buildings to the Nervous Hospital in the spring of 1884.[14] The *Eagle* claimed that when the second Woman's Hospital was organized the following fall, Dixon Jones took the early history of the first institution and made it the history of the second. Dixon Jones thus misused people's good names, and obscured the institution's origins to Reid. The present "Woman's Hospital," run by mother and son, was "getting $2000 under Chapter 666, Laws of 1887, and $866 from the Excise Fund, and is constantly reaching out for more." Readers were left to ponder the implications of this "very strange state of affairs."[15]

In several more articles published over the course of the next week, the *Eagle* continued to highlight the twin themes of misrepresentation and mismanagement. Reid and a team of reporters interviewed most of the men who were cited as hospital trustees. In addition to Brooklyn's District Attorney James A. Ridgway, they spoke with Augustus Van Wyck, a prominent lawyer elected a city court justice in 1884, D. W. McWilliams, former president of the YMCA and the superintendent of Lafayette Avenue Presbyterian Sunday School, lawyers Foster H. Backus and George G. Reynolds, Brooklyn's ex-mayor, the Honorable Samuel Booth, and Howard A. Smith, vice president of the Bedford Bank, whose name was listed in the Hospital's annual report as treasurer of the institution. The latter, a friend of Paul Grening's, had taken over the hospital's books the previous summer only as a favor to Grening, who was obliged to sort out the affairs of a hotel he owned in Saratoga Springs. Smith attended one meeting of the Board of Trustees and, along with "the best in the city," admitted to heartily enjoying the Knapp concert. Though almost all the other men were present at the concert as well, they were nevertheless "astonished" to hear that their names had been listed as incorporators or trustees of the hospital. Ridgway, who would eventually prosecute a manslaughter indictment against Dixon Jones, had given her a $50 contribution, but knew little about the institution, save that some "splendid names" were linked to it. Like Ridgway, Van Wyck vaguely recalled a visit from Dixon Jones "some years ago" asking for permission to use his name. He had declined, but generally responded favorably when contributions to the hospital were solicited. The others recounted a similar story.[16]

Using words like "humbug," while accusing the city of being "completely fooled," the newspaper compared Dixon Jones's manipulations to a "confidence game" that would have given the notorious confidence man "Hungry Joe" pause.[17] Neither the hospital's trustees nor members of its advisory board apparently knew of their office. "Mrs. Jones . . . took a handful of names and juggled them to suit herself and each man thought that all the other men mentioned knew all about the matter. . . ." Those solicited assumed that their patronage was imitated by "some of the best men in the city." "How Mrs. Jones must have smiled," one feature concluded.[18]

Reiterating its charge that the institution was "altogether a private hospital imposing on the public and individuals by pure bluff," the *Eagle* printed the hospital's entire articles of incorporation, dated May 7, 1885. "There are some queer things about this instrument," not the least of which was that the organization "did not follow its own rules," it editorialized.[19] On April 26, Paul C. Grening sent the newspaper a full financial statement of hospital activity for the duration of his affiliation, along with his letter of resignation, effective immediately, as president of its Board of Trustees.[20]

MAD AND BAD IN BROOKLYN: MEDICINE, SCIENCE, AND MURDER

The *Eagle*'s accusations of misrepresentation certainly undermined public confidence in Mary Dixon Jones's personal integrity, but even more shocking were its revelations regarding her surgical practice. On May 2, the newspaper resumed its exposé with the story of forty-nine-year-old Sarah T. Bates, the faithful wife of a U.S. Navy engineer stationed with the Pacific Coast Squadron. Beginning with the Bates incident and continuing for the next two weeks, the themes of lives destroyed by unnecessary surgery and a doctor covering her tracks in senseless and irrational ways recurred like leitmotifs in *Eagle* accounts. In its discussions of hapless patients, the *Eagle* not only hinted at cruelty, but drew a portrait of science gone mad. A private hospital on public funds, a "bogus" Board of Trustees and consulting staff, a president "who only knew what they . . . told him" was "bad enough." But such facts would become "insignificant and altogether immaterial," promised the *Eagle*, when measured against other, more dreadful transgressions. The newspaper then tantalized readers with heart-wrenching narratives of several unfortunate women who "fell into the hands of Dr. Mary A. Dixon Jones."[21]

Bates was "a most lovable woman, member of Rev. Charles Cuthbert Hall's church" and the beloved sister of the *Eagle*'s outraged informant, Mrs. Annie Gale, wife of a local leather merchant. Claiming in its headline that "SHE WAS ALIVE, and the Undertaker Waited for Her to Die," the newspaper told a tale of "the most remarkable hospital case on record . . . the strange story of a surgical operation and the stranger developments which followed it." According to her sister, Bates had consulted Dixon Jones for an ailment Gale described as "not of a serious character": an inability to take long walks. Gale emphasized her sister's continued ability to complete her "everyday duties and occupations." Nevertheless, after several visits to Dixon Jones, Bates announced that the doctor had recommended a "slight and safe" operation with a three-week recovery period. She entered the hospital on June 16, 1888, and Gale was asked not to visit her sister until "she was ready to receive [her]." Seven days later, in response to a note from the doctor, Gale went to the hospital to find Bates disoriented and barely conscious. Informed by Dixon Jones that she had had a cancerous tumor removed, Mrs. Gale was shocked, as were several of Bates's female relatives and friends. All of them came to visit her in the hospital and testified to the *Eagle* that she was in good health when she first consulted Dixon Jones. In addition, added a cousin, "the hospital was a miserable, dirty place, and the room was very forlorn." As Bates lost her grip on life over the course of the next several days, Dixon Jones admitted to Gale that her sister was dying. Gale claimed that during Bates's last moments Dixon Jones "pushed her away" from the room where her sister lay, alleging that Bates had blood poisoning and a malignancy that was "highly contagious." Sending Gale's husband for the undertaker, the doctor forcefully advised that the body be buried as soon as possible, preferably without a funeral.[22]

In an even more bizarre turn, the *Eagle* interviewed Edward Foote, the undertaker's "chief assistant." Foote averred that, when he arrived at the hospital, "Mrs. Jones . . . told me the lady was not yet dead, but said I could go into her room and wait." Foote and his assistant actually stood by the bed for roughly fifteen minutes before Bates expired. In addition, he claimed, Dixon Jones was anxious to have the body removed as soon as possible, citing a hospital rule that the death of a patient must be concealed from other "inmates of the house." Though Foote claimed to have found Dixon Jones's behavior "strange," he complied with all her requests, moving the body in an "ice box" for the purposes of concealment, and parking the undertaker's wagon across the street from the hospital. In fact, the undertaker may have been quite used to this attempt at camouflage: Most hospitals in this period were extremely careful to conceal patient deaths. The Boston City Hospital even built an underground tunnel so that stretchers might carry the dead from hospital to morgue without being observed.[23]

Meanwhile, the *Eagle* interviewed Foote's boss, undertaker George F. Corlis, who saw nothing dangerous in allowing the family to view the body. Bates's relatives had hired Dr. L. H. Barber to perform a postmortem examination. When the *Eagle*'s reporter questioned him about it, Barber revealed that in his estimation Bates was "perfectly healthy." He could find no trace of blood poisoning and no indication that there had ever been a tumor. Indeed, Barber believed Bates died "from the exhuastion resulting from a useless operation."[24]

In the same May 2 article, following the harrowing account of Sarah Bates's fateful death, came a description of the demise of Ida Hunt, whom we have already met. Indeed, in the next several weeks, the *Eagle* recounted case after case of women who endured needless operations, were bullied or cajoled into consenting to surgery, or were kept ignorant of what would happen to them. "Has She A Craze For Hurrying Women to the Operating Table?" asked the newspaper in its May 7 headline, adding that "a mania and a surgeon's knife make a terrible combination."

Oliver P. Miller, assistant cashier in the Williamsburgh Savings Bank and superintendent of the Lee Avenue Congregational Sunday School, paid Dixon Jones $1100 for the removal of a cancerous tumor from his wife that allegedly would burst and kill her instantly. Dixon Jones justified the expense by claiming that the operation was the most difficult she had yet attempted and that the "charge was the smallest she ever made." Mrs. Miller now lay dying.[25] Josephine Steinfeldt and her sister Mrs. Gerry, an epileptic who was not considered mentally competent, both heard from Dixon Jones that the removal of their malignant tumors would make them well. When neither's health improved, they were informed that they would need a second operation. Yet their former physician, Dr. Carolan, told the *Eagle* that neither Steinfeldt nor her sister had operable complaints.[26] Mrs. Elizabeth Bruggeman, the wife of a tinsmith, died during an operation for uterine myoma. Dixon Jones insisted on the death certificate that she had heart disease. Moreover, Bruggeman's body was mysteriously removed from the hospital without a permit.[27]

Dixon Jones told Mrs. Euphemia Tweeddale that she would not live another two years, suffering as she was from a "cancerous degeneration." Tweeddale became alarmed enough to consent to surgery, but when it was not successful in alleviating her symptoms, the doctors proposed another operation. She complained, whereupon Charles Dixon Jones bullied her, raving, she confessed, "until I was frightened and took back all I had said. I was all alone in the house and he looked very fierce." Tweeddale consulted another doctor and was told she had no malignancy.[28]

Most poignant of all were women like Mrs. John McCormick, the wife of a pattern-maker employed at the Brooklyn Navy Yard. Visiting the hospital dispensary for strain and irritation, she too was informed of a tumor that might cause her "to drop dead on the street." Agitated and alarmed, she submitted to surgery, but discovered weeks later that she would no longer be able to have children. McCormick was "shocked and surprised," claiming that Charles Dixon Jones had misrepresented the facts. "What he did was done without my knowledge or consent," she told the *Eagle*. For a time McCormick, who was "very fond of children," tried to conceal her sterility from her husband, but eventually she felt obligated to tell him. The couple wanted to sue, but didn't have the money. McCormick claimed that "many of the other patients were deceived in the same manner as myself and were intensely angry, but the nature of the operation was not one that any woman would like to admit having suffered." Eventually, McCormick, too, consulted another physician who claimed the operation was unnecessary and it was "improbable" that she had ever had a tumor.[29]

Meanwhile, *Eagle* reporters were hard at work interviewing neighbors who lived adjacent to the Woman's Hospital, located on Greene Avenue, in the heart of a mixed-class neighborhood built of brownstone and brick. Many of them were inordinately hostile to the institution, and the information they offered raised even more doubts in the minds of *Eagle* readers as to what kind of medicine was practiced there. John Delany, for example, a saloon keeper whose place of business was located directly across the street, claimed to have seen fifteen or sixteen bodies taken away from the building, generally in the middle of the night. In August, he alleged, he had confronted three men loading a coffin into an undertaker's wagon. "Seeing so many coffins going out," he felt, gave him the right to ask what they were doing and whether they had a permit to remove a body. They admitted to not yet having a permit, but added that Delany better shut up and mind his own business "if [he] did not want to be thrashed." Just then, Dr. A. T. Smith came by on his way home from a meeting held in the neighborhood. When Delany consulted him, Smith advised going directly to the police. Delany did so, and later contacted the officer on the beat, who accompanied him to inquire at the hospital. But by then the wagon had disappeared and the hospital nurse could tell them nothing. Both Smith and Officer Cale of the Ninth Precinct confirmed Delany's account.[30]

Delany was not the only eyewitness to report unsettling experiences with the "slaughter house" at Greene and Sumner. Other neighbors came forward to testify as well. The *Eagle* speculated that according to these informants there were not two deaths at the hospital, as the Joneses claimed, but closer to fifty. Mrs. Henry Hall, an invalid who lived with her husband and daughter next door to the institution, kept a diary of the goings-on at what she called the "butcher shop next door," recording bodies removed and scenes overheard. Claiming that she shared a wall with the hospital, which enabled her to "hear distinctly everything that goes on as plainly as if it happened in [their] own room," she noted several instances of patients groaning, screaming, and begging for water for hours on end. "On June 10 the groans and shrieks were so fearful that I sent my daughter out of the house," she noted. Mrs. Charles A. Dayton confirmed hearing patient moans as well, while several of the husbands grumbled that they had bought homes in the neighborhood specifically because the deed of purchase guaranteed against nuisances such as these. Everyone interviewed complained of "sickening" odors emanating from the hospital yard.[31]

Mary Dixon Jones was giving hospitals and physicians a bad name. Indeed, at one point in a summary of its charges against her, the newspaper invoked the dreaded word "vivisection," a culturally loaded term with connotations of mad scientists performing cruel experiments on live human beings.[32] At the end of its story of neighborly disgust, the *Eagle* transitioned to yet another of its many grievances against the Joneses, closing with the following letter to the editor, dated May 7, 1889:

I have read with interest the exposé of the Woman's Hospital as given in your columns. If a hundredth part of what you have published concerning the treatment of patients at the hands of Mrs. Jones can be proved, her case ought to be placed before the Grand Jury. The community ought to be freed of any party posing under the title of M.D., who will perform laparotomy and remove the patient from the hospital four or five days subsequent to such operation, which itself is sufficient cause to produce demise. Brooklyn is too intelligent a city to allow such conduct to go unpunished. Her diploma should be forfeited.

Physician[33]

UNPROFESSIONAL CONDUCT

In its May 9 story of the death of Elizabeth Bruggeman, whose body was apparently removed from the Woman's Hospital without a proper permit, the *Eagle* reporter, seeking answers to allegations that Dixon Jones had illegally altered Bruggeman's death certificate, paid a visit to the city health department. Meeting with a variety of officials, he received reassurances that the sort of tampering with an official document that such an infraction would have required could not have slipped by them unnoticed. Joseph A. Devin, who issued burial permits, remembered nothing unorthodox in this case. He observed, presumably in self-justification, that Dixon Jones was "a regularly registered physician and her certificates are received without question."[34] It was a remark full of meaning, one that went to the heart of the outraged feelings of many in the Brooklyn medical community. The letter to the *Eagle*'s editor from the physician who thought that Dixon Jones's diploma should be revoked was typical of the uncomfortable response of physicians to her behavior. Indeed, many doctors, the newspaper intimated, were dismayed by the sensational nature of the revelations because, for better or worse, Dixon Jones was a member of their professional community. The *Eagle* made their disquietude good copy, harping on Dixon Jones's lack of professionalism and calling attention to doctors' apparent inability to adequately police themselves.

Undoubtedly aware of the aversion of regular physicians to advertise, the newspaper began by underscoring the pretentiousness in the Joneses' representation of their hospital. The *Eagle* made much of Dixon Jones's boasting in its first article, when, in her interview with Sidney Reid, she compared her Brooklyn institution to the London Woman's Hospital under the direction of the world-renowned ovariotomist Sir Spencer Wells. The newspaper listed the members of the Brooklyn hospital's hugely padded medical consulting staff in full, presenting a collection of some of the most prominent names in gynecology in Brooklyn, New York, and England, a company that even included Lawson Tait of Birmingham, Spencer Wells's rival in operative gynecology.

But self-advertisement and self-promotion were only the beginning. When the newspaper accused her of running a private hospital with public funds, it also implied that Dixon Jones was money-grubbing, reinforcing this motif with careful and detailed descriptions of the fees she charged every patient and the aggressive single-mindedness she displayed when collecting them. For example, before surgery on Mrs. Euphemia Tweeddale, which at the husband's insistence took place at the Tweeddale home, Dixon Jones allegedly spoke quietly to an already undressed patient, explaining that the anesthesiologist, Dr. King, required payment in advance. The doctor insisted that Tweeddale "go into the other room and find [her] purse all unattired." Dixon Jones charged Tweeddale $35 on King's behalf. Yet King told the *Eagle* that he did not require payment in advance and his usual fee was only $10. When the fees patients claimed to have paid to her were added up, it appeared that the hospital was overreporting the number of charity patients or officially documenting some of its paying patients as persons who had been treated for free.[35]

In explanation for Dixon Jones's troubling behavior, the newpaper hinted at a slightly shady background. Alleging incorrectly that she came to Brooklyn from New England around 1870 to start a "water cure mill with allopathic ramifications," the newspaper immediately tainted her with sectarian connections.[36] It went on to claim erroneously that she practiced without a diploma "for years," finally seeking a degree from the Woman's Medical College of Pennsylvania in Philadelphia only because "a law was passed requiring all practising physicians to register."[37] When she returned to Brooklyn she lectured to women on health matters. "She talked well," the newspaper continued, and "gathered about her a large following of ladies" impressed with her qualities as an "eminent Christian" and an "infallible scientist." It was this group, the *Eagle* alleged, who supported her in the founding of the first hospital. "They had a large board of lady managers and a number of eminent gentlemen as trustees, and there was much enthusiasm."

But the institution "only lasted three months," presumably because of Dixon Jones's imperious behavior. The hospital was reorganized and a second group of more "determined" lady managers attempted to apply "some sort of restraint." For the next two years, according to the *Eagle*, there was "a succession of skirmishes." Jones's medical assistants and the nurses complained of her constantly, and eventually there was a "grand flare up" in the fall of 1884. At a fateful meeting, Mrs. Jones allegedly bullied the lady managers into submission, at one point addressing them in a "towering rage" for attempting to interfere with her, the "chief physician." She refused to allow them to elect a new president. The evening ended when Dixon Jones resigned and left in a huff, intentionally leaving the institution's sick patients in the lurch, according to the *Eagle*, and even taunting the group to hire another "physician and pay him."[38]

"Mrs. Jones has always *posed* as a very pious woman," the *Eagle* continued, "even giving it out that she prayed before every operation. She is still a member of Hanson Place Methodist Church and had a young ladies Bible class there about ten years ago."[39] But "it is asserted by those who remember" that she stopped the Bible teaching for two reasons. The first was an allegation that she attempted to convince "many of the young ladies to undergo serious operations." The second was a scandal that arose in 1879 involving a ten-year-old servant girl indentured to Dixon Jones from the Brooklyn Orphan Asylum. Apparently the girl, Annie Phillips, ran away to a neighbor one night, accusing Dixon Jones of beating and mistreating her. The neighbor, A. W. Tenney, just happened to be a prominent Republican lawyer who was then serving his third term as U.S. District Attorney for the Eastern District of New York. According to the *Eagle*, Tenney had observed some of this mistreatment himself and consequently refused to return the girl to the Joneses.[40]

There were also allegations that some members of Brooklyn's medical community avoided consultation or contact with Dixon Jones, reinforcing general suspicions of her bad character. The most damning evidence was that Brooklyn's Saturday and Sunday Association, a committee of physicians and philanthropists that collected charitable contributions and donated them as needed to hospitals that treated the poor, had turned down her request for funds. In her interview with Sidney Reid, Dixon Jones had claimed this occurred primarily because of the unwarranted animus of one particular physician, a homeopath who, out of "jealousy," presented an unfavorable report "to help his own institution."[41] But the chairperson of the association's Committee of Investigation, Dr. Reuben C. Moffat, alleged that the negative information he received came primarily from the testimony of Dixon Jones's "assistant physicians and nurses." That information "reflected so strongly on her conduct as a woman and physician," he continued, "that the committee suppressed my report and merely advised unanimously against admitting her." The Reverend Charles Cuthbert Hall, a distinguished religious presence in the Brooklyn community and the one member of the committee singled out by Dixon Jones for his friendship to her institution, backed up Moffat's, not Dixon Jones's, version of these events.[42]

The *Eagle* complained that Brooklyn's physicians, though quite willing to confirm Dixon Jones's bad reputation when appealed to directly and "glad to see the *Eagle* paying attention to the Woman's Hospital," were too "cautious in their speech." For example, the newspaper learned from Dr. Segur, a member of the Board of Censors of the King's County Medical Society, that the society had rejected her application for admission "four times" on the grounds of "unprofessional conduct." But most doctors "didn't want to get mixed up in it." Mrs. Tweeddale's doctor, Matthew Howard, confessed to an *Eagle* reporter that he had been complaining to other colleagues about the excessive number of ovariotomies Dr. Jones was performing for "more than a year," hoping "that the public attention of the profession be called to the facts." But he himself took no further steps in that direction, not caring to "mix myself up in any wrangle or to appear to wish to make myself notorious." As anxious as he was to help, he didn't feel justified in giving the *Eagle* the names of other patients whose cases had come to his attention, perhaps because of physician-patient privilege.[43] Similarly, Dr. A. W. Shepard, who took over the case of a patient allegedly rendered sterile by Dixon Jones's surgery, felt so frustrated that he blamed the victim. Unable to control his temper after he examined the woman, and perhaps resenting her demonstration of autonomy, he told her that he was surprised to see her alive. "Who ever told you to go to the Joneses?" he asked. "Don't you know they're killing women by the oceans in that place?" When she asked why "they" didn't "put a stop to it," he responded, "We can't. When a woman is so simple as to go to that place it is her own fault if she is ruined for life."[44]

The *Eagle* contacted over a dozen eminent Brooklyn practitioners for their general impressions of Dixon Jones. All of them commented on the unnecessary surgery performed on several patients. A. J. C. Skene, professor of gynecology in Long Island Hospital Medical School and a nationally known figure in the field, first contended that most of what he knew about Jones was hearsay "which he did not want to repeat." After "persistent questioning," however, he admitted that he had been called in to consult with her on one occasion, after a patient of hers sought out his medical advice. When he disagreed with her diagnosis, the *Eagle* continued, Dixon Jones warned that if he ever spoke negatively about the character of her work, she "had a tongue" and would "use it."[45]

Other physicians reported disturbing incidents as well. Z. Taylor Emery recalled that he had initially been so impressed with Dixon Jones's self-reported surgical skill that he agreed to administer ether for her in a laparotomy case. He was dismayed at her slowness, "taking twice as long" as other surgeons, and he expressed his fear to her that the patient had been under ether too long and might die. Apparently Dixon Jones responded by picking up her implements and immediately leaving the room, "saying she would not stay there if the patient was going to die." The "grossly unprofessional" nature of her behavior "settled Dr. Emery's association with her." Similarly, one of Dixon Jones's past female assistants, Dr. Caroline Pease, recalled that at one operation to remove a diseased organ, the doctor extracted it and immediately covered it up so that Pease "could not see whether or not it was diseased." Soon afterward, she left Dixon Jones's employ.[46]

But perhaps the most unsettling of the accusations of unprofessionalism was the insinuation that Dixon Jones performed abortions. In a portion of an article sectioned off with the title "What the Colored Cook Saw," the *Eagle* claimed to have interviewed "Dollie Brown, colored, aged 22," a cook who worked at the Woman's Hospital for eight weeks in June 1888. Brown told a reporter that while she was at the hospital there were three operations performed, "one by Dr. Mary Jones alone," at which she was present. The patient, a "German woman," would not take the ether "until Dr. Mary Jones hit her three or four times." Dixon Jones explained to Brown that she was removing a tumor, and, when the operation was completed, gave her "something wrapped up in cotton" for immediate disposal. "Before throwing it where she told me," the cook alleged, "I opened the cotton and looked inside. I then saw what proved it to be a case of malpractice." Luckily for Jones, the woman died almost immediately.[47]

On May 17, the *Eagle* published several communications from the Woman's Hospital's illustrious list of consulting physicians, including statements from Arthur M. Jacobus, Paul F. Mundé, and H. Marion Sims of New York, stating either no active connection with the institution or a highly tenuous one. No one from New York, it is important to note, disavowed Dixon Jones's surgical or diagnostic skill. The *Eagle* concluded, however, that the hospital's consulting staff, like its Board of Trustees, was bogus. But perhaps it was Dr. Samuel King, the anesthesiologist in the Tweeddale case, who had the last word. He not only had given ether for Dixon Jones, but was at one time connected with the Woman's Hospital's Fleet Street Dispensary. He resigned "two years ago," he told the *Eagle*, because he had numerous opportunities to "witness the result of both doctors' operations." He considered many of them "absolutely unnecessary." Perhaps the most "charitable" way of explaining some of the things the Dixon Joneses had done, he concluded, "is to consider them both more or less insane."[48]

MARY DIXON JONES FIGHTS BACK

During the beginning weeks of the *Eagle*'s exposé, Mary Dixon Jones attempted in vain to counter the image of her and her medical practice fashioned so meticulously by the *Eagle*. It was a difficult task, especially in the face of the newspaper's contention that it avoided hearsay, confined its interviews to persons with "direct knowledge," and printed only evidence that "would be admitted by a court."[49]

Letters of rebuttal written by Charles met with little success, partly because the *Eagle* was always able to contextualize them in ways that undermined their credibility, and partly because they were often full of contradictions. More helpful, perhaps, were testimonials from satisfied patients, which the newspaper was willing to print. On May 14, several of these appeared. The first was a lengthy statement from Mrs. Alfred Strome, recounting seven years of suffering from painful abdominal tumors and frequent visits from practitioner to practitioner. Finally recommended to Dixon Jones, she was advised to go ahead with surgery. The tumors removed from her abdomen were shown to her husband. Hospital after-care was excellent, and she spent eight weeks in recovery, ample time to observe the quality of the institution's nursing. Although one death did occur during her stay and the body was removed after dark, this was done "in order to save the patients from being mentally worried and frightened about their own future uncertainties." Strome was "now enjoying perfect health, which I have not done for the past seven years, for which blessing I owe thanks only to a kind Providence and Dr. Mary Dixon Jones." The *Eagle* discredited this long communication, however, by claiming that a reporter visited Strome's husband, who admitted that the letter had been written for his wife by a gentleman named Alex Andersen. The impression was left that Mrs. Strome did not speak English well and therefore did not even understand what had been written on her behalf.[50]

A second letter from Elizabeth Carter, a patient still residing at the Woman's Hospital when it was printed, testified to the excellent care she and other women received there. She had seen several recover rapidly from serious operations. As for those heard screaming and crying out for water, this was certainly possible, since patients just out of ether often cry and scream for water, because they are not allowed to drink for several hours after surgery until it is medically safe. The letter went on to call into question the testimony of neighbors like Delany, pointing out that, as the windows of the hospital were always kept closed, it would be impossible to see or hear what went on within.[51] A few days later the newspaper printed a third account from a satisfied patient, Mrs.

W. R. Nash, who claimed to have undergone a successful operation for a huge tumor that had plagued her for six years. Like the others, she, too, was discharged a well woman.[52]

Perhaps the most effective defense from the Dixon Jones camp came in the form of a report submitted by the "Committee of Five," a body appointed at a recent "special meeting" of the hospital's newly constituted Board of Trustees. The group organized itself specifically for the purpose of investigating the *Eagle*'s allegations. The committee's findings were published verbatim in the *Eagle* in a lengthy formal statement. Claiming to have investigated all hospital buildings and interviewed medical staff, nurses, and patients, the committee reconfirmed Mary Dixon Jones's version of the institution's history. It went on to allow, however, that there were indeed "many inaccuracies of business details from 1884 down to the present year."[53]

Circulars with the original names of trustees and incorporators were printed up at the hospital's founding, but never updated. It was true that these were widely distributed, though only with the intention of "doing good by calling the attention of the people of Brooklyn to the new charity inaugurated." Until the *Eagle* began its investigation, however, these had "caused no protest on the part of anyone whose name was used."

Indeed, the hospital's worst infractions grew out of its poverty. Though "rich in the work accomplished," the institution had "never gone to the expense of employing any clerk or bookkeeper, and the work of keeping the accounts has devolved upon such of the trustees as were willing to perform the duty."[54] This situation had led to some serious mishandling of funds. Aside from the meager amounts received from the Excise Board and the state legislature, support for the hospital was solicited untiringly by Dixon Jones, mostly from private patients. These "ladies of high rank and social station" gave freely "in appreciation of the services rendered by her to them" to what they termed her "pet charity." Moreover, when funds were low, Dr. Jones paid the hospital's bills on several occasions "from her own bank account, often waiting for long periods for reimbursement." For years she donated the use of her surgical instruments to the institution. Thus was Dixon Jones burdened with the worry of financial affairs, when it should have been the trustees who managed that aspect of hospital business. With the care of the sick a constant burden, it is no wonder that "accounts have not been kept as they might have been." If mismanagement occurred in these instances, the committee suggested, it was on behalf of a good cause.[55]

The report concluded by reaffirming the high quality of hospital care and declaring that the percentage of mortalities measured against the number of patients treated and the "exceedingly difficult operations performed" was "insignificant." It was true that "the affairs of the hospital in a business sense have, undoubtedly, been carelessly administered." But the Joneses should not be required to shoulder the responsibility in that regard, nor do they deserve "blame" that might be better charged to the trustees. Their connection with the hospital has not enriched them; on the contrary, they have been "out of pocket by reason of it." The report, dated June 10, 1889, was signed by five individuals:

the Reverend H. B. Elkins, Esther E. Baldwin, Mrs. M. Lewis, Mrs. S. J. Millett, and J. C. Moss. All but Moss, the president of the Moss Engraving Company in New York, were involved in reorganizing the hospital in 1884.

The report contained some plausible arguments, though based on a central premise that the *Eagle* articles emphatically contravened: that it was indeed possible to separate the hospital and its board of trustees from the Dixon Joneses and treat these as separate entities.[56] But the *Eagle* did not even bother raising such an argument; instead it discredited the entire statement by interviewing the last signatory, J. C. Moss, who allegedly told a reporter that he was pressured by Charles Jones to become a trustee, that he attended three meetings in conjunction with the committee, and that "personally" he made "no investigation at all." He signed the statement because "it seemed straightforward enough" and his fellow trustees "said they had investigated." Indeed, he was not very interested in the case, had not even read the charges against Dixon Jones, but allowed his name to be used because "I was informed the Joneses were not getting fair play."[57]

THE BROOKLYN *CITIZEN* SPEAKS OUT

By this time, the Joneses might well have been in trouble had not Brooklyn's second largest newspaper, the *Citizen*, begun a series of articles and editorials dealing with the controversy on May 19, only three weeks before.[58] By the end of June, the *Citizen* had put itself forward as the champion of Mary Dixon Jones and the avowed foe of the *Eagle*—a newspaper it accused of printing lies for profit. Indeed, in an editorial on May 26, the *Citizen* had thrown down the gauntlet to its competitor, charging that the *Eagle* was "conducted without the slightest reference to truth or justice." Issue after issue contained some glaring lie or other, "the object of which is either to blackmail an individual, promote some corrupt financial venture, or impair the reputation of a political or business opponent."[59] In the next several weeks the *Citizen* continued to offer the doctors sympathy in increasingly melodramatic tones.

To illustrate the point, an article on May 31 covered the convening of a Grand Jury that recommended the indictment of the Joneses for manslaughter. The newspaper hinted that the *Eagle* had perhaps sought to influence the result. The doctors had already filed for libel against the paper, and the *Citizen* speculated that the *Eagle* had made "extraordinary efforts . . . to bring about the finding of the present indictment" in order to protect itself.[60] On June 4, the *Citizen* featured an interview with the Joneses' lawyer, R. S. Newcombe, who insisted that at the pending manslaughter trial he would bring "positive, absolute, irrefragable proof from . . . the most eminent scientists in the world" to show that both the Bates and Hunt operations were necessary and that no surgeon could have saved their lives. Citing an example of the *Eagle*'s nefarious methods, he pointed to the allegation that Ida Hunt's abdominal cavity "was filled with rags impregnated with ether." On the contrary, Newcombe stated, the filling was iodoform dressing, "one of the best active surgical agents known'' to prevent suppuration. "Most prominent practitioners in the country use it."[61]

Two days later the *Citizen* came out in open revolt, burnishing the headline: "Atrocious Lies. The Outrageous Attacks on Dr. Mary Dixon Jones. Exposure of Them Begun." It published a letter from the Reverend S. L. Baldwin, "the Distinguished Secretary of the Methodist Missionary Society." The letter, it claimed, showed the "absolute baselessness of many of the malignant accusations made in the *Eagle*."[62] Declaring that paper's smear campaign to be "one of the foulest conspiracies ever formed in Brooklyn to effect the ruin of an honorable physician," it stated that Baldwin's very "name is a perfect guarantee of the absolute truth of his statements." It went on to assert that the *Citizen* had "from the outset" found the case of Dixon Jones's vilification "remarkable." Presenting its own version of events, it argued that the *Eagle* initially attacked Dixon Jones out of "malice," on the basis of one letter it received assailing the Woman's Hospital. When Mrs. Jones realized she could "obtain no sort of redress through its columns," she resorted to a libel suit. Understanding its vulnerability, the *Eagle* then stirred up enough sentiment to incite the convening of a grand jury by the District Attorney, at which point the newspaper manipulated the outcome of the inquiry *as it had done with other grand juries in the past.* "Finding themselves in desperate peril of exposure before the public and of a verdict that would jeopardize the existence of their property," declared the *Citizen*, the *Eagle* "resorted once more to the desperate device of making use of the prosecuting machinery of the State to crush their victim for their own protection."[63]

The *Citizen*'s editor, Andrew McLean, might well have been speaking from experience. Only two years before, he had left his position as editor-in-chief of the *Eagle* to establish an alternative Democratic newspaper. Born in Scotland, McLean had emigrated to the United States at the age of fourteen, serving in the navy during the Civil War and afterward settling in Brooklyn. He began his career in journalism at the age of twenty, working first for a small paper in Chicago and later returning to New York as a reporter for the *Times*. After a stint at the Democratic Brooklyn *Union*, he joined the staff of the *Eagle*, where he remained for seventeen years, working his way up to city editor. When Thomas Kinsella, the *Eagle*'s fiery and fiercely Democratic editor-in-chief, died in 1884, McLean took over. But St. Clair McKelway also joined the staff in that year, and, two years later, McLean departed to found the *Citizen*.

McLean, a man of letters like McKelway, respected as an essayist, poet, dramatic author, platform orator, and after-dinner speaker, might well have been ousted from the *Eagle* when McKelway began to envision it less as a Democratic mouthpiece and more as an independent newspaper. The evidence only hints at a struggle for leadership and direction, however. Historian Harold Syrett claims that McLean designed the *Citizen* as a reliable machine organ "which would offset the *Eagle*'s independence." With the *Eagle* rapidly exiting the fold, the *Citizen*, according to Syrett, supported the Democrats loyally, even when the machine's self-interested policies required "some preposterous explanation." Thus, personal animosity and political dissent, rather than a passion for the truth, may well account for the *Citizen*'s interest in Dixon Jones. Competitive rivalry granted, however, there is no evidence to conclude that the *Citizen* deliberately distorted its reportage of the Dixon Jones affair.[64]

During the second week in June, the *Citizen* fashioned the central trope of its own melodramatic rehabilitation of Mary Dixon Jones. It represented her as the innocent victim of a malicious, sensationalist rag and set out to expose the "false," theatrical, and gothic portrait constructed by *Eagle* artifice. In its place the *Citizen* offered counterimages that readers were encouraged to understand as more "objective" and "true," specifically because they were familiar and reassuring. Presumably laying bare the subtext of the *Eagle*'s articles to its readers, it complained of a "dark conspiracy." Acknowledging that those who have their information only from the *Eagle* might readily look upon Mrs. Dr. Jones as a "female Jack the Ripper," a "cross between La Choueuse, the bony and bloodthirsty hag of 'The Mysteries of Paris,' and Mere Frochard, the blear-eyed and rum-soaked virago of 'The Two Orphans,' " the paper elaborated on the feminine archetype depicted in the testimonials of her friends. It noted the doctor's "kind and skillful treatment of the sick," her "Christian character and standing," and her "generous services to the poor and lowly." A reporter from the *Citizen* who visited her found her "kindly," a "true gentlewoman in the full meaning of the word." Dixon Jones's only error was "to have given her time and attention . . . to charitable institutions where there was no pay." Had she confined herself to her lucrative private practice, "no trouble would have been raised about her."

But it was her motherly image of respectability that was most noted. Here was a woman, "small in stature, with a still youthful and handsome face, framed by a mass of silvery white hair."

> From her open countenance beam motherly love and womanly kindness, and the gentleness of her manner and the soft tones of her voice at once betoken the lady of refinement and culture. Her home surroundings are much as one would naturally associate with such a woman. Nothing ostentatious or garish, no attempt at display. Everything quiet and subdued, her attire—the plain black silk dress and neat white collar; the arrangement of her parlors—family portraits, a Brussels carpet of homely pattern; the furniture—modest yet substantial.[65]

This lady, the reporter went on, had nothing to conceal, and was fully willing to "permit the light of the most searching investigation" to shine on her home, her history, her children, and her life's work. Dixon Jones had raised two sons and a daughter, all of whom she supported since childhood. Her children stood as eloquent proof of her motherly skills. Dr. Charles Dixon Jones was a graduate of Wesleyan, where he took special honors. Henry, now an Episcopalian clergyman, attended Harvard, where he taught and occupied the Chair of Elocution for some time. Mary, the youngest, a woman of great refinement whose métier was art, studied at the Packer Institute of Brooklyn.[66] Indeed, when Dixon Jones fought back, it was not for herself, but for her children. "The opprobrium of these attacks has not rendered me unhappy," she told the *Citizen*. "I am only grieved and wounded in my feelings as a mother. It is their effect upon my children which causes me sorrow. I thought I had done a noble work and was entitled to praise, not persecution."[67] Thus has "the gentle mother, who has devoted her own talents to procuring the best possible education for her little brood" been "pilloried before this community as a ruthless criminal."[68]

The following day the *Citizen* bolstered its construction of itself as "objective" and "truth-telling," by launching an attack on "sensational journalism." Hinting cryptically that part of the *Eagle*'s motivation could be understood only by the reader who was familiar "with the internal affairs of that paper's publication office," the newspaper proceeded to denounce scandalmongering. When a journal is losing ground, the *Citizen* continued, "and finds its circulation cut to pieces," its recourse is often "to stimulate the public appetite with the most highly seasoned variety of information they can give. It is the old case of the dreary story teller who supplements his own dullness with lies." The inevitable and unhappy outcome of such mendacity, the *Citizen* concluded, was to give all newspapers, even those who printed only the "truth," a bad name.[69]

For the rest of the month of June, the *Citizen* dedicated its columns to retelling the *Eagle*'s distorted narrative, offering to its readers what its bold June 10 headline proudly declared were "Facts vs. Fiction." The newspaper opened with a critique of the *Eagle*'s description of the Ida Hunt case, calling it a "gruesome" tale "of butchery and blood" written by a reporter "who parts company with the truth the moment he dips his pen in gall." As proof, the *Citizen* claimed that, at the moment such distortions were being written, the *Eagle*'s city editor had on his desk a reprint of an article by Charles Dixon Jones, describing the operations performed at the Woman's Hospital in 1887 and 1888, complete with mortality statistics. Making a case for the resonant cultural power of statistical science, the *Citizen* went on to cite mortality statistics and charts taken from other experts in ovariotomy, demonstrating most clearly that, when measured alongside the leading specialists in the field, the Woman's Hospital's record was exemplary. Indeed, the editorial noted, not only have Dixon Jones's surgical "conclusions in many departments of that science . . . been adopted as authoritative," but her statistical record as published by her son Charles is "more brilliantly successful than some of the most eminent practitioners in the United States." And still the *Eagle* reporter insisted on painting the institution as an "inferno, on whose gates hung the inscription 'All ye who enter here leave hope behind.' "[70]

Nor did the *Citizen* miss the valency of the *Eagle*'s grave intimations that Mary Dixon Jones performed abortions. This, too, the newpaper identified as a vicious attempt at defamation, exacerbated by its understanding of the *Eagle*'s manipulative use of racial tropes. Yet the *Citizen*'s own racism reminds the modern reader of the embeddedness of links between the racialized other and various forms of depravity. "A further distortion of the truth," the *Citizen* editorial pointed out about the *Eagle*, "was to make the public believe that under the pretext of laparotomy she was actually engaged in criminal practice." "And *as usual,*'' the editorial went on, revealing to the modern scholar a good example of the ways in which the Dixon Jones affair conceals layers of possible meanings, the *Eagle* produced the ''inevitable colored'' woman to verify the accuracy of these allegations. ''What this ignorant or malicious creature knew about surgery,'' the *Citizen* protested, ''the intelligent reader may conjecture.''[71]

To the reporter's insinuations that there ''was a perpetual dance of death going on'' within hospital walls, the *Citizen* offered affidavits from satisfied patients, testimony it claimed the *Eagle* deliberately suppressed. Mrs. W. H. Anderson, originally a patient and then a trustee of the first Woman's Hospital, wrote all the way from California, stating emphatically that Dixon Jones's surgical skill had not only cured her, but her sister and a close friend as well.[72] Others had equally glowing stories to tell. Clara Hartisch recovered from surgery for ''tumors filled with pus'' that Professor William Polk of Bellevue helped Dixon Jones diagnose and Dr. A. M. Jacobus, another New York specialist, attended as Dixon Jones's assistant. Mrs. Mary Huck was relieved of uterine hemorrhaging and ''incessant and unbearable pain'' by a very dangerous operation successfully performed by Dixon Jones. Mrs. Mina Emerich, with abdominal pain that led her to consult five or more physicians in Brooklyn and New York who told her she had cancer spreading beyond the uterus, was ready to undergo ''anything that would relieve me, either by cure or death.'' Now, two years later, she claimed to be ''a new woman and perfectly well.'' Anna Brown told how her little girl, Lizzie, whose deformed limbs prevented her from walking, was cured by an operation for which she paid nothing. Margaret Walsh testified to Charles Dixon Jones's solicitous after-care on the occasion of three different operations, and Professor C. H. Edwards, a photographer who was now assisting Dr. Charles by photographing his many cases of deformed limbs, had first come into contact with Jones when his surgery cured Edwards's ailing wife.[73] All of these patients paid minimal fees for their medical care; indeed, many even alleged that Charles Dixon Jones gave *them* money for food or clothing!

One informant told the *Citizen* the story of a woman named Mrs. Jones who earned her living as a seamstress. Forced to enter the hospital for a serious operation that eventually cured her, she was unable to make payments on her sewing machine, and it was eventually repossessed. ''I know for a fact,'' the speaker continued, ''that Dr. Charles Jones went to Wheeler & Wilson, and if you go there they will tell you so, and paid out of his own pocket for the machine and had it sent to the apartments of Mrs. Jones.''[74] A strikingly new element in the *Citizen*'s reportage was its emphasis on the Joneses' kind treatment of children and their extensive pediatric orthopedic practice, which the *Eagle* hardly mentioned.[75]

When speaking of the neighborhood reception of the Woman's Hospital, this time referring to its branch on Tillary Street and its dispensary on Fleet Place, the *Citizen*'s portrait stands in striking contrast to the *Eagle*'s depiction of neighborhood snoops who kept track of the pine boxes leaving the building at midnight and deplored the foul smells emanating from inside. For example, the atmosphere at the hospital's outpatient branch, the Fleet Street dispensary, is described as bustling with efficiency and the resounding cheerfulness of grateful patients. Said one teary-eyed old lady, addressing the reporter, "If you go down to Hudson Avenue and take a pencil and paper with you, you will find hundreds of people, blacks and whites, to speak of the goodness of the doctors."[76]

The *Citizen* covered the vindicating "Committee of Five" report with great fanfare. In addition, it accused the *Eagle* of trying to suppress the statement, on evidence that while *The Citizen, The World, The Tribune*, and *The Standard-Union* all ran the committee's conclusions on June 13, the *Eagle* delayed until the following day! Indeed, the *Citizen* observed in an editorial, the *Eagle* had intentionally concealed many letters written to its editors defending Dixon Jones and her son.[77] Following up on this accusation the next day, the *Citizen* attacked the *Eagle*'s effort to undermine the credibility of the signatories to the Committee of Five testimony, printing letters from John C. Moss, H. B. Elkins, and S. L. Baldwin deploring the *Eagle*'s distortions in reporting their interviews. In an insightful editorial of the same day, the *Citizen* proceeded to deconstruct the *Eagle*'s misrepresentations with the enthusiasm of a literary critic, pointing out not only narrative inconsistences, but ways in which such devices as deliberate misspellings of names were used to undermine public trust.[78]

In a final attempt to discredit the *Eagle*, the *Citizen* reviewed some of that newspaper's earlier allegations in the controversy, revisiting articles published in May and retelling the narratives by restoring crucial details it claimed the *Eagle* had maliciously left out. An interview with Alfred Strome, for example, husband of the Swedish lady whose letter praising Dixon Jones had been discredited because it was written by a friend, revealed that both Strome and his wife understood and spoke English quite well, "though not good enough to put our ideas in writing." The Stromes reiterated their wholehearted satisfaction with Dixon Jones's treament, as did Mrs. Hulten, another patient whose story the *Eagle* allegedly misrepresented.[79] But even more convincing were the host of letters the *Citizen* printed from leading New York physicians, letters that ranged in date from 1880 to 1887 and written by such acclaimed practitioners as Abel Mix Phelps, John A. Wyeth, Robert Tuttle Morris, Paul F. Mundé, William M. Polk, and Benjamin F. Dawson, accepting the honor of appointment to the hospital's consulting staff. These stood in direct contradiction to the *Eagle*'s claim that most doctors knew little to nothing about the hospital.[80]

Last, the *Citizen* devoted two days to reconstructing the case of Mrs. Oliver P. Miller, printing what it termed the *Eagle*'s "bogus" interview with her husband and its own "true" version in double columns side by side. In the *Citizen*'s account, Miller complained about the *Eagle*'s faulty reporting, characterizing that newspaper's version as a "grossly garbled and in many instances absolutely false statement of what was said by me." His wife had been recommended to Dixon Jones by Dr. Wheeler. He admitted to paying Dixon Jones $1100 for his wife's surgery, but believed sincerely that the doctor had been justified in the charge because it was a difficult operation. The amount was agreed upon beforehand. Although Dixon Jones was unsure of the diagnosis, a microscopic examination of the tumor she removed proved it to be cancerous. The doctor informed Miller that his wife "could not be saved" and told him what to expect. She left the case in the hands of Dr. Wheeler, not because she didn't want to treat a dying patient, but because Dr. Wheeler was Miller's family physician and lived near enough to give the constant attention and administer the pain relievers his wife would need as the end came near. Miller went on to acknowledge the aggressiveness of the *Eagle*'s reporter, who told him that the newspaper planned to "run her out of this town" and urged Miller not to pay the remainder of his bill.[81] Moreover, the reporter did not seem to understand that Dixon Jones was entitled to place several private, paying patients in the hospital, and "consequently the money did not belong to the hospital." Indeed, Miller observed, "the deliberation with which words are put into my mouth by the *Eagle* reporter in his so-called interview with me, which I never uttered, is simply astounding." Miller voiced his initial reluctance to speak publicly about such matters, a sentiment that he felt "compelled" to set aside "when confronted with the wrong which has been done Dr. Jones by the report of the interview with me as published in the *Eagle*. . . ."[82] A few days later, the *Citizen* told of Mary Dixon Jones's $150,000 suit for libel against the *Eagle*, printing in full the complaint filed by her lawyers with the state supreme court. The document occupied all four columns and several pages of the newspaper.[83]

On Monday, June 24, the *Citizen* offered a synopsis of its arguments. The Dixon Jones case, the newspaper believed, was "one of the most extraordinary in the history of American journalism," a most "glaring" instance of "journalistic prostitution." It exemplified how far a newspaper would go in the "gratification of personal malice" and how successful it could be in distorting the facts. Little wonder the state legislature had recently refused to modify the laws of libel in favor of the newspapers. Fortunately for all involved, the *Citizen* was ready to expose the truth, marking the "limit of the liberty of the press to run to the most infamous licentiousness."[84]

In the end, however, the *Eagle*'s articles left a powerfully negative impression of Dixon Jones. Nothing, it seemed, not even the *Citizen*'s chivalrous and self-satisfied apologia, could stem the tide of public disfavor. On May 31 a grand jury indicted her and her son on two counts, murder in the second degree for the death of Sarah Bates, and manslaughter in the second degree in the death of Ida Hunt. Mother and son were arrested and arraigned, pleaded not guilty and were held over for trial. Bail was set at $7500 for Dixon Jones and $5000 for Charles. It took two days to raise the money. Mrs. Maria Robbins, the wealthy widow of the Fulton Fish Market merchant Eli Robbins, came to court in person to offer bond. After a night in jail, the Joneses were released.[85]

At the arraignment, their lawyer, R. S. Newcombe, of Donohue, Newcombe and Cardoza, echoing the themes developed in the *Citizen*, claimed that the Joneses had been persecuted by the newspaper. District Attorney Ridgway, who only months before had been a friend of the Woman's Hospital, replied, "The articles published in the *Eagle* had as much to do in procuring this indictment as had the King of Siam. Mrs. Jones and her son were indicted on the evidence presented against them and on that alone."[86] For better or for worse, the Joneses would have their day in court.

2

A City
Comes of Age

Brooklyn is the only female among our cities—the sister city to New York. Like a good woman, she offers little to the chance visitor, impelled to come by idle curiosity, and nothing to the roué, But if you live in her house, as one of her family, you are well off indeed.
—*JULIAN RALPH,* Harper's Magazine, 1893[1]

On Thursday, May 24, 1883, the Brooklyn *Eagle* published a special issue to herald the opening of the Brooklyn Bridge. As was frequently the case in turn-of-the-century Brooklyn, a spirit of self-promotion and civic-mindedness spurred the city's elite to celebrate its connection to but independence from the urban Goliath to their north. Since the idea for a bridge to New York had been a dream of prominent Brooklyn citizens for decades, they were justly proud. Most agreed with the editor of *Harper's*, who praised its "simple graceful span" and proclaimed the structure both a "triumph of human skill" and "one of the wonders of the world."[2] The newspaper marked the event by featuring eight pages of encomium to human ingenuity and mechanical genius, identifying itself and the city with the pathbreaking feat. Imbricated in the laudatory testimonials, the columns of statistics on the bridge, and the dramatic stories of the twenty deaths and various cripplings from caisson disease that had occurred in the thirteen years of hard labor was a carefully crafted history of Brooklyn and its development, emphasizing the city's independence from New York and detailing its unique combination of cosmopolitanism and hospitality. For decades afterward, the *Eagle* faithfully marked this important anniversary. Some editors and employees came to "consider themselves the spiritual custodians" of the bridge's traditions, a task that entailed nourishing the city's sense of historical continuity by the repeated retelling of this symbolic achievement.[3]

In this chapter we will digress from accusations and counter-accusations, manslaughter charges, medical malpractice suits, and court proceedings in order to make the point that context is critical to understanding and judging trials and verdicts. I will argue that the Dixon Jones affair had as much to do with the city of Brooklyn, its history, geography, and social development, as it did with Dixon Jones's character, changes in medicine, the emergence of new surgical techniques, or the status of women in the medical profession. Indeed, it is not likely that an event of this nature would have occurred in New York, Boston, or Philadelphia. When Mary Dixon Jones settled in Brooklyn in 1864, the city was already beginning to occupy a unique place in the narrative of late nineteenth-century urban development, and its special characteristics are essential to our story.

From the very beginning, Brooklyn's attraction for all classes arose in part from its proximity to New York. Especially during the second half of the century, the accessible residential and commercial wards in King's County were offered in stark contrast to those of Manhattan, across the river, which was increasingly perceived as a degenerating center of urban corruption, rife with disorder and decay, replete with extremes of wealth and poverty. In contrast, Brooklyn in the 1850s had come to be known as "the city of churches," because of its favorable ratio of religious congregations to population. Three decades later, when a second wave of immigrants from southern and eastern Europe discovered the city's virtues, choosing, according to one commentator, "cozy homes" over "crowded tenements," Brooklyn became the third largest city in the nation.[4] It displayed much of the vitality of the modern urban center, yet was seemingly more manageable, safer, and considerably more pleasant in its order and cleanliness.[5]

While the image of a refuge prevailed among the city's promoters until at least the end of the century, Brooklyn also suffered an inferiority complex that could have been overcome, noted one historian, "only by widening the East River to the proportions of an ocean or by the destruction of its elephantine

neighbor."[6] Brooklynites resented the frequent allusions to their city's dependence on New York, especially when its attractions were reduced solely to its
cheap housing.[7] To be sure, Brooklyn's leaders were quite proud of its commercial expansion, which catalyzed the growth of city services, such as a ma-
turing police force, a professionalizing fire department, and boards of education
and health.[8] Also welcome was the augmentation of urban transit, including
railroads, ferries, elevated street cars, and new roads.[9] The flourishing of business at the docks, stimulating the erection of new warehouses, grain elevators,
and other buildings, proved an additional source of satisfaction, leading one
historian to quip that Brooklyn became the storehouse as well as the bedroom
of New York in these years. Indeed, by the early 1890s, the receiving and
exporting of grain from Brooklyn's harbor exceeded that of New York, Jersey
City, and Hoboken combined, while, adjacent to the waterfront, stood the city's
famous sugar refineries, marking Brooklyn as the greatest sugar refining center
in the world. In addition, lumberyards, machine shops, and oil refineries lined
the area. Manufacturing also flourished, and the census of 1880 placed the city
third in the number of factories, fourth in invested industrial capital, fourth in
the value of products produced, and second in average wages. In truth, Brooklyn's industrial economy was "remarkably diversified."[10]

So, too, with increasing visibility, was its population and class structure.
Although Brooklyn boasted some exclusive neighborhoods, like Brooklyn
Heights and the Hill, mixed-class and poor immigrant working-class areas prevailed, especially in the most industrialized sectors of the city, stretching along
the East River and the harbor, from Williamsburgh to Bushwick and Greenpoint.
Poles, Jews, Slovaks, and Slovenian workers predominated, but Williamsburgh
was also home to Brooklyn's greatest concentration of German immigrants,
comprising 94,000 souls by 1890, the largest immigrant group in the city. According to Harold Syrett, the filth and poverty in which they lived was surpassed
only by the Irish. Germans were not all poor, however, and an article in the
New York *Tribune* of 1893 describes not only laboring families, but "German
lawyers, German doctors, German professors and musicians" who "could be
found on every block."[11] The Irish distributed themselves all over Brooklyn,
but the largest communities were still crowded into the tenements and flats south
of the Navy Yard through the City Hall district and South Brooklyn. Even the
African-American community, which "had the good fortune to rent small two-
family houses rather than tenements" and lived in the City Hall district proper,
apparently managed better housing than their Irish neighbors. The neighborhood
south of Prospect Park boasted a thriving settlement of Swedes, and a lively
Syrian enclave nestled on the edge of Brooklyn Heights.[12]

Thousands of workers were employed in the garment industry, baking and
confectionery, glass and gas-lamp production, and carpentry. The 1890 census
revealed that over 2500 masons lived in the city, and more than 3000 laborers,
including women and children, toiled in the Navy Yards. Another 8000 peopled
the industrial sections that dotted the coastline. Nevertheless, wages were low
and unemployment rife, with roughly 25 percent of the work force without jobs
in any given year. The situation was so desperate that "dependent people were

regularly thrown onto the local charity rolls, or alternatively, into charity hospitals when illness was added to unemployment. Small community hospitals, organized by local merchants or religious or other civic and moral leaders, were overwhelmed by a needy and increasingly impoverished population.''[13]

Dixon Jones's hospital and several dispensaries, for example, were originally established in Brooklyn's City Hall district, which insured a mostly poor and lower middle-class clientele. After 1884, her private hospital, the dispensaries, and the gynecological department, where much of the surgery took place, relocated to Bushwick and the 16th Ward in Williamsburgh, also mixed-class areas. Both locations were close enough to wealthy residential districts, especially Brooklyn Heights, the Hill, and Prospect Park, to draw in occasional patients from the upper classes as well. Ida Hunt, for example, lived in Bushwick with her husband and parents, whereas Sarah Bates, the other patient whose surgery the *Eagle* accused Dixon Jones of botching, resided in Brooklyn Heights.

In addition to emphasizing homes and churches, orators, especially after the completion of the Brooklyn Bridge, were fond of describing Brooklyn as the "bride of New York."[14] The domestic imagery imbricated in these sobriquets, alluding to a feminized, kinder, and gentler city, in which marriage and middle-class family values still held absolute sway, speaks eloquently to the power and directedness of Brooklyn's self-definition. "If one city calls up the idea of commercial eminence," wrote an editor at the Brooklyn *Eagle*, "the other represents a special emphasis on those principles which are symbolized by the word 'home'."[15] Indeed, one of the "attractive features" of the city, according to one commentator, was the custom of holding a yearly parade composed entirely of school children and their instructors, winding energetically down Brooklyn's tree-lined streets. Beginning with the Sunday schools, and eventually extended to the public schools as well, "Saint Children's Day" was a regular feature of the May calendar. "A more inspiring scene can hardly be imagined," noted this observer, "than that presented by those myriads of hopeful, fresh young faces, looking eagerly forward, a prophecy and full of promise to the city of the future."[16]

Thus was Brooklyn's self-image fashioned very consciously in binary relationship to the perceived unmanageability of the adjacent metropolis to the north. Indeed, negative representations of the latter, an urban center that, in the minds of many, increasingly came to symbolize what was wrong with city life in general, had special resonance for Brooklynites. Henry Ward Beecher's famous rhetorical query in a sermon, "Who owns the city of New York?" to which his response was "The Devil," was typical of the attitudes of many of his parishioners at Brooklyn's notoriously celebrated Plymouth Church. Indiscriminate fears of "the city" as an emblem of disorder became a powerful subtext lurking just beneath the surface boosterism of Brooklyn's many admirers, creating a kind of rivalry in the minds of residents, one generously giving their city the upper hand in any serious moral accounting.[17]

PROFESSIONAL AND ENTREPRENEURIAL ELITES: ORDER AND
TRADITIONAL VALUES

Commercial expansion fueled Brooklyn's institutional, cultural, and social life, leading to the development of exclusive suburban neighborhoods, such as Brooklyn Heights and the Hill, and later Park Slope, Bedford, and the East End, where a growing entrepreneurial and professional elite resided in middle-class comfort.[18] Until the 1880s, however, the best men and women of the city preferred to maintain their distance from local politics, free to do so by their unwavering commitment to a belief in Brooklyn's small-town atmosphere and the increasingly misguided sense that Brooklyn remained insulated from the vexations of urbanization. Instead, they devoted their efforts to the rich associational life that had become the hallmark of a middle-class community ethic, one that contributed to the shaping of a more diversified public realm in the second half of the century. Evangelical societies, supplemented by countless other organizations—lyceums, literary gatherings, music and choral groups, cricket clubs, brass bands, lodges, benevolent and charitable activities—all flourished in Brooklyn in abundance. They shaped new constructions of taste, respectability, manners, domestic space, social interaction, child-rearing, and family life, marking social identity in novel ways.[19]

The professional and mercantile elite whose careers kept them in Brooklyn proper formed the backbone of middle-class group life in the city, with clubs like the Brooklyn, Hamilton, Lincoln, Oxford, Union League, Montauk, Hanover, and Algonquin dominating the scene. Though these organizations were "admirable and important," one contemporary felt, none was "decidedly prosperous in the degree which marks the prosperity of clubs in the more masculine great cities." Indeed, some displayed a "peculiarity" typical of the city's "character." This was the habit of members referring "to their wives . . . and personal servants, with the knowledge that these personages are known to the other members." A few clubs, noted this reporter, actually admitted ladies to designated spaces—four establishing "restaurants and rooms" for women. " 'Interest your wife, and she will let you join,' is the principle upon which this evolution is working," he advised. In Brooklyn, it seems, the new bourgeois heterosociality so characteristic of the shopping and mercantile centers and other sumptuous commercialized urban spaces of midtown Manhattan did not include the ratcheting up of erotic female display or the loosening of sexual norms.[20] Indeed, Brooklyn's intelligent and public-spirited classes, forming the core of its citizenry, considered it their good fortune that Brooklyn was dominated by a bourgeois culture more unified and more pious than most cities of its size.

The *Eagle* acknowledged Brooklyn's bourgeois amicability in its celebratory volume on the city's history, published in 1893. Moreover, it argued, distinctions between different social circles had "rapidly" diminished in the last decade, and "society is massing itself into one body." Indeed, "in characteristics, little if any difference is to be noticed between the members of the various sets."[21] Traditionally there were three ways to enter Brooklyn society: "church, charity, and grandfather." As to the last, the city most definitely had its share of descendants of the colonial "merchant princes." And lineage had often taken precedence over wealth, to the degree that wealth has not had "the slightest value to the young man or the debutante" with family connections among the older elite of Brooklyn Heights. Whereas elsewhere "the evolution of society has been along very different lines," with a social pecking order increasingly structured by money alone, even in Brooklyn's newer, fashionable neighborhoods, it was the church that still "brought people together." Sociality began with Sunday school classes, "the church sociable in private houses continued it," and, finally, "the step from this to little dances of an independent order was very slight." At present, this author believed, "the surest way for a young man to gain his *entree* into social life is to join the young people's association of some energetic church congregation." Emphasis on church membership set Brooklyn's bourgeois public culture apart from that of New York City in ways that would become crucial, I will argue, to Mary Dixon Jones's career in the city. As we shall see, during the libel trial prominent ministers, their wives, and pious congregants appeared as character witnesses for both sides.[22]

Churches fostered private charity, which played a central role in solidifying social relations, and the city boasted of benevolent activity in abundance. Such institutions emerged as part of the larger movement of cities toward the development of the public sphere and served as "experimental testing grounds" for new kinds of services and novel forms of social welfare fully developed in the progressive era and beyond.[23] Men and women affirmed their charitable inclinations in public by donations of time—sitting on institutional Boards of Directors, for example—as well as money. Organized charities in Brooklyn were also allotted sums from the city itself, which distributed excise funds according to the number of individuals receiving aid from a particular organization. Social clubs performed the work of providing efficient venues for the information-gathering necessary to intelligent decision-making in the realm of public welfare, and women's groups played a special, heuristic role in schooling members in the minutiae of management. Interest in better health care facilities and increased cultural amenities within these clubs was palpable.[24]

In Brooklyn, as in other cities, women were particularly visible in the work of benevolence, and the interest that Dixon Jones generated among prominent city wives was typical of these larger impulses. Institution-building of this type proved an outlet for ambitious and talented women, giving them a sense of purpose and identity as well as a "platform from which to criticize the masculine world." In many respects, medical charity seemed an extension of their natural sphere. Collaborating physicians, of course, were as much motivated by professional as by charitable aims. Hospitals served the poor, but they also provided direct clinical experience to young medical students and nurses. Because Boards of Lady Managers devoted themselves as much to the moral as to the physical regeneration of patients, tension often arose when professional and charitable aims came into conflict. Thus, clashes between physicians and hospital trustees were not uncommon in this period. One of our tasks will be to determine whether the controversy involving Dixon Jones's hospital represented normal stresses and strains, or matters more serious.[25]

Stimulating Brooklyn's need for charity and hospital services was the expansion of manufacturing, which multiplied the number of work-related injuries. This growth, combined with an increasingly diversified population of immigrant poor living in unhealthy conditions, put pressure on already overcrowded institutions to expand. In response, the 1880s saw the establishment of a number of small neighborhood hospitals, differing in "religious and ethnic orientation, source of financial support, size, medical orentation, and the type of service provided." The formation of such institutions was a reaction not simply to the increase in need, but to geographical change that promoted the migration of private physicians out of the center city and its adjacent poorer areas into the newer, mixed- and middle-class neighborhoods. Much like Dixon Jones's establishment, which was, at least on the surface, a typical example, many were homes that had been "quickly put to use when a need arose." As one historian has noted, "the community-supported charity hospitals were an indispensable resource for the ... dependent poor," particularly before notions of organized public welfare took hold.[26] Indeed, middle-class philanthropy and working-class needs remained so intertwined that Dixon Jones tapped easily into an eager and enthusiastic female charity culture when she first proposed organizing her hospital in 1881.

According to contemporaries, Brooklyn was "a woman's town."[27] Boosters were visibly proud of the city's lack of prurient urban amusements, and emphasized the city's "elbow-room and a hush at night," where residents "see trees and can have growing flowers." Indeed, it was primarily "the home of the married middle people of New York," and whereas husbands were "far more interested in New York than in Brooklyn," Brooklyn's wives kept alive the city's powerful sense of superiority and "look[ed] down on the metropolis." Though they shopped there, they despised it "as a 'shoddy' town and a Babel." New York was not simply "cold and monstrous"; its materialistic social boundaries were "un-American." In contrast, Brooklyn's middle-class women displayed an ambivalence toward consumption. Attracted by the increasing availability of goods, they nevertheless worried about the corrupting influence of excessive conspicuous display. They took pains to distinguish themselves from the very rich.[28]

While husbands commuted to work in New York, Brooklyn women were left alone. According to one commentator, they "rule over the children, maids, nurses, shade trees, flowers and pretty door-yards. Thus encouraged, each studies her own neighborhood. Each remembers how the other called on her when she moved to Brooklyn, and each calls on those who come after her."[29]

The sense of safety in Brooklyn, the absence of men during the day, and the ability to live well on a modest budget combined, suggested one writer, to "widen" women's "freedom." But while some genteel women in New York City developed the reputation for expressing their newly fashioned public agency by strolling provocatively down "Ladies' Mile," a commercial district replete with lavish luxury department stores and elaborate window displays, Brooklyn's middle-class women took comfort in the "self-improvement" of reading and literary societies, feminine piety, and noblesse oblige. Not oblivous to New York fashion, "always provided that it does not cost too much or require going to the theatre," Brooklyn women were "the very backbone of the churches, in which they sing and hold fairs, and by means of which they figure in circles that are proud of them."[30] "Is it any wonder," asked this commentator rhetorically, "that they cannot tolerate New York, where the shopkeepers won't send a purchase around the corner without pay in advance, where the pews are private property in the best churches, and where a lady feels herself of no account in the hurly-burly?"[31]

Thus did Brooklyn's middle class deliberately represent itself as distinct from that of New York's. Moreover, this self-representation worked as a powerful backdrop to the Dixon Jones affair—a public trial in which a woman physician was accused of behavior that was decidedly out-of-bounds. Extremely useful in helping us to understand why this might be so is David Scobey's provocative work on the subject of sex and the bourgeois public sphere.[32] Scobey shows that the character of public space was shaped by an intricate and eloquent performativity that historians need to consider seriously in their elaborations of middle-class culture. This point is illustrated in powerfully suggestive ways in his examination of the cultural implications of "Ladies' Mile," located in a Manhattan Scobey characterizes as "the national center . . . of elite amusements, genteel fashion, luxury consumerism, and commercialized refinements." Important for our purposes, particularly when we consider the ramifications of Brooklyn's relationship to New York City, is Scobey's argument that the latter led the nation in "matters of style, sociability and leisure," representing the "benchmark for respectable taste about what to wear, sit on, eat, and see."[33] It was within this contested public landscape that conflicts over changing standards of female behavior were acted out, with the elites of New York City and Brooklyn winding up, not surprisingly, in opposing camps.

Scobey's work suggests that the last third of the nineteenth century produced competing images of bourgeois female respectability—the eroticized and free-wheeling shopper and the pious and selfless reformer—that troubled middle-class commentators on social life until the end of the century. His speculations gain credence when we contemplate the meaning of Brooklyn's elaborate representation of itself as a morally conservative counterweight to Manhattan. We shall see that several themes in the Dixon Jones trial help elucidate how, with the aid of its many entrepreneurial boosters, the city stubbornly and with considered judgment resisted repeated threats of unwelcome and morally compromising change.[34]

MEDICINE AND THE TRANSFORMATION OF PROFESSIONAL VALUES

Even Brooklyn's professional life, with its attendant organizational activity that flourished at the end of the century, bore the stamp of the city's distinct self-characterization as a refuge for women, families, and bourgeois civilized morality. To be sure, just as in other cities, the emergence of values based on individual expertise, faith in the authority of "objective" science and technology, and business administration in government contributed powerfully to the shaping of Brooklyn's middle-class culture in these years. But however much professional ideology in Brooklyn reflected standards developing nationally, however much it was a product of social, economic, and technological change, and however thoroughly it was stimulated by the emergence of new forms of knowledge, Brooklyn–New York tensions colored even these factors in unique and instructive ways. In Brooklyn, the practice and appreciation of medicine, and the trajectory of surgical gynecology as an emerging subspecialty, took a particular course, one reflected eloquently in the heated medical debates for which the libel trial provided a particularly public platform.

General anxieties regarding specialization and professionalization in medicine provide an important context for understanding Dixon Jones's reception as a surgeon by her Brooklyn colleagues. Specialization challenged an older conceptual framework and gave rise to heated discussions over the meaning of medical science. The relevance of this development to our story will be examined in more detail in the next two chapters, where we focus on Dixon Jones's medical career and the growth of the specialty she helped to promote with such vigor. For the moment, however, we want to ask how such growing pains meshed with the other anxieties plaguing urbanizing Brooklyn—especially those linked to the administration of charity and benevolence, the legitimate distribution of public funds, and the transformation of institutions—particularly the hospital—to accommodate the needs of both medical professionals and the collective community.

Linked to debates over the emergence of the specialties was an undercurrent of fretfulness around economic issues, which Brooklyn physicians shared with colleagues elsewhere across the country. From mid-century on, doctors began to complain about overcrowding in the profession, and, indeed, the physician-patient ratio dropped in the first half of the century from about one doctor for every 950 patients to one in 600. The loosening of professional restrictions, especially in educational standards and licensing, contributed to the situation for much of the nineteenth century, and, especially for urban physicians, the trend was exacerbated by increasingly disproportional geographical distribution. In large cities in the years between 1870 and 1910, the number of physicians per 100,000 people grew from 177 to 241, while in other areas that figure actually fell, from 160 to 152.[35] Brooklyn's statistics were no different, and the economic insecurity expressed by some of its physicians was acute.

Many physicians blamed increasing specialization. For example, in 1888, Willard P. Beach complained in an article published in the *Brooklyn Medical Journal* that the proliferation of specialists and specialties was making it difficult for the young physician starting out to establish a financially secure practice. Part of the reason for this, he argued, was that too many were poorly trained, and when presented with even a "simple" case for diagnosis, they became so "alarmed" that they called in a specialist "at once." The result, that the general practitioner "becomes the feeding reservoir to keep the offices of the specialists filled with patients, and their pockets distended with money," was disastrous for even the *skilled* "family doctor," who was forced to eke "out an economical existence, working night and day for miserably small pay."[36]

Others feared that doctors were being exploited by the public and participated too freely in the administration of gratuitous medical services to the poor, "*The physician's first duty to society is to make a living and keep out of the poor-house,*" asserted one angry Brooklyn practitioner in 1893.[37] Though not everyone agreed that medical men were in dire financial straits—an editorial in the *Brooklyn Medical Journal* in 1888 claimed that "the doctor is no worse off than the rest"—the fact that the debate took place at all testifies to the salience of the issue.[38]

Sometimes this discomfort took the form of hostility to dispensaries and suspicions that they were abused, by both unscrupulous doctors and deceitful patients. Dispensaries, both free-standing and attached to hospitals, were earmarked for the ambulatory care of the sick poor, and fees were either minimal or nonexistent. Given the overcrowding in the profession and alleged financial insecurities physicians expressed, many viewed dispensaries as part of the problem. One Brooklyn doctor noted, for example, that they had a tendency "to educate the people to be dependent and pauperish," and that "patients without number" obtained free advice and medicine from them "when they are abundantly able to pay a reasonable amount to a physician for his services."[39]

Mistrust of dispensaries also generated another form of tension, namely, between practitioner and practitioner. Not only did some physicians fear that *patients* defrauded them out of rightful financial compensation, they worried that *fellow physicians* used dispensaries to attract clients. Louis F. Criado pleaded with his professional brethren to recognize the necessity of hospital and dispensary reform, asserting that at least 60 percent of the people who received medical advice from dispensaries were "*well-to-do impostors.*" But even more rankling to Criado and many of his colleagues was the possibility that physicians would steal patients from each other. Dispensary doctors were advantageously positioned to do that, he believed, suggesting in a series of proposed reforms that "any physician convicted of soliciting dispensary patients for his private practice should be dishonorably discharged, and henceforth disqualified from serving *in any dispensary or hospital.*" Criado extended his suspicions to ordinary colleagues as well, some of whom, he feared, were capable of being "summoned to attend others' patients" and "unhesitatingly" prove "themselves at variance with the original diagnosis" with a mind to soliciting the patient's future patronage. Were not financial exigencies driving members of the profession to dishonesty and intrigue, "notwithstanding the *falsity* of our most apparent courtesy and pleasing etiquette towards one another?"[40]

Collegial mistrust also manifested itself in worries about the counterfeit medical charities that, according to Dr. Reuben Jeffrey, "unfortunately glut the market." In a letter to the *Brooklyn Medical Journal*, he complained that too many of these in Brooklyn were used "as a side-door to . . . private practice" or to "prop up some weak physician who dare not take his stand upon his own merits.''[41] Anxieties about this kind of fraud would become intertwined with support for Brooklyn's reform mayor, Seth Low, who in 1881 turned his attention to streamlining a number of city services, not the least in importance were its medical charities. Echoes of all these themes can be heard in the *Eagle*'s exposé of Dixon Jones in 1889.

Adding to such concerns was a real disparity in talent within the Brooklyn medical community, generated, many felt, by the dearth of hospitals as teaching institutions and a dangerous reluctance to recognize their relationship to advances in medical education. In 1888, Lewis Pilcher, a well-respected Brooklyn physician and surgeon, gave a paper to the King's County Medical Society on the development of surgical practice in the city. In assessing the triumphs and disappointments of the last decade and a half, Pilcher was especially anxious to emphasize the crucial relationship of up-to-date medical institutions to medical innovation.[42]

This was particularly true of surgery. Acknowledging that advances in the field in the period under review were more remarkable in other parts of the country than in his own city, Pilcher did not hesitate to voice his disappointment with developments in Brooklyn. In the early 1870s, for example, when antisepsis was just beginning to be accepted among American physicians, ''the complete antiseptic idea'' was particularly ''slow'' to take hold there, due to the ''natural conservatism of men who by their age and experience have justly been intrusted [*sic*] with the control of hospital interests.'' Indeed, improvements in surgery were especially hampered by the city's inattention to hospitals. Pilcher viewed Brooklyn's record of hospital-building with dismay. This was a significant source of regret to enlightened physicians, he confessed, because on the number of hospitals, ''their character and organization, and . . . the spirit which characterizes their management depends much of the tone of the profession throughout the community.'' Hospital-trained doctors would not only relieve the suffering of the poor, but in ''wards and post-mortem rooms,'' they would test new medical theories.[43]

Pilcher blamed past inadequacies on ''a lack of public spirit'' among the city's wealthy citizens. Brooklyn's neglect of its hospitals had persisted far too long. The one public hospital serving the county had inadequate facilities, while the work of ''all the other hospitals of the city'' was ''greatly circumscribed and embarrassed by want of means.'' Indeed, until the city's hospitals measured up, Brooklyn's medical profession could not claim ''that meed of respect which is their due.''

Happily, the situation was being remedied, and Pilcher was pleased to report that his ''reproach is being rapidly wiped away.'' Brooklyn's elite had responded positively to the city's needs, and hospital building was already being stepped up. ''The newer hospitals with their younger workers, untrammeled by long established usages'' were ''bringing the general surgical work of the city up toward the plane of achievement found in other places.'' He concluded with an exhortation: Benevolent good works were never ''merely places where charity is dispensed'' but ''training schools'' of the future ''in all matters of professional advance.''[44]

As if heeding Pilcher's call, Mary Dixon Jones established the first Woman's Hospital of Brooklyn in 1882, in the midst of the city's general stock-taking and excitement over new possibilities. In an atmosphere generating increasing clarity of understanding as to the city's specific medical needs, her own plans proved attractive to supporters. Dixon Jones's institution boasted of an exemplary medical consulting staff, including several Brooklyn physicians, and a prestigious assembly of female officers, the wives of a handful of Brooklyn business and professional men.[45] Contemporary observers, indeed, had nothing but praise for the institution and its founder. One reporter emphasized that Dixon Jones's motive in establishing the hospital was to help the city's "*poor* women" who, though "burdened with the same physical ills" as those patients in her "extensive practice," who "could command the best medical skill, and surround themselves with every comfort that love and money could supply," were "wholly unable to command medical help" in the manner of their "more favored sisters." When an attempt to secure a bed for a Brooklyn woman in the New York Hospital for Women failed, Dixon Jones spearheaded a drive for a hospital and dispensary closer to home. "The Mission of the Dispensary and Hospital is to help suffering women and children," concluded this writer. "During the past year over 1,500 visits of the sick have been made to the Dispensary."[46] It seemed, indeed, that Dixon Jones's timing was perfect. The city's need for new hospitals, coupled with the obvious worthiness of targeting poor women and children for public largesse, boded well for a future filled with the success, public gratitude, and respectable middle-class connections. We will soon learn more about why such status proved important to her.

Seven years later, Dixon Jones and her institution would become the focus of anxieties regarding medical fraud and the abuse of charities that colored the public discourse of citizen concern in the 1880s. [47] The remarks of Pilcher and others were fairly typical of the discussions that took place among Brooklyn physicians. They reveal that, like the city's business elites, the local medical profession also grappled with the urban disquietude generated by rapid social change, while struggling as well with insecurities particular to medicine's changing professional status and structure. Many Brooklyn doctors shared the conservative and family-oriented self-image cultivated by hometown boosters. They responded with appropriate alarm to the various professional tensions their brethren struggled with in other cities, and those pressures, as we shall see, thread through as subtext in Mary Dixon Jones's two very public trials.

MIDDLE-CLASS CULTURE FINDS LOCAL POLITICS

Politics also played a part in the *Eagle*'s targeting of Dixon Jones and her institution, especially where accusations of fraud were concerned. Delving briefly into the city's political history can suggest a partial motive for the newspaper's involvement, while helping us to understand the resonance of accusations concerning the misappropriation of public funds. Since the 1850s, Brooklyn had come to be dominated by an immigrant machine government resting primarily on the voting strength of the immigrant Irish. Elected and appointed local officials were almost all retainers of "Boss" Hugh McLoughlin, originally a foreman at the Brooklyn Navy Yard, who rose through the ranks and, by the early 1870s, dominated Democratic policy in the city. These developments gave Brooklyn's respectable classes a convincing excuse to shun local political contests, and they concentrated instead on national issues. In so doing, they were not unlike elites in other cities who lost power and interest in local government in these years.[48]

By the 1880s, however, Brooklyn's progressive-thinking businessmen and professionals began to understand that the corruption, widespread graft, and endless inefficiency geared to line the pockets of members of the McLoughlin coterie hurt business interests and intruded on the ability of middle-class residents to live in the material comfort that should be proffered by a well-run city. Continued population growth meant that municipal services were not keeping pace with Brooklyn's self-image of genial habitability, and it became increasingly apparent that the disorder and inefficiency of local government was at fault. Brooklyn voters' habit of deciding local issues along national party lines was also an irritating deterrent to the logical consideration of municipal problems, and many residents understood that it was time for a change.[49]

Indeed, the situation had grown so acute that Brooklyn developed a certain notoriety for its subordination to patronage and party. Even mayors who wanted reform were unable to dissipate the narrow partisan spirit that dominated city management. Partially to blame was Brooklyn's charter of 1873, which guaranteed a decentralized governing system so diluting the power of the mayor that few with a forward-looking program could be elected, and those successful were hamstrung. But in 1882, a "single-head" law, strategically managed in committee by a former mayor who had been elected to the state senate, was miraculously passed by the New York legislature. Brooklyn's mayor gained veto power and direct responsibility for the management of affairs. The change revolutionized municipal government, not only in Brooklyn, but elsewhere as well, as cities across the nation began to imitate its provisions.[50]

This dramatic alteration in Brooklyn's governing structure lured segments of the city's progressive middle class into politics. Indeed, the spirit of professionalism that prevailed nationally led to the emergence of a group of independent reformers loosely associated with the Republican party, who had already begun to criticize political corruption on the federal level. Calling themselves Mugwumps, they pressed for civil service reform and a public ethic that could transcend "the language of interests and practicality," stymie the use of partisan politics to foster the advancement of personal wealth, and promote scientific objectivity and specialization—already watchwords in business and the professions—in a thorough-going overhaul of political life.[51]

In Brooklyn, these developments coalesced in a movement to oust Hugh McLoughlin from the leadership of the Democratic party, a campaign spearheaded by Thomas Kinsella, the editor of the Brooklyn *Eagle*. The *Eagle* had been a passionately partisan Democratic newspaper from its inception in 1841, but in the mid-1870s under Kinsella's guidance it began occasionally to take stands that were independent of the machine. Though Kinsella had been a personal friend of the "Boss," a feud developed between the two men in 1880, fueled by differences over presidential politics. The *Eagle* began to launch attacks against the Democratic machine, and in the 1881 mayoral election, the newspaper backed Seth Low, a handsome, thirty-two-year-old Republican lawyer with pronounced reform leanings, who rapidly became nationally known as a Republican reformer.[52]

Low's family traced its origins back to the Massachusetts Bay Colony, and his ancestors had flourished in business in New England before his grandfather settled in Brooklyn in the early 1800s. Low identified strongly with his Puritan heritage and demonstrated an early interest in Brooklyn's municipal problems.[53] One contemporary described him as "a young man who against all the inducements that wealth offers to lead a life of selfish pleasure, has developed a most laudable public spirit and acquired an intimate acquaintance with public affairs." According to Lincoln Steffens, Low "always gave more than he took."[54]

When he entered the mayoral race in 1881 and won, he had widespread backing from the progressive middle class of both parties. A combination of Republican vigor and Democratic disorganization gave him a majority of over 4000 votes. Indeed, Brooklyn's political historian characterized this election as a watershed of sorts, marking the city's "emergence from the stone age of municipal government." Low promoted the "Brooklyn Idea," a philosophy of municipal management that insisted on a strong executive, made watchwords of business administration and efficiency, and instituted a system of responsible home rule.[55] Low served two successful terms before going on to become president of Columbia University and mayor of New York. Historians credit him with "revolutionizing" Brooklyn's city administration. Indeed, his name became nationally known for efficient, responsible city government, and Brooklyn was viewed as an "oasis in the desert."[56]

Perhaps more important than his substantive accomplishments was his ability to infuse the city with the spirit of reform and galvanize support from respectable middle-class voters who, until the decade of the 1880s, had deliberately stayed out of local politics.[57] Low had been interested in the inefficiency of the city's Board of Health and the "mal-administration and abuse of the city and county charities" even before he became mayor. Disgusted by the corrupt system of outdoor relief in Brooklyn and by the partisanship of the charity commissioners, he helped found an association of private charities and became its first president in 1879. This group sustained a central office and a salaried superintendent who fostered cooperation between various church and private agencies, discouraging fraudulent claims and offering various social services in addition to temporary relief.[58]

When he took office, Low continued to demonstrate interest in charity reform, extending his concerns to the area of health as well. One of his most effective appointments was that of Dr. Joseph Raymond, whom we meet again at Dixon Jones's libel trial, as commissioner of the Board of Health. Under Raymond's supervision, the board tightened health standards in the city's manufacturing sector, developed a corps of vaccinating physicians who kept winter epidemics at a minimum, and updated and codified health laws. These activities dovetailed with the concern expressed by members of the King's County Medical Society, which, as we have already seen, had its own slant on a number of these issues, including the abuses of medical charity and the neglect and mismanagement of Brooklyn's hospitals. Thus, the *Eagle's* initial questioning of the financial and governmental policies of Dixon Jones's institution was already well within the bounds of public discourse when the articles first appeared in 1889.[59]

Though Low retired after a second term, the changes he had wrought were difficult to dismantle completely, and in the decade after 1885, "Brooklyn's government, like its press, was characterized by a conflict between the ideas represented by Hugh McLoughlin and Seth Low."[60] Indeed, Low's message of optimism, reform, honesty, and good government generated a powerful sense of boosterism among some of Brooklyn's respectable professionals throughout the 1880s and into the next decade.

"HONEST AND MANLY JOURNALISM": NEWSPAPERS AND THE POWER
OF DISCOURSE

Throughout the decade of reform struggles in Brooklyn the *Eagle* kept a watchful eye over events. The newspaper's support had been crucial to the election of Seth Low, and that campaign represented as well the gradual refashioning of the *Eagle's* self-image. In the 1880s, the newspaper transformed itself from a party organ to a more modern, independent-minded daily. Historians have credited nineteenth-century newspapers with providing city readers with a crucial sense of belonging, and in many respects, the Brooklyn *Eagle*, a paper "intensely local in spirit," but with excellent general news coverage, superior editorial skill, and boasting by 1890 a large circulation and a national reputation, stands as a vivid example of this phenomenon.

Indeed, it is possible to argue that the *Eagle* played a critical role in representing the coherent community that Brooklyn was struggling to become in the 1880s and 1890s, as the whole essentially emerged as more than the sum of its parts. Unlike other cities, Brooklyn had attained maturity "literally overnight." In 1854, it was only the seventh largest city in the nation. A year later, a consolidation act that annexed Bushwick and Williamsburgh moved Brooklyn from seventh to third place in the nation. In 1886, the town of New Lots was incorporated as the city's 26th Ward, and in the mid-1890s, Flatbush, Gravesend, New Utrecht, and Flatlands were gobbled up by the city as well. The *Eagle* devoted itself to reinforcing the community identity of this urban space in rapid flux. In effect, over the last two decades of the nineteenth century, the *Eagle* enacted a partially conscious aspiration to capture Brooklyn's complex process of identity formation. It reproduced public discussions of class, status, education, and politics, accomplishing important cultural work in the circulation of ideas and serving as an accessible and centralized communication hierarchy that provided common intelligence for the community as a whole. An apostle of what was known as the "Brooklyn Spirit," the *Eagle* kept the faith, even during the times when radical change called feelings of commonality into question.

We have already noted the *Eagle*'s origins as a Democratic party newspaper in the 1840s. Four decades later it was undergoing most of the changes experienced by the news industry in this period, when the dailies, as they were called, became an integral part of a competitive, industrializing society. Newspapers, like other industries, expanded at an unprecedented rate. In 1870, for example, there were 489 English-language general circulation papers; by the turn of the century the number had almost quadrupled to 1,967.[61] Newspaper work at the *Eagle*, like most of its competitors, became increasingly segmented, as publishers became less involved with day-to-day production, and editors, now themselves becoming specialized, parceled out the news-gathering process to staff reporters. This phenomenon occurred throughout the United States, but it was particularly apparent in New York, the nation's largest city and the site of the most innovative changes in late nineteenth-century journalism.[62]

Along with innovations catalyzed by structural, technological, and economic change, newspapers increasingly began to play a more significant cultural role in city life. Many scholars have written about how the disorder, complexity, and unmanageability of city life led to a lost sense of control that probably hastened the decline of regularity, predictability, and the familiar, face-to-face routines characteristic of rural existence.[63] Alan Trachtenberg, for example, has argued in particular that newspapers served to dramatize what he believes was a central paradox of urban life—that "the more knowable the world came to seem as *information*, the more remote and opaque it came to seem as *experience*." The city allegedly deprived its inhabitants of authentic experience, replacing it with spectacle and vicarious spectatorship—primarily in the guise of reading and looking. But I want to suggest that the city offered a different type of experience as well, one that combined distance and community, intimacy and numbers. The dailies, in their invention of a novel kind of news, emphasized the sensational and the dramatic, often creating an "urban form of village gossip, designed to make the lives of distant others seem near and 'human'." Certainly, face-to-face relationships declined in the city, but what arose in their place was an imagined community that connected diverse neighborhoods with a unifying set of images and representations.[64]

My use of the term "imagined" in this context does not necessarily connote imaginary or inauthentic. Indeed, newspapers surely helped to create alternative conditions of commonality, and the Brooklyn *Eagle*, particularly because of its attention to local news, was especially adept at this. Newspaper readers thus often experienced life in their city in mediated fashion, but a sense of the city's unity, the connections between neighborhoods through associational life, through community celebration and spectacle, and through the daily reportage of familiar aspects of neighborhood existence was always a part of the *Eagle*'s renderings of Brooklyn. It was surely at this moment in the late nineteenth century that tradition itself would become, as John B. Thompson has recently pointed out, "increasingly interwoven with mediated symbolic forms." Though newspapers began this process, movies, radio, and television would continue it into the next century; experience would be taken up and reshaped, and traditions, reenacted and elaborated over time, would be reinvented for new public venues. Yet to argue that these experiences cannot thereby be rooted in the day-to-day lives of individuals and are *merely* impositions from the outside—by political elites, media gurus, over-enthusiastic reporters, or hungry advertising agents— represents a variation on a familiar historical fallacy: the idea of a past golden age in which life was better, more "authentic." "Traditions," Thompson reminds us, "which rely heavily on mediated symbolic forms are not *ipso facto* less authentic that those which are transmitted exclusively through face-to-face interaction. In a world increasingly permeated by communication media, traditions have become increasingly dependent on mediated symbolic forms; they have become dislodged from particular locales and re-embedded in social life in new ways."[65]

For all its mawkish extravagance, the antebellum penny press anticipated some of these major innovations in post–Civil War journalism. Challenging the monopoly of the partisan dailies, usually mouthpieces for party politics or the mercantile elite, penny papers were the first commercial enterprises bent on making a profit. In this sense, they were linked to the development of a free market economy and underscored the rising emphasis on individualism. Michael Schudson notes that they represented for the first time a press oriented toward a readership with which it had no face-to-face connections. Competition reigned, as various dailies contended over both readers and advertisers, accepting and acting out the ideas of the new capitalist elite. In terms of their efforts to broaden the public knowledge base and break through the traditional privileged domination of political parties, repeatedly stressing in their message the superior importance of factual news over opinion in a democracy, these papers helped structure a decidedly more egalitarian public discourse. Advocating objectivity, which in the 1830s merely meant autonomy from party control and not the scientific rendering of "truth" that it would come to mean later in the century, the penny press began to represent itself as a champion of the common people.[66]

Part of that task entailed a dramatic increase in the human interest story, the reportage of local events, and sensationalist accounts of "crimes, disasters, sex scandals, and monstrosities."[67] The penny press did not invent this genre, but they made it a staple of their news. They deliberately wove their stories into a pattern expressive of basic class tensions and antagonisms. Especially hostile to the moral weakness and unjust privileges of the wealthy, they relied on "the artisan-republican ideology of equal rights for all citizens," even as the trajectory of their economic organization and commercialization embedded them deeper and deeper in the capitalist relations imitative of the new industrial elites. For example, population growth alone permitted increased newspaper circulation, which, in turn, demanded larger investments and expanding operating expenses and, with these developments, structural differentiation.[68]

In addition to the quadrupling of the number of newspapers, including dramatic increases in foreign-language dailies, other changes are worth noting. Evening journals began to replace morning editions as the most important one of the day, as audiences were increasingly made up of "shopping crowds, homeward bound workers, and theater fans.'' The evening papers were also specifically targeted to women, evidenced especially by the dramatic increase in department store advertisements that fattened the later editions considerably. Some newspapers were so intent on attracting women readers that their Sunday editions carried full-page news and features designed especially for them, prototypes of what eventually became the woman's page.[69]

More significant than format, however, was the changing nature of news reporting. Increasingly after the Civil War, sensational journalism, pioneered by the penny press, became a daily staple. The first to develop what newspaper historians have called ''story journalism'' into an art form was Joseph Pulitzer, an Austrian Jew who moved to the United States in 1864, invented and perfected his techniques in the 1870s as publisher of the St. Louis *Post and Dispatch*, and brought the ''new journalism'' to New York City when he bought the floundering New York *World* in 1883. By the late 1880s the *World* was the largest daily paper in the country; its Sunday edition alone reached 250,000 people. Scholars agree that Pulitzer's innovations ''affected the character of the entire daily press of the country.''[70]

One factor in Pulitzer's success was his recognition that there were large numbers of New Yorkers who were either not interested in the news or could not afford to buy a paper. He priced his paper at one cent, and unabashedly targeted immigrant readers by demanding of his reporters the simple sentences and language that even ''greenhorns'' learning English could comprehend. Not surprisingly, immigrants comprised a significant segment of the *World*'s readership. But the *World* also appealed to a cross-section of the newspaper audience, attracting middle-class readers because, according to one scholar, Pulitzer understood not only their desires for ''effective leadership reflecting progressive attitudes,'' but also their craving for entertainment. Key features of the *World's* attractiveness were colorfully presented news items, an editorial page acclaimed for its high quality, and crusades and stunts geared to attract the credulous and over-curious.[71]

For example, Pulitzer put a high premium on news reporting. His writers ''scoured the city for incidents, events and situations which could be made interesting. These were presented as colorfully as possible,'' with headlines that could not fail to attract attention. But it would be a mistake to suppose that ''trivial sensationalism'' was all that the *World* strived for; according to Frank Luther Mott, ''important and significant news was by no means neglected; it was the backbone of the paper.''[72] Moreover, Pulitzer was more interested in the editorial department than in any other aspect of the newspaper. He thought of it as the heart of the publication, the paper's chief reason for existence. In the early years especially his careful editorials gave him a reputation for responsible leadership somewhat at odds with the more prurient aspects of the *World*'s offerings.[73]

Nevertheless, it was the *World's* extravagance and melodrama that had the greatest impact on the press in New York, the nation, and the world. Mott cites sensationalism and the way it fueled the feverish competition in the New York press after Pulitzer's arrival in 1883 as one of the primary features of late nineteenth-century journalism. Indeed, when the streets did not provide enough news for Pulitzer, he sent his reporters out to create copy by devising self-promoting crusades and stunts that kept the newspaper in the limelight. It was Pulitzer, for example, who sent the female reporter Nelly Bly around the world, beating the record of Jules Verne's fictional hero in *Around the World in Eighty Days*. The increase in readership resulting from the stunt marked the Bly incident as one of the paper's most successful escapades. In addition, crime news, political corruption, and social scandal, long the gristmill of the penny press, became important insofar as these events were discovered, exposed, or even created by the newspaper. Within such a framework, timing was key. As the historian Bernard Weisberger noted, "a paper achieved rank and readers by being first with the news. If the stories it furnished could be not only early, but exclusive, that was even better."[74]

One way to achieve exclusivity was to manufacture news, and Pulitzer accomplished this feat by launching extravagant news crusades that ran the gambit from unveiling political corruption to exposing white slavery, and pulling readers in with exciting installments, much as television soap operas did a century later.[75] While creating news gained additional readers and cemented the loyalty of the regulars, newspapermen and women also believed that these exposé served a social good. Sidney Kobré argues somewhat idealistically that Pulitzer's crusades helped make newspapers a type of social agency capable of carrying out the functions of investigation and exposure. Certainly Pulitzer himself believed that these moments of social responsibility were especially meaningful to many of his readers, especially those who were marginalized and thereby excluded from mainstream social respectability.[76]

Also worth noting is that, by the latter decades of the nineteenth century, the press increasingly defined itself as a distinct entity with a duty to the public to observe, investigate, and report public proceedings, monitor the actions of public officials, and reveal all matters of public interest.[77] This newly crafted sense of professionalism was particularly apparent in the way the commercial press defended itself in libel proceedings, which multiplied appreciably as the new notions of journalism introduced by the penny press took hold. Ironically, throughout the century, judges remained unresponsive to publishers' attempts to shape a condition of special privilege for the institutional press, one that built on the common law and emphasized its public role. The bench continued to distrust the argument that the press should be free of legal constraint, and exhibited extreme displeasure with the kind of sensational crime reporting that included the insertion of editorial comment into crime and trial stories. In spite of this wariness, however, libel laws did tend to become somewhat less onerous through state enactments and the occasional liberal court decision. Newspaper crusades continued to generate a multitude of private actions for libel, but often these individuals found the libel suit an ineffective weapon of defense.[78]

On the other hand, Michael Schudson notes that reporters increasingly viewed themselves as "scientists uncovering the economic and political facts of industrial life more boldly, more clearly, and more 'realistically' than anyone had done before. This was part of the broader Progressive drive to found political reform on 'facts.' ''[82] These new approaches to the meaning of the news resulted in some tensions over writing style. For example, reporters and editors disagreed about how much imaginative writing should dominate a news story. Language was, after all, one of the most powerful tools the reporter had at his or her disposal. Although the New York *World* exhorted its employees to pay attention to accuracy, it assumed that there would be no contradiction between "facts" and "color"—good reporters attended to both. But in tandem with the story journalism pioneered by the penny press and perfected by Pulitzer, an alternative form of newspaper reporting emerged, exemplified by the New York *Times*, a publication that steadfastly renounced the melodramatic in favor of what Schudson calls "information journalism." Associated with "fairness" and "scrupulous dispassion," this style of reporting was less tolerant of creative embellishment, and some young reporters chafed under the rigid distinction between news and opinion. Lincoln Steffans, for example, complained bitterly of the training he received on E. L. Godkin's *Evening Post*:

> Reporters were to report the news as it happened, like machines, without prejudice, color, and without style; all alike. Humor or any sign of personality in our reports was caught, rebuked, and, in time, suppressed. As a writer, I was permanently hurt by my years on the *Post*.[79]

Newspapers generally became identified with one form of journalism over the other, although it would be an exaggeration to argue that any individual paper adhered exclusively to a single style. A publication like the *Times* could easily be seduced into launching an occasional crusade or to offering up human interest stories written in colorful language, while the *World*, as we have already pointed out, always maintained a thoroughly reputable and well-regarded editorial page. Both forms of writing emphasized the importance of facts, and, notes Schudson, information journalism was "not necessarily more accurate than story journalism." Rather, "the moral division of labor between newspapers" paralleled "the more respectable faculties of abstraction and the less respectable feelings." Yet in the 1890s, the proponents of the two journalisms remained antagonistic to each other, with the *Times* taking the lead in a high-minded attack on "yellow" newspapers.[80]

Indeed, Schudson characterizes the tensions between the two modes of journalism as primarily a moral dispute, not unlike "the moral wars of the 1830s," which were in effect "a cover for class conflict."[81] Thus Pulitzer's hyperbolic appeals to immigrants stand in sharp contrast to the New York *Times*'s emphasis on decency *marketed* as accuracy and geared to attract respectable readers. The latter advertised itself with the slogan "It does not soil the breakfast cloth," implying of course that "yellow" journals did. The *Times*'s editor, Adolph Ochs, promised a nonpartisan newspaper, one devoted to sound money and tariff reform, opposed to waste and corruption, and wary of too much government. Politically, the newspaper appealed to the wealthy, who were attracted by its conservatism and business orientation. In its coverage of politics it was characteristically Republican, somewhat belying its nonpartisan self-description, while many of the more sensational journals were nominally

Democratic. Not only the wealthy read the *Times*, however, and the readership of the sensational press hailed from all social strata as well. Indeed, E. L. Godkin grudgingly complained that "the grumblers over the wicked journals are often their most diligent readers."[82]

In the end, the reading audience may have been divided more by their class-structured subjectivities than strictly by the more familiar material markers of social status. In an essay written in the *Atlantic* in 1926, the critic Benjamin Stolberg argued that the *Times* attracted not only the elite, but those who desired to emulate the elite. Ochs himself had commented of his newspaper that "no one needs to be ashamed to be seen reading" the *Times*.[83] Though the educated and the wealthy also read the story newspapers and magazines, they may have done so with some embarrassment and a great deal less pride. In short, newspapers that concentrated on information journalism, sponsored by and for the economic and cultural elite, offered readers a mantel of respectability. In contrast, readers of the *World*, more dependent and nonparticipant in city affairs, read newspapers for the sense of immediacy and personal involvement their human interest stories offered.[84] Pulitzer himself understood this phenomenon well. "Please impress on the men who write our interviews . . . the importance of giving a striking vivid pen-sketch of the subject," he wrote to his managing editor. "Also a . . . picture of his domestic environment, his wife, his children, his animal pets. . . . Those are the things that will bring him more clearly home to the average reader than would his imposing thought, purposes or statements."[85]

By the 1890s, the Brooklyn *Eagle* had experienced all the various substantive changes in the newspaper industry just described and, in the process, had managed to craft for itself a strikingly unique personality in the exciting world of New York journalism. Because the *Eagle* played a crucial role in the most cataclysmic moments of Dixon Jones's career, we must ask how it came about that the paper envisioned itself as a principal actor in this drama, a drama partly of its own making. What sort of a community was Brooklyn in the *Eagle's* imagination, and what relevance did its image of the city have to the libel trial and the events that set it in motion?

THE *EAGLE* AND BROOKLYN: HOLDING FAST TO THAT "BROOKLYN SPIRIT"

By the middle of the 1880s, especially after the opening of the Brooklyn Bridge, Brooklynites found themselves more integrally linked to their unruly sister metropolis to the north. It hardly needs mentioning that eased access between the two cities fueled Brooklyn's commercial, industrial, and real estate development, but it also served as an additional stimulus to new immigrants to settle in the community. By 1890, roughly one-third of Brooklyn's citizens were foreignborn.[86] It was also at this time that business leaders, politicians, and newspaper editors in both cities began to speak more seriously about the benefits of consolidation. Indeed, the *Eagle* remained the only newspaper in the city to oppose merging with New York until the bitter end.[87] Perhaps the most revelatory short summary of the community imagined by the *Eagle*'s editors was the daily leader the paper ran in 1897, stating its reasons for why consolidation should be rejected:

> Brooklyn is a city of homes and churches.
> New York is a city of Tammany Hall and crime government.
> Rents are twice as cheap in Brooklyn as in New York and homes are to be bought for a quarter of the money.
> The price of rule here is barely more than a third of what it is in New York.
> Government here is by public opinion and for the public interest. If tied to New York, Brooklyn would be a Tammany suburb, to be kicked, looted and bossed as such.[88]

Despite these confident assertions, urbanization in Brooklyn continued to belie the city's image as a "safe haven," producing a metropolitan culture increasingly "torn by philosophical, class, ethnic, and religious factions." Modernized and eager to boast of many of the new journalistic trends, the *Eagle* nevertheless resisted many of the implications of these larger social and economic changes. Indeed, according to one historian, "the *Eagle*'s Brooklyn remained stable, homogeneous, business-oriented, and Protestant." In its special issues and brief biographies of prominent citizens, Raymond Schroth has observed, the *Eagle* promoted "the image of a particular type of successful man, the professional man who . . . personified long-established Brooklyn institutions, owned an imposing private home, belonged to the Crescent Club and the Riding and Driving Club, invested in real estate, and saw Brooklyn as the heart and capital of Long Island, if not the center of the universe."[89]

At the helm in the editorial office was St. Clair McKelway, who took over from Andrew McLean in 1886. McKelway, the son of Scotch and Irish immigrant parents, had grown up in Columbia, Missouri, coming east to New Jersey to be educated by a grandfather in 1853. He began writing at seventeen, read law, and was admitted to the bar in 1866. After working for a number of New Jersey and New York papers, he became the Washington correspondent for the New York *World* and the Brooklyn *Eagle* in 1868. From 1870 to 1878 he wrote editorials for the *Eagle*, and worked a six-year stint as editor of the Albany *Argus*, returning to the *Eagle* in 1884. When tension ensued between McKelway and Andrew McLean, the man who had replaced the deceased Kinsella as editor only two years before, McLean left the *Eagle* to found the Brooklyn *Citizen*. McKelway, an anti-machine Democrat, was reputed to be an intellectually brilliant editorial writer. He was a hands-on editor who continued to shape policy, write editorials, and share the ownership of the paper until he died in 1915.[90]

McKelway could not have had a more congenial partner in Colonel William Hester, nephew of the newspaper's founder Isaac Van Anden, who succeeded his uncle in 1875 and remained the *Eagle*'s publisher, managing its business affairs until 1921. Hester, like McKelway, was self-made despite his middle-class origins and had a reputation for being forceful, though broad-minded, pragmatic and decisive, though tolerant. He consulted with McKelway "almost daily" on policy, often displaying superior logic and sounder judgment. Though his interests were primarily the business end of the newspaper, Hester had tried his hand at writing as well, and in 1878 he published a domestic comedy about journalism, *That Husband of Mine*. Like McKelway, Hester was a social conservative with a reputation for gentlemanly dignity. He directed several of the borough's financial institutions in addition to running the *Eagle*, and promoted real estate development on Coney Island, taking a special interest in the Brighton Beach Hotel. Like McKelway and the many Brooklyn leaders whom the *Eagle* celebrated, Hester was a club man, boasting of membership in some of the most exclusive in Brooklyn, including the Nassau Country Club, the Riding and Driving Club, the Metropolitan Club, and the Brooklyn Club.[91]

Both of the men at the *Eagle*'s helm were well suited to the nonpartisan reform-oriented political stance the newspaper took throughout the 1880s and 1890s. Nominally Democratic, the *Eagle* stood increasingly independent of party, preferring instead to continue to promote the reform critique of city corruption begun by Seth Low, of whom the paper was justly proud. The *Eagle*'s journalistic style might be viewed as one that achieved an interesting balance between information and story journalism, and we shall see that the Mary Dixon Jones affair and the way it was reported in the newspaper reflected the *Eagle*'s philosophy in this regard in decisive and enlightening ways.

It seems apparent that the Brooklyn imagined by the *Eagle*'s leadership and projected onto its pages was decidedly not a growing metropolis torn by urban strife and increased diversity, but a community peopled by responsible, cultured, family-oriented, and respectable self-made businessmen and professionals, of which group its own editor and publisher were representative models. Indeed, when the newspaper celebrated its seventy-fifth birthday in 1916, Arthur M. Howe, the man who had just replaced the deceased McKelway, reiterated in emphatic tones the philosophy of journalism these two men had fashioned. "Newspapers and communities grow side by side," Howe wrote. "They are in the truest sense interdependent. The newspaper advertises the community. The community sustains the newspaper." This is how it had been in Brooklyn since the *Eagle* was established. It is true, Howe admitted, that the city had grown, and that pessimists riveted upon the past worried that "the advent of this huge population, due largely to our bridges, subways and tunnels," had led Brooklyn to lose much of what had made it special. But Howe denied that "the old qualities of citizenship that gave Brooklyn its distinction as a city of churches and of homes, that put a premium upon education, cultivation, thrift and clean living" had passed away completely. Nor had the *Eagle*'s task diminished. The *Eagle*, Howe concluded, had been wrongly accused "of being a class newspaper." Rather it was "a newspaper of class." The distinction was important: "The *Eagle* serves no class except the constituency of readers it has created, a constituency in which are represented all grades of society. . . ." Proud to count itself among the "conservative journals," Howe identified his newspaper with the papers who did not find it necessary to manufacture "sensation where none actually exists," but "find sensation only where sensation is, and that appeal to people whose preference in reading is dictated by their intelligence and not by their emotions."[92]

It is not that the *Eagle's* editors were willfully immune to innovation. On the contrary, they were sensitive to the revolution in American journalism that had occurred in last decades of the nineteenth century and watched the growth of the *Eagle's* New York counterpart, the New York *World*, with increasing interest. Indeed, Schroth claims that Joseph Pulitzer's influence on the *Eagle* was "profound." Only one year after the *World* moved its operation into the largest, gilded-domed building in New York, the *Eagle* settled its production offices in sumptuous new quarters in downtown Brooklyn, inspired by Pulitzer's. Like the *World*, the *Eagle* called itself a "public service newspaper," and, like the *World*, it was not above sensational reporting or an occasional campaign. But in selecting its targets, the paper would never be as daring as its New York rival, and its coverage of mayhem and murder was usually confined to the last page. By 1891, with a circulation approximately half that of the New York *Times* and *Tribune* and 13,000 more than its closest rival, the Brooklyn *Citizen*, the *Eagle* was a "prosperous, handsome, and dignified paper."[93]

Indeed, Joseph Pulitzer admired the newspaper's accomplishments, calling it "among the foremost newspapers of the Nation" and praising it not only for its "courageous, non-partisan" editorial page, but for its reflection of "the moral sense and public opinion" of Brooklyn, "which it largely creates." Foreign visitors also took note. Lord Northcliffe, who visited the *Eagle*'s plant in 1905, described it as "the only non-metropolitan newspaper . . . that is known in England and France." Likewise admiring its editorials and remarking that McElway was a "man who is known to newspaper men wherever our language is spoken," Northcliffe thought the publication "unique" in its "hold on Brooklyn itself," especially "on the minds and hearts of Brooklyn people."[94]

Throughout the 1890s and into the next century, the *Eagle* did its best to preserve the image of the city it projected in its massive commemorative volume of 1893, *The Eagle and Brooklyn,* put out on the occasion of its move from its quarters on lower Fulton Street to its new, modernized plant at the corner of Washington and Johnson streets, near Borough Hall. In this volume, as well as in subsequent commemorative issues published in the following decade and a half, the *Eagle* held fast to its representation of the city with whose history the newspaper's own was so intertwined. We need not dwell particularly on this publication, because it repeated all the various themes regarding the city that we have already noted throughout this chapter. It included feature articles on Brooklyn real estate, club life, neighborhood spirit, charity work, the bench and the bar, social welfare associations, churches, schools, and cultural institutions. Biographies of representative men and women, now a familiar tactic and an unwitting guide to prominent trial participants, peppered its pages.[95] Noticeably absent was the Brooklyn of growing class divisions, the Brooklyn of mounting labor strife, the Brooklyn of blighted tenements and urban poverty. Absent as well was any notion of the complex economic and social pressures pushing the city toward amalgamation with New York. Conspicuously present, however, and quite fascinating for our purposes, was a reference embedded in a long section on the history of the newspaper to the *Eagle*'s role as "A Defender of the People." The evidence offered up in substantiation of this claim was an eloquent, self-congratulatory account of the recently concluded Dixon Jones libel trial.

At first glance it perhaps seems odd that the newspaper would choose this incident to advertise its role as a public service newspaper. It surely tells us that in the *Eagle*'s lexicon of significant events, the Dixon Jones affair had top billing.[96] Clearly the paper felt that important precedents were being set regarding the ability of newspapers to defend themselves in court, and it expressed satisfaction that at the trial the "methods of a responsible newspaper in the careful investigation of facts before making a serious publication" could be revealed to "most of the community." In attempting to expose Dixon Jones's wrongdoing, the paper believed that it was conserving "public morals" and defending "the integrity of public institutions." Dixon Jones was represented as a powerful adversary. "She came into court supported by a formidable array of counsel, and by her sons and a group of women friends who had stuck by her through evil report and good report since her difficulties with hospitals began in the town." In the end, the account continued, the *Eagle* proved successful "in its demonstration of the necessity of such a press as the champion of the lured, the credulous, the illiterate, and the self-defenseless for protection and preservation." The verdict, *The Eagle and Brooklyn* concluded, "was the best thing justice has done for life, home, truth, the suffering and the unwary."[97]

Yet we must ask: How often did accounts of the trials and tribulations of the "illiterate" and "self-defenseless" appear on the pages of the newspaper? *Which* individuals composed "the people of Brooklyn" on whose behalf the *Eagle* proved such an assiduous and loyal champion? The *Eagle*'s Brooklyn was composed of upwardly mobile, hardworking, business-oriented citizens. Of what possible threat was Mary Dixon Jones, herself a hardworking, business-oriented, woman professional? We begin to see that the entire affair was laden with numerous tensions wracking the city and the newspaper in the last two decades of the century. It began as a tale of urban corruption, but quickly moved to a more disturbing narrative of self-promotion and the violation of professional ethics through dishonesty and deceit. Dixon Jones's story made most physicians and, by extension, professionals in general, truly uncomfortable, undermining trust between doctors and patients. As the voice of the respectable classes, the Brooklyn *Eagle* seized the right to police the boundaries of the public sphere, with questions about character and gentlemanly professionalism obscuring the more crude and stark tensions over class. Philanthropic elites closed ranks when the cracks in a carefully designed system of behaviors were exposed to public view.

David Rosner emphasizes the contingent and inefficient nature of private philanthropy in these years, helping us to understand why Dixon Jones's exploits could so easily have passed unnoticed. Care often depended on "the good will and idiosyncratic decisions of local elites," making the system haphazard and difficult to penetrate. While some neighborhoods had an abundance of hospital services and dispensaries supported by activist churches or individual benefactors, others, disabled by the centrifugal forces of urbanization, suffered severe shortages: "People could not expect to be cared for but could only hope that someone would come to their aid."[98]

City leaders were certainly aware of these inadequacies and probably did not want them exposed to public view. But what may have rankled most was the vision of a woman physician who had infiltrated the respectable middle classes in order to prey upon them from within. Dixon Jones was represented by the newspaper as a social counterfeit, the female counterpart of the "confidence man," a figure enormously disturbing to Victorian middle-class sensibilities because of the ambivalent feelings around success and its personal price that such a symbol could evoke. "In the fragmented and shifting world of the nineteenth century city," John Kasson has insightfully observed, "social detection was not always so easy." This was because the demands of the marketplace often prompted individuals to deliberately elude discovery. "Unstable" and "illegible" identity, coupled with the ambivalence respectable elites displayed toward the blatant pursuit of economic gain, colored social interaction. "Despite attempts by various popular writers to formulate a science of character based upon outward expression and to establish a system of stable meanings between outward signs and inner substance, social counterfeits did a brisk business—and one with an occasionally disturbing kinship to putatively legitimate activities."[99]

Perhaps Dixon Jones held up a mirror to a society not willing to admit that it, too, was on the make, reflecting an aggressive, self-satisfied image that notables in the Brooklyn community preferred not to see. The fact that she was a woman not only enhanced these anxieties but exacerbated others about middle-class women's entrance into the public sphere. As a woman surgeon, Dixon Jones appeared to be doubly out of bounds.

We will return to these themes toward the end of this book. In the meantime, we need to know more about the development of surgical gynecology as a specialty and about Dixon Jones's remarkable career. Who was Mary Amanda Dixon Jones, and how did such a woman orchestrate her own emergence into the public limelight in such a flamboyant and dramatic way?

3

Becoming
a Surgeon

Mary Dixon Jones had much to lose
when the Brooklyn *Eagle* undermined
her credibility with its damning series
of articles in 1889. She had painstak-
ingly built an admirable reputation
among the respectable middle class in
Brooklyn and had gained membership
in a very male world: an international
group of elite surgeons currently in the
process of creating gynecological surgery. Certainly she was one of the
most ambitious female surgeons of her
generation. Pioneering operative innovations, she demanded that male
colleagues recognize her contributions.
In addition, her published work on the
cellular pathology of the female reproductive system took risks in countering prevailing medical theories of the
female body. Dixon Jones attained a
professional status unique to her sex at

the time, but one that was bound to be challenged, particularly in a conservative city like Brooklyn, struggling not only with complex social changes but also with the various challenges to the medical status quo raised by her chosen specialty. No wonder her achievements were gained at high cost.

To appreciate how Dixon Jones managed to compete with the best medical men of her generation, we need to understand the strategies she used to garner such success. This chapter will explore her career as a physician and surgeon. We will learn that she accomplished her goals both through raw talent and an acute professional sensitivity to the kind of conduct that could advance her career. In the next chapter we will see how her finely tuned antennae helped her negotiate the uncertain waters of a new specialty in the making.

DIXON JONES'S EARLY CAREER: CHOOSING SURGERY

Dixon Jones was born into a comfortable Methodist family of shipbuilders on Maryland's eastern shore on February 17, 1828. Her parents had been married for twenty-one years before she was born, and she had several siblings. She claimed to be the granddaughter of the Reverend James Dixon, a prominent British Wesleyan Methodist minister, but little is known of her childhood until her teens.[1] By then, Mary Amanda Dixon had received a better education than many southern girls, and in 1845 she graduated from Wesleyan Female College in Wilmington, Delaware. There she taught physiology and literature for a couple of years, and then moved to the Baltimore Female College before becoming the principal of a girls' seminary in southern Maryland.[2] In 1845, she began reading medicine with two established Maryland practitioners, Henry F. Askew, president of the American Medical Association in 1846, and Thomas E. Bond, Jr., who helped found, and then became dean of, the Baltimore College of Dental Surgery.[3]

In 1854, Mary Dixon married a lawyer, John Quincy Adams Jones, and for a time the young couple resided in the West, first in Rockford, Illinois, and then in Madison, Wisconsin. During that period Dixon Jones gave birth to two sons and a daughter.[4] The westward venture must have failed, however, because by 1860, the couple had returned to Baltimore, where John resumed the practice of law with his cousin Isaac Dashiell Jones, a two-term Whig member of the House of Representatives, elected state Attorney General in 1867.[5] In 1862, Dixon Jones left her family in Maryland to study medicine in New York City, where she received a degree from the Hygeio-Therapeutic Medical College, an irregular, coeducational medical school. When the Civil War ended, Dixon Jones settled in Brooklyn with her children, leaving her husband behind in Baltimore. Although he occasionally lived with his wife and family in New York for ex-tended periods, Jones maintained an active law practice in Maryland and, by the end of the 1870s, ceased being a part her daily life. The marriage continued as a long-distance one. Such separations were uncommon in this period, but not unknown.[6] Jones attended the manslaughter trial in 1890, dying shortly thereafter. Two years later, Dixon Jones still dressed in ''deep mourning.''[7]

Dixon Jones practiced successfully in Brooklyn for almost a decade, working along the same lines as other sectarian women physicians. While studying in New York, she was introduced not only to water cure but also to reform, abolitionism, and women's rights. She lectured to ladies on the "laws of health," hoping to attract patients through public exposure. She advertised in the radical women's rights journal *The Revolution*, edited by Elizabeth Cady Stanton and published by Susan B. Anthony. She both benefited from and contributed to the female reform community that historians have associated with nineteenth-century women's culture. Meanwhile, her practice flourished. Between 1862 and 1872 her income rose from $1000 to $5000 a year, at a time when male physicians in New York earned an average of $1500 to $2000.[8]

One suspects that she began to encounter patients with severe gynecological problems and increasingly felt the deficiency of her medical preparation. Moreover, if she was reading the medical journals as avidly in the 1870s as she did a decade later, she was bound to have come across the exciting experiments in ovariotomy published by the Atlee brothers and the work of E. R. Peaslee on ovarian tumors. "In 1876," A. J. C. Skene recalled of the period, "gynecology appeared like a young and brilliant member of the medical profession, well versed in all that was known at that time, but not the mature expert, well trained by long experience, yet enthusiastic and very anxious to push onward to new and higher attainments."[9] Most dramatic of all were the surgical successes of J. Marion Sims and his protégé, Thomas Addis Emmet, performed in the newly established New York Woman's Hospital. The first of its kind in the United States, it was located only a short distance across the river from Brooklyn. It is likely that, like many other New York physicians, Dixon Jones attended one or more of Sims's highly publicized operative demonstrations.[10]

In 1872, at the age of forty-four, she made a decision that eventually altered both her status and collegial relationships within the profession and her therapeutic world view and management of patient care. She became a student again, entering the Woman's Medical College of Pennsylvania for a three-year course. We have no record of why she returned to formal study, but it was not unusual for a sectarian woman practitioner to seek an additional, orthodox degree.[11] In Philadelphia, she learned the principles and practice of surgery from Benjamin B. Wilson and attended the weekly surgical clinics at Blockley Hospital. She heard lectures from Emmeline Horton Cleveland, the Paris-trained Professor of Obstetrics and Diseases of Women, who eventually became dean of the school. Beloved by her students, Cleveland was the first woman surgeon to perform an ovariotomy in Philadelphia.[12] But it was Wilson who impressed her the most, and she engaged him as a private tutor.[13] Equally memorable was Rachel Bodley's up-to-date chemical laboratory, and work in microscopy under John Gibbons Hunt, the newly appointed professor of histology and microscopy. Though he never studied in Germany, where laboratory work was flourishing, Hunt was a skilled technician and Dixon Jones would eventually apply what she learned from him to her work in surgical pathology.[14] During 1873, Dixon Jones passed a three-month preceptorship with Mary Putnam Jacobi in New York City, probably continuing her work in pathology and diagnosis.[15]

Until this moment in her medical career, Mary Dixon Jones had negotiated her professional identity by following pathways into the profession particularly amenable to women physicians at mid-century. Beginning as a teacher of biology in a female seminary and easing into the study of medicine at an institution and under the auspices of a medical sect that was particularly proud of its receptivity to women, she did not, like Elizabeth and Emily Blackwell, who trained at regular, coeducational medical schools, have to deal immediately with the culture of orthodox medical professionalism or directly confront the deep ambivalence many male physicians felt toward women doctors. Moreover, studying water cure techniques linked her to traditional female health reform networks. Evidence about her gleaned from *The Revolution* suggests that Dixon Jones anticipated the patronage of the nineteenth-century women's reform community for success in her practice.

Even after her decision to retrain herself, Dixon Jones remained comfortably ensconced within a medical subculture that was predominantly female. To be sure, in 1872 she had few other options for further study: The University of Michigan was the only coeducational medical school that offered training comparable in quality to the two women's schools in closest proximity, the Philadelphia college and the newly established New York Infirmary for Women and Children. But women students in Philadelphia got something more than a good medical education; they received a kind of nurturing that proved particularly useful to the first generations of women physicians.[16]

It is difficult to know for certain how Dixon Jones responded to the female professional culture she found in Philadelphia, but her reminiscences suggest that she appreciated the support of women. Of the Professor of Anatomy, Mary Scarlett-Dixon, she had nothing but praise. Dixon Jones judged her superior to the two male professors she had studied with previously at the Hygeio-Therapeutic College, celebrating her ability "to give us science and facts, and at the same time . . . [show] us the beautiful qualities of love, patience and charity." Rachel Bodley, Dean and Professor of Chemistry, also won Dixon Jones's loyalty. She, too, balanced rigorous science with "the most kindly consideration" for the "personal welfare of each graduate."[17]

Whatever satisfaction Dixon Jones derived from her links to female physicians' professional networks, however, was not enough to entice her to accept the offer of a faculty position in Philadelphia. She nurtured a powerful ambition for success as a surgeon among her male peers and a genuine interest in the newest frontiers of medical science. Believing that she could better fulfill these aspirations in private practice, she returned to Brooklyn to pursue a set of strategies different from those of the other women physicians she knew, one that would be less constrained by the predominately female world she would have lived in had she stayed.[18] Indeed, for the rest of her career Dixon Jones would remain largely indifferent to the female networks that were developing among women practitioners and turn her attention instead to means of self-advancement readily being utilized by men.[19] She reopened her practice armed with a letter from her professor of surgery at the Woman's Medical College, averring that she had graduated with high standing and had "especially" made "very great progress" in the "department of surgery."[20]

We know comparatively little about the individual negotiation of professional identity in the late nineteenth century. What little we do understand suggests that aspiring doctors within the New York medical world worked within what one historian has described as "an intricate web of patronage and training, of medical practice and laboratory procedure, of personal services and nascent bureaucracy."[21] What is certain is that, in the years between 1880 and World War I, a new kind of scientific medicine pervaded teaching, practice, research, and the burgeoning world of public health. Institutional changes in the hospital and medical school, the development of organized medical philanthropy, shifts in caregiving facilitated by the rise of professional nursing, new drugs, novel technologies, and the move from rational, monistic pathologies to empirically oriented concepts of specific, localized infection—all these developments altered ideas about science in medicine and created new notions of the good practitioner. This is the world in which Mary Dixon Jones made her way.[22]

Given our ignorance of the personal dimensions of this emerging professionalism even for young men, we are especially unclear about how women forged their careers. Certainly institutional constraints required them to use a variety of success strategies and nurture more divergent goals of individual aspiration. Comparing and contrasting career opportunities for men and women helps illuminate the professional milieu. Moreover, focusing on the career of the one woman who made it in the elite world of gynecology brings the various strategies used by men and other women into bolder relief, telling us something about the development of the specialty in the process.

Working in Dixon Jones's favor was the fact that the newness of gynecology as a specialty opened it to criticism from traditional practitioners and the public, exposing its vulnerability. An unintended by-product of this professional weakness was that relatively flexible boundaries of entry prevailed in the early years. Male gynecologists' willingness to accept Dixon Jones reflected a desire to encourage all practitioners capable of advancing the work. Moreover, Dixon Jones was assiduous in her energetic self-promotion. This ease of entry did not last. Accessibility declined with gynecology's maturation and enhanced status. Its institutionalization in formalized courses of study, internship, and residency programs, coupled with the emergence of specialty societies that deliberately screened new members, eventually excluded or at best marginalized women. But the latter decades of the nineteenth century represented a unique moment, when gynecology, and especially aggressive surgical treatment, still needed justification and advocacy both therapeutically and as a separate specialty. As long as gynecology struggled for legitimacy, increasing its ranks was strategically desirable, even if it occasionally meant muting traditional gender antagonisms in the interests of professional solidarity.

Among the women surgeons of the period, Dixon Jones was exceptional in her careful attempts to connect herself with male professional networks. Certainly she was not the only woman doctor interested in ovariotomy, nor was she the first to perform it. Between fifteen and twenty other women physicians were known to have carried out abdominal surgery during this period. Some were based in women's hospitals with private practices on the side; others were entirely in private practice. Perhaps five or six had the opportunity to complete as many laparotomies as Dixon Jones had in her surgical career: roughly 100 or more. Emmeline Cleveland and Anna C. Broomall, both of whom, like many others in this group, had European training, were surgeons at the Woman's Hospital of Philadelphia. Elizabeth Keller and Mary Smith operated at the New England Hospital for Women and Children.[23] In New York, Emily Blackwell, a student of James Y. Simpson's in Edinburgh, was reputed to be skilled with the knife, as was her partner, Elizabeth Cushier. Both women practiced at the New York Infirmary for Women and Children. Mary Thompson, Marie Mergler, and Lucy Waite had active hospital practices in Chicago. In 1880, an ovariotomy in private practice was performed in Rhode Island by Anita E. Tyng, the first woman to be admitted to the Rhode Island Medical Society. Tyng, like Dixon Jones, a graduate of the Woman's Medical College of Pennsylvania, was assisted by no fewer than four other women physicians, all fellow graduates of the school, who traveled to Providence especially for the operation.[24]

Two factors stand out in distinguishing the careers of these women from Dixon Jones's. First, none of them published as extensively or engaged in such vigorous or direct debates regarding diagnosis and technique. Nor did any of the others represent themselves as pathologists as well as surgeons. Second, the *tone* of their publications appears more deferential and modest than hers.[25] None of this should be surprising given the circumscribed opportunities for expanding their skills. Even finances proved an obstacle: For example, at the New England Hospital for Women and Children, which was founded by women physicians explicitly to give themselves hospital training, advances in surgery were severely constrained by the reluctance of the Board of Directors to erect an expensive surgical pavilion and pay for surgical instruments.[26]

Women's chances for advancement in surgery were severely limited not only by their limited access to training and to the easy professional exchange characteristic of male networks, but also by the small number of female surgeons who could serve as mentors. Like Dixon Jones, some fortunate few were aided by enlightened men who took an interest in promoting women in medicine. William H. Byford, Charles Warrington Earle, and F. Byron Robinson in Chicago and B. B. Wilson and W. W. Keen in Philadelphia were among several generous individuals who contributed their time and knowledge. But in the 1880s, only a handful of women specialized in surgery.[27] So few were they, indeed, that when Elizabeth Blackwell, the founder of the New York Infirmary for Women and Children and the first woman to earn a medical degree in the United States, wrote her colleague Mary Putnam Jacobi in 1888 about the "problem" of gynecological surgery, proposing to rally the women doctors of the United States against it, Jacobi cut her off. "When you shudder at 'mutilation,' " she wrote impatiently, "it seems to me you can never have handled a degenerated ovary or a suppurating Fallopian tube. . . ." Given the constraints on women's opportunities, she complained to Blackwell, "why should not women be delighted if they succeed in achieving a difficult and useful triumph in technical medicine?"[28]

While they may have privately regretted and publicly protested their narrow opportunities, the reference groups of most women practitioners emerged primarily from female professional communities linked to the various women's institutions.[29] None sought out the recognition and approval of her male colleagues with the persistence and energy of Dixon Jones, neither did any suffer the notoriety heaped on her when she sued the Brooklyn *Eagle* for libel. But the professional recognition she wrested—through a complicated set of ingenious strategies—was also hers alone.

One advantage Dixon Jones had working in her favor was that all nineteenth-century pioneers, regardless of sex, were largely self-taught. Only after the turn of the century did surgical training come to embody formal, postgraduate residency service. From the 1870s on, leading practitioners began to organize professional societies and establish specialty journals, venues where they might enjoy fellowship and trust while discussing and debating technique, diagnosis, pathology, and treatment. Individuals honed their skills through a loose system of apprenticeship, intellectual exchange, and mutual observation. The institutional informality of this training allowed Mary Dixon Jones to rely on her own resources in much the same way as her male colleagues. But in terms of access to the informal networks available, networks that were overwhelmingly male, her options, like those of other women physicians of her generation, were severely constrained.

By the last third of the nineteenth century, both male and female medical students learned some surgery, which was taught by lecture, demonstration, dissection, and sporadic clinical experience.[30] At Harvard in the 1870s, Dr. Henry J. Bigelow lectured on the principles and practice of surgery and allowed medical students to accompany him on hospital rounds at least once a week. John B. Wheeler recalled the frequent frustration of that experience, however, as forty or fifty students crowded around a single patient's bed. Arthur E. Hertzler had similar memories of the operative clinics that were given a prominent place in the Northwestern University Medical School curriculum in the 1890s. "These were really shows or rest periods for us students," he recorded. "All we saw were the backs of the professor and his assistants. . . ."[31]

The aspiring male surgeon hoped to catch the attention of the professor of surgery at his medical school, thereby gaining clinical experience through apprenticeship. Some women were similarly encouraged by male mentors. The lucky few won hospital appointments. John Allen Wyeth, who eventually married the surgeon J. Marion Sims's youngest daughter, came to New York City with a medical degree from the University of Louisville. Hoping without success to find special courses for graduates, he was eventually forced to enroll at Bellevue Hospital Medical College, where he took an *ad eundem* degree in 1873 in surgery, medicine, and obstetrics. To improve his technique, he devoted most of his time "to the clinics and surgery in the hospital and chiefly to dissecting." With graduation came the fortunate offer of a position as assistant demonstrator of anatomy in the college from D. G. Janeway, one of the foremost clinical teachers and consultants in pathological anatomy of his generation. Under Janeway's tutelage, Wyeth joined the New York Pathological Society, thereby making contacts with most of the leading clinicians in New York.[32]

The Chicago gynecologist Franklin H. Martin, one of the founders of the postgraduate Medical School of Chicago and the journal *Surgery, Gynecology, and Obstetrics*, quite unexpectedly received aid from the professor of surgery at Chicago Medical College. Edmund Andrews's influence and tutelage eased Martin's adjustment to a hospital internship at Chicago's Mercy Hospital in 1880. During this year, he gained enough clinical experience to be offered a position as a part-time clinical instructor in the Chicago Medical College gynecology dispensary, where he continued to acquire the experience and reputation necessary to successful private practice.[33]

In 1876, E. C. Dudley, only a year after setting up practice in Chicago, returned to New York, where he had graduated from the Long Island Hospital Medical College, to secure a hospital appointment. "Such service," he remembered, "were [sic] obtainable only after rigid competitive examination, and were so desirable that applications by senior students were made months in advance." Preparation for the examination took the form of quiz groups, led by the brightest and most enterprising young medical graduates, known as quiz masters. Usually men with connections, these instructors intensively prepared aspirants. "So great was the rivalry among the New York colleges," according to Dudley, "that students in order to make the hospitals were excused from lectures and permitted to substitute the quiz."[34]

Eventually Dudley won a coveted position at the New York Woman's Hospital, but not without invoking the influence and support of Alexander J. C. Skene, his much-admired Professor of Gynecology at Long Island Hospital Medical College. Years later, he still reveled in his good fortune. "Invitations to the operations at the Woman's Hospital were much in demand among doctors," Dudley recalled, "because the work there at the time was novel. . . ."[35]

As E. C. Dudley made clear, hospital experience was particularly welcome, but the young men and women who were fortunate enough to attain it were few.[36] Even with hospital training, however, no one was fully prepared for the complicated gynecological cases inevitable in private practice. In the 1870s and 1880s, gynecology was only just beginning to distinguish itself from general medicine, and the lines between general surgeons, gynecological surgeons, and obstetricians remained ill-defined, creating tension among them as to who should most logically perform surgery on women.[37] Many of the leading gynecologists had not initially intended to specialize in surgery and the diseases of women, and their own professors of gynecology were first-generation. Franklin Martin, for example, initially chose ophthalmology, another embryonic specialty that was beginning to engage the interest of the curious. Before he left Chicago and won an internship at the New York Woman's Hospital, E. C. Dudley had planned to be "an old-fashioned family doctor." Howard Kelly was initially drawn to anatomical research. Though as an intern at Philadelphia's Episcopal Hospital in Kensington he built up a fine gynecological clinic, much of what he learned he acquired on his own and through reading.[38]

Similarly, in 1881, after barely a year in practice, Franklin Martin began to read gynecology and obstetrics in his spare time. "Due to Byford, Emmett, Sims, Battey and others," he reflected years later, "obstetrics and gynecology" began to be regarded as a separate specialty.[39] Like most of his surgical contemporaries, Martin learned to operate by practicing on patients. On Sunday mornings, he performed surgery on people who could not gain admittance to Mercy Hospital's free wards. He worked without compensation, for the experience. Usually the surgery took place at the hapless individual's home, where the kitchen or sitting room was converted into an operating room, "using the kitchen table as the operating table, the wash boiler on the kitchen stove as a sterilizer, and the cooking utensils as receptacles for instruments, sponges, etc."

Although Martin did most of the surgery—ranging from emergency amputations to laparotomy—he rarely operated alone. His "neighbor doctors"— older and more experienced practitioners or medical faculty whose offices were close by his own—"gladly volunteered as assistants, anesthetists, orderlies and operating room nurses." In the beginning, he took only those cases in which "the diagnosis was self evident" and did not require "superior judgment." Surgeons in those days "were not made to order as in more recent times," he recalled tellingly. "Surgical cases were not a matter of selection":

> There were very few transcendent surgeons whose operations one could witness. . . . They wrote books and papers, illustrated their articles by drawings, and clearly described their technique; or they reviewed the cases and indicated those in which operation was advisable. Those of us who were interested in gynecological surgery literally learned it by operating on patients; and only a few of the group perfected a technique and became skilled in this specialty.[40]

BUILDING A CAREER AND CONSTRUCTING A PROFESSIONAL IDENTITY

Mary Dixon Jones learned her surgery in much the same way as these men did. Her published articles indicate that she increasingly saw patients suffering from serious and life-threatening gynecological problems, including fibroid tumors, various forms of uterine and ovarian cancer, and infected tubes and appendages.[41] It is possible that her training in Philadelphia encouraged her focus on these ailments. By this decade surgical fashion dictated that practitioners were reporting such conditions with increasing frequency. Indeed, as we have already seen, during the last two decades of the century, the number of individuals whose practices were devoted almost exclusively to gynecology grew. In the 1870s, specialists began to organize professional societies, such as the American Gynecological Society, and to establish journals like the *American Journal of Obstetrics and Diseases of Women and Children*, venues where they might find fellowship and debate technique, diagnosis, pathology, and treatment. Still, even at the end of the century, the boundaries between surgeons, general practitioners, and gynecologists were more permeable than they would become even a decade later.[42]

Especially in urban practice, women physicians concentrated on gynecology by default: The patients who sought them out were overwhelmingly female. As we have pointed out, women did not have open access to developing male networks, and they were additionally constrained by cultural assumptions that surgery was men's work. For example, when she accepted the position of Chief Resident Physician at the Philadelphia Woman's Hospital in 1875, Anna Broomall, a graduate of the Woman's Medical College of Pennsylvania, who obtained postgraduate training in obstetrics and surgery in Vienna and Paris, was ordered by the Board of Directors to have a male surgeon assist her at all laparotomies.[43] After a few instances of monitoring, the practice was discontinued when her male colleagues insisted that she was more skilled than most of them. But the incident illustrates that, even as the woman physician became more accepted by the public, her specialty choices continued to be delimited by powerful conceptions of femininity.[44] As a result, women tended to form their own professional networks and maneuver primarily within them.[45]

It is difficult to know whether Dixon Jones consciously shunned this trammeled road to achievement; I believe that she did. In declining the invitation to join the faculty and female community of the Woman's Medical College of Pennsylvania, she chose a more individualistic, more aggressive, indeed, for her social context, a more "masculine" route to successful practice. As far as I know, no other woman of her generation followed a similar path with such perseverance. Her case is instructive in part for being unique.

In 1876, she began studying pathology with Dr. Charles Heitzman, a Hungarian-born immigrant, expertly trained in surgery, and a skilled microscopist with degrees from the universities of Pesth and Vienna. Heitzman, one of the founders of the American Dermatological Association, had only just settled in Brooklyn in 1874 and was to become her mentor in pathology for the next several decades. Much of her research in the 1880s and 1890s was carried out under his guidance.[46] In the fall of that year she also made a trip to Europe, observing various surgery clinics, including Theodor Billroth's in Vienna.[47]

It made perfect sense for an ambitious woman like Dixon Jones to seek additional training at the newly established Post-Graduate Medical School and Hospital in New York City. Spearheaded by John A. Wyeth, the young doctor who had despaired of finding postgraduate training when he arrived in New York in the early 1870s, a group of physicians organized the school to offer graduate M.D.s specialized courses on a par with the best European universities. Male and female practitioners were welcome, and Mary Putnam Jacobi joined the faculty as clinical lecturer on children's diseases.[48]

Benjamin Franklin Dawson, a thirty-five-year-old obstetrician who had graduated from the college of Physicians and Surgeons in 1866, served as an acting assistant surgeon in the Federal Army during the last year of the Civil War, and established a practice in surgery, gynecology, and obstetrics, took charge of the gynecology department. In 1868, Dawson founded the *American Journal of Obstetrics and Diseases of Women and Children*, one of the earliest specialty journals in obstetrics and gynecology, remaining active as its editor until 1874. Also an assistant surgeon at the New York Woman's Hospital and a founding member of the New York Obstetrical Society, Dawson nurtured an abiding interest in the pathological anatomy of the female reproductive system.[49]

In 1882, Dixon Jones, at the age of fifty-four, assumed the position of chief medical officer at the Women's Dispensary and Hospital in Brooklyn, a charitable organization whose Board of Lady Managers included some of the most prominent matrons of the city. Running her own hospital provided her with the clinical setting to pursue her interest in gynecological surgery. Taking an object lesson from the Woman's Hospital of New York, which for more than a decade had offered unique opportunities for gynecological work to its attending staff, Dixon Jones understood, as did many others in this critical period, the increasing significance of women's specialty hospitals to advancing careers and technological skill.

Within a couple of years, a dispute with the Board of Lady Managers resulted in the disbanding of the first Woman's Hospital of Brooklyn. It is difficult to be certain of the nature of the quarrel, because the only evidence available comes from testimony at the libel trial. The president of the board, Cornelia W. Plummer, averred that in the fall of 1883, rumors and complaints began to circulate about "illegal practices in Mrs. Jones's professional career." Plummer and the Lady Managers were particularly disturbed by the story of an abortion performed allegedly at Dixon Jones's home on a woman named Mrs. Lindsay. The woman, who died before she could testify in 1892, was moved to the hospital after the procedure and admitted the operation to Plummer. The situation was exacerbated by two inflammatory letters to the board criticizing Dixon Jones for maltreatment of patients, one written by a member who had undergone an operation of indeterminate outcome. After a confrontation with Dixon Jones, which Plummer remembered with extreme discomfort, repeating several times that the board "avoided as much as possible . . . having any unpleasant or heated discussions," the women withdrew their support. Dixon Jones then reincorporated a second institution five months later without Lady Managers and with a new, predominately male, Board of Trustees, which seemed content to let her run the hospital without interference.[50]

She promoted her hospital with the rhetoric of uplift and charity common to hospitals founded by other women physicians in the years after the Civil War, but there were marked differences. While other women's institutions founded by women physicians served as training centers where young graduates could attain much needed clinical experience, Dixon Jones felt no obligation to teach others. The medical staff for most of the hospital's existence consisted of herself and her son, Charles N. Dixon Jones. Nor, like other women's establishments, did the hospital involve itself in nursing education. Finally, although Dixon Jones claimed to be dedicated to treating poor women, the Brooklyn *Eagle* cast some doubt on her concern for the poor, suggesting that she was running a private hospital with public funds.[51] Of course there were plenty of hospitals run by male gynecologists as personal fiefdoms, which also received local and state support. J. Marion Sims intended to manage the Woman's Hospital of New York in such a manner, and like Dixon Jones, he eventually clashed with the Board of Governors and the Board of Lady Supervisors; Sims resigned in 1874.

Soon after she took up her hospital position, Dixon Jones began a course of study with Benjamin F. Dawson at the Post-Graduate Medical School. We do not know what he saw in her, perhaps her maturity: In 1882 she was already fifty-four years old. Possibly her hospital appointment impressed him, or the imprimatur she bore from Charles Heitzman and her former preceptor, Mary Putnam Jacobi. Her sheer enthusiasm for operative treatment—a still controversial course of action among practitioners, one that would be heatedly debated over the next decade—might also have pleased him. What is certain, however, is that it was Dawson who came to Brooklyn to be at her side, aiding and encouraging her when, in 1883, she performed her first laparotomy. Also present to assist were her son, Charles N. Dixon Jones, a recent graduate of Long Island Medical College Hospital, and two prominent local members of the King's County Medical Society, J. H. Hobart Burge, who administered the ether, and Frank W. Rockwell.[52]

In the next decade, Dixon Jones performed between 100 and 300 laparotomies.[53] In the beginning, in addition to Dawson, whom she continued to consult, she sought the advice and assistance of other experienced practitioners in New York and Brooklyn. Several of these men, themselves in the process of building careers, attended her operations. W. Gill Wylie, C. C. Lee, Henry Clark Coe, Arthur M. Jacobus, and Robert Tuttle Morris were notable New York surgeons who operated with her at least once. In Brooklyn, she received assistance from Samuel King, John Merritt, and J. W. Ingalls, all three of whom were graduates of Columbia College of Physicians and Surgeons and members of the local medical society. Moreover, Dixon Jones continued to attend operations at the New York Woman's Hospital and at Bellevue, where she undoubtedly met Lawson Tait, the renowned British ovariotomist, and saw him operate during his trip to the United States in 1884.[54]

PUBLISHING: THE FRUITS OF SELF-PROMOTION

Even more remarkable than Dixon Jones's early identification with the leading male gynecological surgeons of New York was her meticulous construction of an international professional identity. She achieved this by reaching out, hardly an invited guest, to as many professional networks as would have her and by strategic placement of her medical work. Her articles found their way into leading specialty journals at home and abroad.

Clearly, Dixon Jones understood the importance of publishing. Musing somewhat sardonically about his own discovery of the merits of writing for an audience, Arthur Hertzler, a younger surgical contemporary, spoke self-deprecatingly about his first experience with it in the 1890s: "The chief value . . . lay in that after the book was published it brought me much consultation practice. . . . I learned here the professional as well as the intellectual value of authorship. For some strange reason the general opinion among doctors is that if one writes a book he must have superior knowledge of the subject.''[55]

Unlike Hertzler, a relatively well-connected male doctor who could perhaps afford a little self-irony, Dixon Jones took publication quite seriously. Thanks to the openness of gynecology to interested practitioners, she had learned to operate. Now she must make her achievements known. Publishing provided the most effective avenue for attaining this goal. She not only offered her articles to important journals but also served for periods from several months to several years as an associate editor of the *Philadelphia Times and Register*, the *American Journal of Surgery and Gynecology*, and the *Woman's Medical Journal.*[56]

Editing, too, was a route to self-advertisement. Nineteenth-century medical editors, co-editors, and assistant editors, W. F. Bynum and Janice Wilson have found, were ''an ambitious crew,'' whose editorial posts promoted their success. Though the journals Dixon Jones identified with as an editor were not as prestigious as the specialty journals in which she placed her articles, she demonstrated remarkable skill at keeping her name in print.[57]

Dixon Jones published approximately fifty papers, wrote several letters to editors of various medical journals, and received numerous journal notices for presentations she made at the New York Pathological Society, where she attained membership in 1887. Her articles were of three types, all typical of the published work of the prominent male practitioners she sought to emulate. Surgical case reports highlighted accomplishments in the operating room and innovative technique. A second set of case reports drew attention to her diagnostic abilities, deliberately engaging the heated debates then going on in the field between ''radical'' and ''conservative'' interventions.[58] A third collection of writings ventured into surgical pathology, substantiating malignant cell formations and identifying new diseases. Each kind of narrative called attention to a different dimension of her talent; taken together they painted a portrait of an experienced, innovative, and up-to-date surgeon and diagnostician who, as she herself never hesitated to remind her readers, was a recognized authority among the international surgical community.

This meticulous self-advancement began in November 1884, when her first clinical case report appeared in the prestigious *American Journal of Obstetrics*. Even the choice of a title for the piece displayed audacity. ''A Case of Tait's Operation'' invited readers to associate her work with that of the famous ovariotomist from Birmingham, England, Lawson Tait. By the mid-1880s, this ambitious, talented, outspoken, and somewhat uncouth man from the English provinces had successfully maneuvered among the various elite interest groups that traditionally constrained the fortunes of aspirants to success in the English medical profession. Now a prosperous and accomplished gynecological surgeon, Tait helped to create a new specialty as he forged his own medical career. Known and admired by leading surgeons in the United States, to Mary Dixon Jones he was not only a hero, but a role model after whom she clearly patterned her career.[59] Gynecology had made Tait famous; it could do the same for Dixon Jones.

In this first article, Dixon Jones played out many of the themes that were to become standard in her surgical case studies. She introduced a classic case of "hystero-epilepsy due to reflex irritation" in the person of Mrs. Alice Mc., a twenty-seven-year-old, twice-married woman, who had long suffered intense pain in the area of the ovaries, and had endured spasms, fainting spells, convulsions, and recurring hysterical fits, especially during menstruation. Addicted to morphine for the pain, Mrs. Mc. had visited several physicians over the years, the last of whom had not given her long to live. An examination revealed a retroverted uterus, inflammatory adhesions and infection of the Fallopian tubes, and a suspicious mass of tissue located at the upper end of the cervix. Dixon Jones concluded that diseased ovaries and tubes were doubtless the cause of the nervous symptoms. Upon hearing the diagnosis, the patient urged an operation, declaring that dying under the knife would be better than the living hell that had been her lot. This recurring theme is typical of almost all of Dixon Jones's case reports: By her account, it was usually the patient, not the doctor, who was most eager for the surgery.[60]

Not wishing to represent herself as someone who would resort to surgery too soon, Dixon Jones reported an attempt at palliative treatment for over a year, and, in consultation with Dr. B. F. Westbrook of Brooklyn, a trial of massage. Nothing worked. She finally brought the patient to B. F. Dawson in New York. He urged an immediate operation, declaring that it was the only hope: Without surgery the woman might well end her life living in an insane asylum. On May 14, 1883, the abdomen was opened in the presence of several physicians, including Dawson, who "helped liberate the organs," which were matted together in "one inflammatory mass." The left ovary and Fallopian tube were removed. Though the patient seemed to recover nicely, septicemia set in on the morning of the sixth postoperative day. Dawson was called in, but he could do nothing, and Alice McC. died that afternoon.[61]

The article concluded with a discussion of the results of the postmortem, at which Dawson, Dixon Jones, and her son, Charles, were present. According to Dixon Jones, the ovaries and tubes presented in a state of advanced, chronic infection, and skillful surgery and good healing could deliver no one from such a condition. The specimen spoke volumes about the sad fate of this patient, whose organs were eventually exhibited by Dawson at the Post-Graduate School and at the Obstetrical Society of New York.[62]

Subsequent articles deployed a formulaic style that was refined during the next two decades. The interpretive narrative, considerably elaborated in later accounts, was often accompanied by pathological data and reprints of microscopical slides. It told of patient suffering, followed by Dixon Jones's keen diagnosis, and then the proposal of radical surgery. Often her advice of removal was accompanied by regret that disease had progressed for so long. Implicit was the accusation that the doctors whom the patient had previously consulted had allowed her to deteriorate while they fiddled with ineffective treatments and improper diagnoses.[63]

Elaborating on antiseptic precautions and surgical technique, Dixon Jones typically involved a host of distinguished colleagues in her work, presenting herself by default as part of their community. For example, she had sponges prepared "according to the process described by Weir in the *New York Medical Journal*, modified by the method described by Pilcher in his work on 'Treatment of Wounds'." She massaged the abdomen and pelvic region with sweet oil for two days preceding according to Frisch's suggestions. She followed Wylie's habit of packing the pelvis with cotton soaked in alum and glycerine to soften the adhesions. After removing one ovary and tube, she closed the abdominal wound with silver sutures, following "Goodell's suggestion in *The Medical Times*." The wound was dressed with a "small piece of Lister's oil silk protective," and "a layer of McIntosh's thin adhesive strips."[64]

Dixon Jones developed the habit of quoting other practitioners' letters to her, which became a familiar attention-getting device. In her second published piece, she dramatically concluded with correspondence from Lawson Tait. A few weeks after the publication of her first case study, she noted, he wrote to her, praising her work and agreeing with her conclusions "absolutely." "That poor girl's life," he opined, "would have been saved had the operation been done months or perhaps years before you were courageous enough to undertake it." Graciously, she gave Tait the last word. "There can be no doubt," his letter asserted, "that the only regret about all such cases is that they are allowed to go on so long without operation."[65]

In an 1888 article she published a letter from Paul F. Mundé, then editor of the *American Journal of Obstetrics and Diseases of Women and Children*, not only to call attention to the fact that such "an eminent authority" had taken a moment to acknowledge and praise her work, but to make a point regarding the difference between "Tait's" operation and "Battey's." Though Tait's emphasis was on the removal of the appendages as the seat of disease, the American Surgeon Battey, like Spencer Wells, Tait's rival in England, removed only the ovaries. Moreover, though Tait accepted the diagnosis of reflex irritation, unlike Battey, he was deeply resistant to the removal of "normal" organs unless they were attached to diseased appendages. While many practitioners regarded the two operations as interchangeable, Dixon Jones not only took care to distinguish between them, but remained even more emphatic than Tait that only diseased organs should be removed. How she determined disease was another matter. Here she was somewhat disingenuous: If we read her articles carefully, we see that her decision to operate when patients presented with hysterical symptoms was wholly subjective.[66]

Male surgeons who published in the same journals also cited the techniques of colleagues, and frequently drew attention to themselves. But I believe Dixon Jones's efforts were noticeably excessive. Perhaps she was insecure about her authority as a woman. Whatever her motives, the strategy worked. A number of prominent practitioners stood ready to cite her in their own publications; others corresponded with her. Indeed, aside from Mary Putnam Jacobi, she was the only woman physician of her generation whose medical activity received this level of recognition in print, publishing more articles than any other woman surgeon of her time.[67]

She especially cherished Tait's attention. In his mention of Dixon Jones in an 1888 article on the removal of the uterine appendages, Tait appeared delighted with the advantages of having a woman surgeon on his side, especially when we realize that some women doctors denounced the excesses of surgical gynecology. Clearly Dixon Jones represented a bridge to female patients as well as to more skeptical male colleagues. Responding to critics that decried the sterility resulting from Tait's operation, he offered Dixon Jones's argument (also his own) that it was the disease, not the operation to cure it, that caused the condition. Prefacing his reprinting of her comments with the remarks, "I have a great belief in the opinions of women upon all matters concerning their own sex. Here is the opinion of a very clever woman on this subject, Dr. Mary Dixon Jones of Brooklyn," he used Dixon Jones to take a swipe at his rival Sir Spencer Wells. "He will see," he observed of Wells, directing him to one of Dixon Jones's recently published articles, "how a woman can understand, recognize, and successfully treat the troubles of these out-of-the-way organs when the subject of irreparable disease."[68]

Such effusive recognition from the men led Dixon Jones to respond in kind. In an article recounting achievements in laparotomy on two continents from 1879 to 1889 and defending the collective record of mortality statistics, she concluded:

> They [gynecological surgeons] have labored unceasingly, and with clearer and clearer light, and with unfaltering firmness to secure the best results. No body of men are more self-sacrificing, more generous, or labor more courageously or more faithfully for the good of humanity, and ofttimes without pay or recompense except, perhaps, blame and persecution for their excellent work.[69]

Dixon Jones undoubtedly counted herself among these "men."

Indeed, she found herself occasionally defending male surgeons against the accusations of female physicians. A couple of years after the libel trial was over, she received a letter from a female practitioner indicting some male laparotomists knew to be reckless who had "escaped unscathed by lucky accident." How could this woman possibly know them to be reckless? responded Dixon Jones. "How could she speak thus of these great, good and eminent surgeons? I have seen many of the distinguished laparotomists in New York operate, I have never seen anything but the most careful and painstaking efforts . . . faithfully and zealously trying to be the best for each and every patient. . . . 'Escaping unscathed': who can escape from evil tongues?"[70]

In 1886, Dixon Jones and her son Charles toured European operating theaters, where she cemented relationships not only with Tait, but with other leaders in the profession, including August Martin and Karl Schroeder of Berlin, Christian Leopold of Dresden, Theodor Billroth of Vienna, Franz von Winckel of Munich, Alfred Hegar of Freiberg, and several members of the British Gynecological Society. Part of the reason for her cordial reception in Germany was that her M.D. degree commanded respect in spite of the fact that she was a woman, and, since American physicians stood outside the German status hierarchy, the attention proffered them did not compromise an individual's standing with German colleagues, while it did enhance one's reputation in the United States.[71] Women were not admitted to the British Society at the time, but Charles Dixon Jones became a member, undoubtedly standing in as his mother's proxy. Here she also met Robert Barnes, Mendes de Leon, and Henry MacNaughton Jones, who, in his 1898 presidential address to the society, took a moment to single out her work in pathology, commenting that "her researches into the nature of endothelioma of the ovaries, gyroma and the origin of cancer in the connective tissue and lymphatics have been of the highest order."[72] The Brooklyn *Citizen* made much of the visit in 1889, describing it as a professional triumph, a "constant round of receptions at the houses of the most distinguished surgeons, and invitations to the most famous hospitals of Europe." All the surgeons she visited were listed by name and location, and the paper claimed that she was treated with extraordinary hospitality, admiration, and respect.[73]

A year after her return from Europe, Dixon Jones performed the first successful total hysterectomy for fibroid tumors ever to be attempted in the United States. She presented the case at the New York Pathological Society meetings in December 1888, and the operation received notice in a number of medical journals, including an elaborate reference by the Boston gynecologist Ernest W. Cushing in his long article on the evolution of abdominal hysterectomy in America published in the *Monatsschrift für Geburtshilfe und Gynakologie*. In the next few years, she fought several small skirmishes in the medical press to retain credit for this "first," even accusing one hapless southerner of plagiarism. Bold, radical, and successful, the operation was generally given the credit it deserved by Dixon Jones's contemporaries, and even Kelly and Burrage highlighted it in their discussion of her career in the *Dictionary of American Medical Biography*.[74]

SPEAKING THE LANGUAGE OF SCIENCE

Though clinical case reports and exercises in diagnosis comprised the bulk of her early work, it was of her writings in cellular pathology, so generously recognized by Henry MacNaughton Jones, that Dixon Jones was especially proud. This work testified to her identity as a clinician who understood the new science and could use it at the bedside.[75] And here we come to the third category of subject matter in her articles, her work in cellular pathology. As we will see in the next chapter, Dixon Jones's pathology was characteristic of a transitional stage when pathological theory and the role of the microscopist evolved in interaction with each other.[76] Much of this aspect of her career flourished in the 1890s. An enthusiast for the microscope, she solicited slides and specimens from fellow practitioners, including her longtime colleague and operating partner W. Gill Wylie, and William M. Polk and James Ewing, both clinicians connected to the pathology laboratory at Cornell. She pored over these and her own extensive collection of material, diagnosing and rediagnosing, refining and redefining "diseases" she had begun to identify early in her surgical practice.[77]

JoAnn Brown's work on the language of professionalization helps to explain some of Dixon Jones's enthusiasm for pathology. Brown argues that surgeons deployed the vocabulary of pathology to underscore the legitimacy of new technology. Brown shows how carefully chosen language both mystified knowledge and enhanced public respect for professional expertise. Surgeons founded institutions, journals, and other venues not only to speak to each other but also to collectively claim their competence in the public sphere. They searched for the effective rhetorical expression of esoteric knowledge that could underscore their authority to prospective clients while helping patients to properly value the uniqueness of their professional achievement. In Dixon Jones's case, language not only validated her work, but attracted the attention of male colleagues. There is little doubt that she had a penchant for the scientific and technical aspects of surgery, but her ability to "do" pathology also gave her a respected place among an elite group of men.[78]

It is difficult to judge the quality of Dixon Jones's pathological work. Russell Maulitz has emphasized that virtually no one in the United States in this period was doing systematic academic pathology; it was still something clinicians involved themselves in to bolster the authority of their clinical decisions. What is clear from reading her articles, however, is that she remained current with the debates in the field. She comfortably referred to an international community of researchers in her work, demonstrating at least an awareness of publications in both German and French.[79]

Dixon Jones had a reasonable grasp of histopathology and used it rather deftly in many of her publications. Little of what she had to say was original, although she incessantly claimed originality for her work and unabashedly identified her complicated "discoveries" of new diseases. Perhaps much of what she published can best be described as falling into the natural-historical tradition, which consisted primarily of classification and description. She did not keep good statistics, nor did she appear to follow up patients systematically. In pathology, she worked with concepts that were accepted in the literature: vascular tumor, endothelial cells, carcinoma, hematoma. Kelly and Burrage credit her with the description of two diseases, "endothelioma," and "gyroma," both allegedly states of extreme tissue inflammation and degeneration that warranted the removal of ovaries and tubes.[80]

Though Dixon Jones's pleas for early and frequent operations incurred criticism from conservatives still ambivalent about the relevance of laboratory science to work at the bedside, not everyone who questioned her medical judgment was suspicious of the new science. Joshua Van Cott, an associate of Skene's at Long Island Hospital Medical College and Professor of Pathology there, spent 1888–89 studying in the laboratories of Koch and Virchow. The thirty-year-old Van Cott, an aspirant to an academic career in pathology and fresh from Germany, a fact that rendered him thoroughly up-to-date as no mere clinician could be, voiced muted contempt for Dixon Jones's assiduous self-promotion by appearing at the 1892 libel trial as an *Eagle* witness. Testifying that he did not consider the specimens presented by her as evidencing an advanced state of disease, he also asserted that gyroma and endothelioma were actually normal variants of healthy organs. "The only pathologists he knew who believed in the existence of the two Jones diseases," he stated, giving voice to generational tensions between older and younger pathologists, "were the Drs. Heitzman, in whose laboratory they were said to have been found."[81] Thus the controversy over diagnosis reflected not only anxiety over how to use the new pathology but also the tentativeness of pathological wisdom at this early stage, when clinicians presented with cystic, sclerotic, or hyperplastic organs were unable to distinguish the diseased from the normal.[82]

Within a decade of the turn of the century, microscopical diagnosis would be used routinely for its predictive significance in screening patients for surgery. Although a few cancer cases among Dixon Jones's numerous reports indicate that she occasionally took biopsies before surgery, her pathology, like that of her surgical colleagues, was offered primarily as post hoc confirmation of the decision to operate. The slow pace of this change is typical of many technological innovations in medicine at the time.[83] Yet Dixon Jones and her fellow radicals deserve credit for playing a key role in transforming medical practice by benefiting from and hastening the clinical use of insights derived from nineteenth-century pathology regarding the localization of disease.

Examining Mary Dixon Jones's career strategies helps us to understand how a woman made it in a world of men, even as it tells us a great deal about that world, including how male surgeons learned to prosper in a field still in the early stages of establishing itself as a separate specialty. Dixon Jones used as many of the avenues to advancement as were open to a woman. All of them were available to men on a grander scale. As a surgeon, she was bold, radical, and innovative, quick to criticize the temporizing of more conservative colleagues and anxious to advertise her innovations in technique. In this she mirrored the behavior of many of the leading men she most admired.

Her contributions to pathology were also respectable for a clinician. These publications, so crucial to advancing her career, accomplished two things. First, they allowed her to speak the language of the new science and establish the intellectual credentials necessary for her to be taken seriously by the relatively small group of academic surgeons she chose as her audience. Though she elbowed her way into their drawing rooms by initiating dialogues with them in print that they most likely did not invite, once the conversation began, they felt obliged to respond. She orchestrated a relationship with Lawson Tait and other European practitioners and publicized those connections assiduously in her medical articles. She corresponded with the great men in the field, offering them specimens and theories that were plausible enough to generate a response. Scientific professionalism as well as gentlemanly courtesy demanded that they listen, for the world of science was allegedly a meritocracy, where no one who could contribute to the expansion of knowledge would knowingly be turned away. And, as we will see, in 1892, when Dixon Jones's operative judgment and surgical technique was exposed to public scrutiny in a sensational libel trial, many of these men traveled to Brooklyn to testify in her defense.

Conversely, Dixon Jones's pathology validated not only her own clinical behavior and decisions, but those of her male reference group as well. It justified, in every logical detail, their surgical procedures. Her opus is long-winded, discursive, and filled with self-referential asides. But it also displays a therapeutic logic that is revelatory, not just of Mary Dixon Jones's surgical career, but of surgical careers in general. Her banner of attainment was the surgical knife and her uncanny command of newly formed professional venues for self-promotion: specialty journals, pathology societies, laboratories. Her weapon of defense was the microscope, a reigning symbol of advanced, up-to-date science.

Chronicling her efforts explains her success. Her career also affords us an interesting and somewhat unique perspective on how individuals negotiated the effects of medical professionalization, reminding us that the careers of women physicians—even unconventional ones—can often offer important insights into broad historical changes in medicine. Yet we also understand better why other women were unable to duplicate her accomplishments. The recognition that she attained took bluster, resourcefulness, and an extraordinary gift for self-advancement. Pushy, and perhaps even aggressive, Dixon Jones displayed none of the collegiality her medical colleagues, especially those in Brooklyn, had come to expect from fellow practitioners. Moreover, most women physicians, choosing not to behave as she did, remained safely ensconced on the margins of medicine. She, in turn, kept aloof from their networks. Yet her striving for recognition did not lead Dixon Jones to shun the cause of women. As we shall see in the next two chapters, she was willing to disagree with male colleagues in defense of women's health, and she developed a set of ideas about the female body in health and disease that earned her the right to be counted not only as a premiere gynecologist and surgeon, but also as an advocate on behalf of her sex.

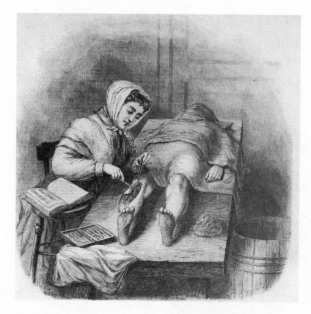

Dissection at the New York Medical College for Women. From *Frank Leslie's Illustrated Newspaper*, April 16, 1870. This sketch, along with several others, accompanied an article featuring women doctors. Courtesy of the University of Chicago Library.

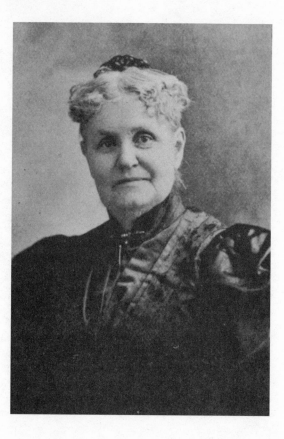

Dr. Mary Amanda Dixon Jones. Courtesy of the New York Academy of Medicine Library.

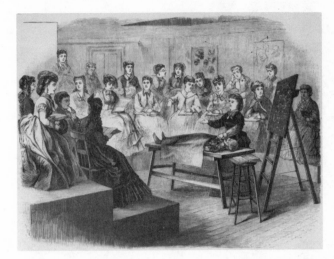

Anatomy lecture, New York Medical College for Women. From *Frank Leslie's Illustrated Newspaper*, April 16, 1870. Courtesy of the University of Chicago Library.

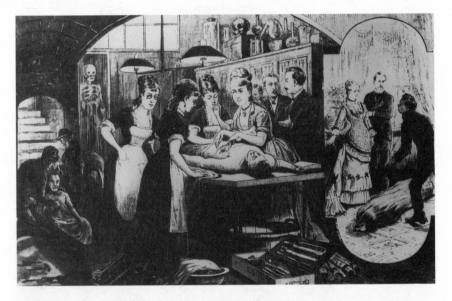

Gentle caricature of women medical students examining a male cadaver. The left and right corners of this drawing depict grave robbers procuring a body and laying it before the feet of a fashionably dressed female student and her male escort. The caption reads, "finding out with the aid of a lancet the peculiarities of the masculine heart." Attributed to *Frank Leslie's Illustrated Newspaper*, date unknown. Courtesy of the Archives and Special Collections on Women in Medicine, Medical College of Pennsylvania Collection, Allegheny University of the Health Sciences.

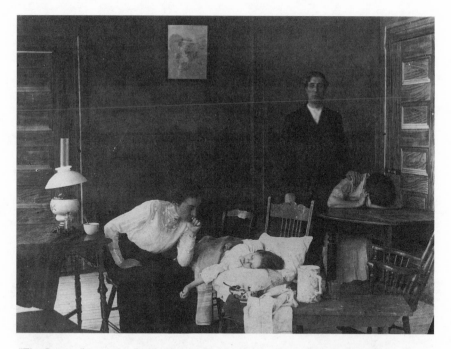

"The Doctor," ca. 1920. Dr. Agnes Hockaday of the Woman's Medical College of Pennsylvania poses as a late nineteenth-century physician visiting a patient. Courtesy of the Archives and Special Collections on Women in Medicine, Medical College of Pennsylvania Collection, Allegheny University of the Health Sciences.

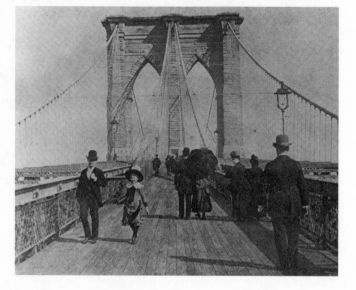

On the Brooklyn Bridge Promenade, ca. 1892. From Henry W. B. Howard, ed., *The Eagle and Brooklyn*, 1893. Courtesy of Dartmouth College Library.

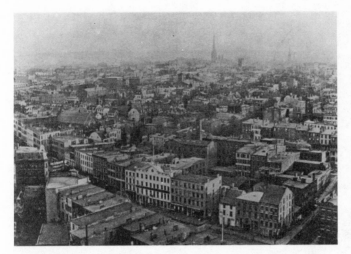

Birds-eye view of Brooklyn from the top of Bridge Tower, 1880. From Henry W. B. Howard, ed., *The Eagle and Brooklyn*, 1893. Courtesy of Dartmouth College Library.

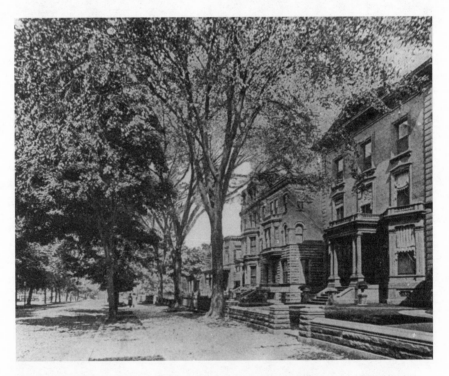

Typical street scene (Clinton Avenue, looking north from Lafayette) in Brooklyn's comfortable Hill district. Dixon Jones lived approximately six blocks away. From Henry W. B. Howard, ed., *The Eagle and Brooklyn*, 1893. Courtesy of Dartmouth College Library.

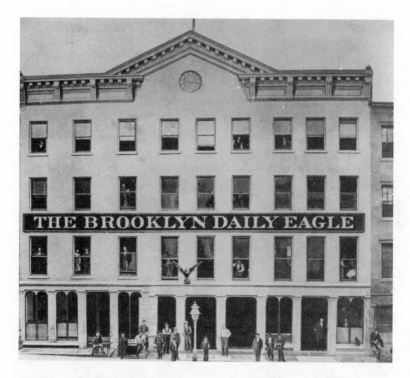

The Eagle Building until July 1892, when the newspaper relocated to a larger and more modernized structure. From Henry W. B. Howard, ed., *The Eagle and Brooklyn*, 1893. Courtesy of Dartmouth College Library.

King's County Court House. From Henry W. B. Howard, ed., *The Eagle and Brooklyn*, 1893. Courtesy of Dartmouth College Library.

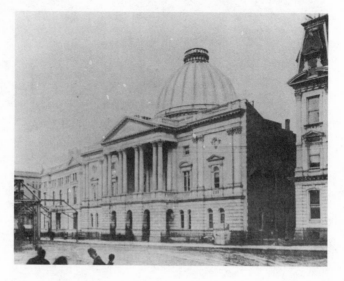

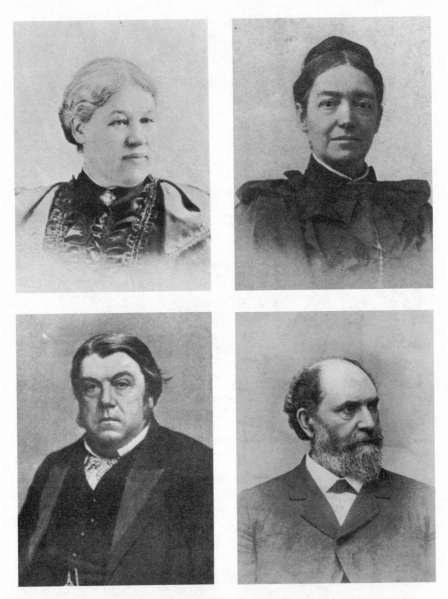

Top left: Eliza Mosher received her M.D. degree from the University of Michigan in 1875. She questioned Dixon Jones's "character," both in a letter to Elizabeth Blackwell and on the witness stand in 1892. From Irving A. Watson, *Physicians and Surgeons of America*, 1895. Courtesy of the University of Michigan Library. Top right: Dr. Mary Putnam Jacobi. Highly respected among male and female colleagues alike, Putnam Jacobi was the only woman physician to testify on behalf of Dixon Jones. Bottom left: Dr. Lawson Tait of Birmingham, England. Tait was a world-renowned ovariotomist. Bottom right: Dr. Alexander J. C. Skene, professor of gynecology at the Long Island College Hospital and Medical School. Last three photos courtesy of the New York Academy of Medicine Library.

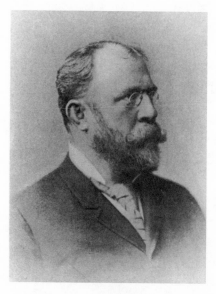

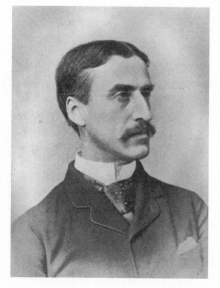

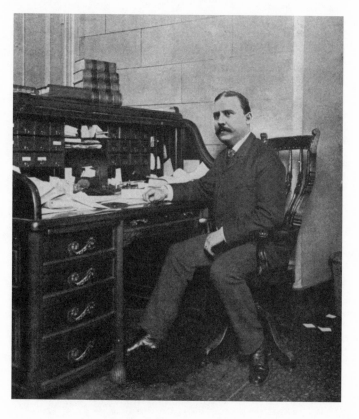

Top left: St. Clair McKelway, editor of the Brooklyn *Eagle*; top right: Judge Willard Bartlett; right: James W. Ridgway, prosecuting attorney for both trials. All photos from Henry W. B. Howard, ed., *The Eagle and Brooklyn*, 1893. Courtesy of Dartmouth College Library.

4

Gynecology Becomes a Specialty

Readers familiar with the struggle of women to enter the professions at the end of the nineteenth century may find remarkable the very existence of a nationally and internationally known female ovariotomist. By 1900, fewer than a handful of women physicians had achieved comparable status. Dixon Jones negotiated her professional identity over a period of thirty years in the practice of medicine, at a time when boundaries, behaviors, techniques, and ideologies of practice were in flux. But resistance to women doctors was heated at times, and even successful practitioners faced chronic discrimination. Signs of hostility are present in various and subtle forms throughout the unfolding of her case. For example, the presiding judge at the manslaughter trial was chagrined by how long it took to gather a jury—most of the men interviewed disapproved of female physicians. But if discrimination were the *primary* precipitating factor in this tale, it would not be worth telling. What is more intriguing about Mary Dixon Jones's difficulties with the Brooklyn *Eagle* is that they were linked as much to her penchant for gynecological surgery as to her sex. What was the cultural meaning of the normalization of such operations in late nineteenth-century Brooklyn? How did Dixon Jones come to support such radical treatment procedures, defending her surgery even against the assaults of other women physicians? What led her to become embroiled in a public battle over medical therapeutics with the Brooklyn *Eagle*? We can begin to understand why female surgery raised eyebrows not only in the public arena, but among physicians themselves only by returning to the eighteenth century, when science and medicine altered its traditional conceptions of the human body.

Until that time, common belief inherited from the Greeks held that male and female bodies were essentially the same. Superior structure and the presence of greater heat explained why men's genitals were visible *outside* the body; otherwise, they were believed to be analogous in every way to women's hidden organs. Male and female differences, in other words, lay not in biology. In the late 1700s, however, this was challenged by a new paradigm of divergence.[1]

Associated with novel ideologies about gender, these changes were useful to the developing social and political relationships that emerged with the decline of religious and metaphysical authority. No longer confident of concepts like "divine right" and "the great chain of being," Enlightenment thinkers interested in answers turned to positivistic science, which, with its passion for seeking evidence "in nature," its belief in reason, empiricism, and the possibility that knowledge could be both objective and value-free, proved eager to rise to the occasion.[2]

The "science of woman" was a by-product of these developments. It rested on the notion that women's bodies were in some measure a case apart, and that man was the physiological norm. Thus has gynecology's emergence correctly been characterized as a culmination of two centuries of shifting scientific thinking on the subject of sex differences.

This chapter will concentrate on three themes. First, it will offer an overview of the development of gynecological surgery. We cannot know how Dixon Jones approached her task as a physician without a more detailed picture of the disagreements over surgical and other treatments that troubled practitioners of gynecology, still a relatively new specialty in the last third of the nineteenth century. Second, we will attempt to understand how Dixon Jones came to favor radical surgery in the treatment of female ailments, especially at a time when many leaders of the women's medical movement, such as Elizabeth Blackwell, stood in vocal opposition to such solutions. Finally, although I am sympathetic to previous historical characterizations of radical surgeons as biased toward surgical solutions and overly willing to perform unnecessary operations, I will show that there were other developments that contributed to gynecological surgery's acceptance at this particular time. These included the very real suffering of nineteenth-century women, the perceived lack of alternatives to surgery for doctor and patient, the exciting advances in surgical techniques arising out of trial and error, and the extraordinary courage of certain women who chose an often dangerous procedure as an alternative to chronic, debilitating pain. Each contributed substantially to the growth of the field.

Thus, surgical gynecologists had other motives than victimizing women, and their patients often came to them suffering from grave, sometimes fatal, physical handicaps. These ailments presented both as palpable cries for help as well as intellectual and technical problems demanding to be solved.

GYNECOLOGY MEETS SURGERY: THE EARLY YEARS, 1850–80

In the 1830s and 1840s, crucial innovations in clinical research and medical theory emerging from clinics in Paris paved the way for the expansion of surgery and indirectly for the development of surgical gynecology as well. New technology, such as the stethoscope and the thermometer, and innovative techniques, such as auscultation, percussion, and palpation, trained practitioners' attention on specific organs and abnormal internal structures. New knowledge of the body was generated out of this clinical and diagnostic innovation, yielding novel approaches to treatment that encouraged specialization. Once the surgical point of view pictured internal pathology as local, "the body became a surgical object *in potentia*." Practice logically followed.[3]

This period of medical expansionism represented a gradual shift from art to science, from general practice to specialization, from medical to surgical solutions. These changes generated anxieties that paralleled problems already vexing the society at large, namely, the difficult transition from craft traditions, where unique products were fashioned holistically by a skilled workman, to mass production, where identical goods were mass-manufactured in a reductionist manner by a series of "specialists" created by the new, more modern division of labor.[4] Lawson Tait, the British ovariotomist rivaled only by Spencer Wells in his many contributions to the field, accounted for the emergence of gynecology in terms social scientists would find familiar. The new gynecology was "inevitable," he enthusiastically explained, "so soon as the advancement of medicine was great enough to admit of the division of labour."[5]

Tait's considered opinion aside, however, the new gynecology was *not* inevitable, and it is only with historical hindsight that its emergence "makes sense." Part of the reason it evolved slowly was that specialization itself was hardly automatic, nor was the process of medical specialization necessarily destined to play itself out in the manner that it did. Specialties could just as easily have been systematized otherwise: by tissue type, for example, or race, class, age, or disease etiology. None of the explanations historians have offered for the present organization of Western medicine, neither the argument that the specialties followed naturally from research in pathological anatomy, nor that they represented a division of labor modeled on industrial capitalism, completely satisfies. The social context must be explored as well, because gynecology is "a specialism which is underpinned by a historically contingent notion of woman." It is not impossible to imagine a time, one scholar reminds us, when "the rationale for differentiating gynaecology to the present degree may cease to exist," leading to its "disappearance . . . from the medical cosmology."[6]

In spite of cultural and scientific pressures, gynecologists separated themselves off from generalists gradually, cautioning us to remember that events in social ideology and in medicine parallel each other only imperfectly. Most physicians still regarded specialization as a form of quackery, and, in medical schools, the diseases of women were tellingly subsumed under the rubric "Diseases of Women and Children." Though Gunning S. Bedford (1796–1872), professor of obstetrics at the University Medical College in New York, established the first gynecological clinic in the United States in 1841, and J. Marion Sims founded the New York Woman's Hospital in 1855, the gynecologist Ely Van De Warker lamented as late as 1888 that gynecological instruction in medical schools was still primitive and inadequate. Indeed, in the 1850s, Sims was deeply discouraged by the initial response of New York's medical community to his idea of a special hospital for women. Even two decades later, Henry O. Marcy recalled, those wishing to concentrate in surgical gynecology in Boston in the 1870s were "shunned" by the medical community.[7] Thus, though later in this chapter we will note the increasing *popularity* of gynecological surgery in the last two decades of the century, developments in the field remained haphazard and uneven well into the twentieth century.

During the early stage, much of the physician's role was palliative. Doctors encountered women suffering from huge ovarian cysts and other types of abdominal tumors, their distended abdomens, excruciating pain, and emaciated bodies indicating unspeakable suffering. Before anesthesia and antisepsis, however, surgery terrified patients and was justly regarded by practitioners as a last resort. The physician who attempted it needed brute strength, manual dexterity, speed, and a strong stomach. Confining themselves largely to amputations and setting bones, surgeons performed harrowing procedures on semi-conscious persons whose senses had been dulled by alcohol and whose bodies were held down by strong male assistants. Patients often went into shock. The surgeon, one commentator remarked, needed to be willing "to cut like an executioner."[8] Indeed, surgeons' metaphors led them to compare their work to the conquest of the frontier, where "darkness was giving way to light and civilization was taming the 'primary terrors' of pain and suffering."[9]

Determination and a steady arm aside, worry about the consequences of invading bodily cavities meant that, before the 1850s, most practitioners diagnosed serious female illnesses as incurable. They confined themselves to the repeated tapping and draining of fluid-filled sacs, removal of labial growths, minor plastic procedures in the form of perineal repairs, and curretting and topical treatments for a variety of inflammatory indications. Sponge tents and pessaries inserted at the mouth of the cervix were also favorite devices for treating uterine displacements. Without any means of alleviating pain, early gynecologists were reluctant to operate on female patients, especially those of the white middle class.[10] And yet, real suffering led a few bold practitioners to try. As early as 1809, Ephraim McDowell of Danville, Kentucky, performed the first successful ovariotomy on a willing patient, Jane Crawford, who survived the surgery and lived in good health until her seventy-eighth year. But the dangers of the operation were readily apparent; McDowell attempted it only twelve more times, with eight recoveries and four deaths. After McDowell, a few in the United States and abroad tried ovariotomy with varying degrees of success.

The Atlee brothers, for example, John Light (1799–1885) and Washington L. (1808–78), were particularly proficient operators, achieving notice in the 1840s and 1850s. Other pioneers in the United States included Edward R. Peaslee and T. Gaillard Thomas, by the 1860s both associates of J. Marion Sims in New York, and Robert Battey of Rome, Georgia, and H. T. Byford of Chicago, both of whom became active in the 1870s. Between 1701 and 1851, according to Washington Atlee, a total of 222 recorded ovariotomies were completed in Europe and the United States combined. The high death rate—about 66 percent, from shock, infection, and hemorrhage—however, warned most practitioners off, in spite of the fact that these operations were usually desperate efforts to save sick women from certain death.[11] Still, surgeons made progress in the period before 1850, and we might well mark the years between 1850 and 1880 as a turning point in gynecologic practice. It was in these years that the use of anesthesia, first invented in the 1840s, and experiments with antisepsis urged on colleagues by the Scottish gynecologist James Y. Simpson in the 1860s and 1870s, became more widespread.[12]

American physicians greeted the work of pioneer ovariotomists with a mixture of respect and suspicion. In the medical world, surgery always had dramatic appeal, and the early ovariotomies, sometimes performed without anesthesia and before antisepsis, were no exception. Harvard's Henry J. Bigelow admitted that surgery received "undue appreciation" because it was gory, exciting, and intense.[13] Ovariotomy certainly lived up to these expectations and more: It was bold, radical, and life-threatening. Precisely for these reasons, many leading spokesmen, in the United States and abroad, actively opposed the new techniques. Philadelphia's Charles D. Meigs, arguing that removing women's ovaries was both immoral and ineffective, attempted to have the operation legally prohibited, and British surgeon Robert Liston labeled it "belly ripping." The French were even more reluctant to perform it, pointing to the inaccuracy of diagnoses and the experimental nature of treatment. Ectopic pregnancy, for example, was occasionally misconstrued as a tumor or cyst.[14]

The best explanation for why some practitioners resisted the new techniques is that surgical knowledge was not necessarily objective and competed with other ways to describe the body. Surgeons, Mary Dixon Jones included, were not merely revolutionizing treatment; they were altering traditional understandings of body parts and their diseases in a manner that led to "the desirability of surgical intervention." Moreover, how medical problems were defined or redefined as surgical, privileging one route toward solution over another, is the story of "conflict between different communities with differing interests." Surgical practice is never merely empirical. Restating a point first made in the 1930s by Irwin Ackerknecht, the historian of surgery Christopher Lawrence reminds us that "the simplest of surgical procedures are complex cultural phenomena."[15]

The conquest of vesico-vaginal fistula by J. Marion Sims is a perfect case in point. Usually honored as the "father of American gyecology," Sims's work muted some of the criticism of early medical skeptics and generated more confidence in the potentialities of improved technique. An unlikely candidate for fame in his youth, Sims attended medical school primarily because he demonstrated little aptitude for anything else. A southerner, he began his experiments in 1845 after a fairly undistinguished career as a general practitioner in Montgomery County, Alabama. Because of his developing interest in surgery, several plantation owners in the area requested that he treat slave women suffering from various injuries sustained during childbirth. Particularly frustrating were cases of vesico-vaginal fistulae, holes in the vaginal wall created by the pressure of the fetus that demolish bladder and sometimes rectal control and render young women incapable of work or future reproduction. It is not known whether slave women, perhaps because of poor nutrition and back-breaking physical labor, suffered inordinately from this condition, but the problem was familiar to practitioners in Europe and America, and doctors had struggled with it "from the earliest days of recorded medical history."[16] Women afflicted with fistulae lived anguished lives, and their torment knew no racial or class boundaries. Their plight was described vividly in an oft-quoted passage written by Dr. John Deiffenbach, a German practitioner:

> A sadder situation can hardly exist.... A source of disgust, even to herself, the woman . . . becomes in this condition the object of bodily revulsion . . . everyone turns his back repulsed by the intolerable, foul uriniferous odor. . . . The labia, perineum, lower part of the buttocks and inner aspects of the thighs and calves are continually wet, to the very feet. . . . Intolerable burning and itching torment the patients. The refreshment of a change of clothing provides no relief, because the clean undergarment, after being quickly saturated, slaps against the patients, sloshing their shoes as if they were wading through a swamp. . . . Even the richest are usually condemned for life to a straw sack, whose straw must be renewed daily. One's breath is taken away by the bedroom air of these women. . . . Washing and anointing do not help; perfume actually increases the repugnance of the odor. . . . [17]

Although a few surgeons in the United States and abroad had experimented with reparative procedures, Sims, unaware of this work, at first refused all fistula cases, despairing of possible solutions. Then, quite unexpectedly, while treating a local white woman for internal injuries incurred when she was thrown from a horse, he was literally struck with a new technical idea for approaching the problem of fistulae, which grated on his consciousness in spite of his attempt to avoid it. But when, how, and under what circumstances could he test out the procedure? As long as he operated without anesthesia, it was inconceivable to try it on white patients. Female slaves offered a ready-made patient population, and nineteenth-century theories regarding the lesser sensitivity of black women to pain gave Sims added incentive.[18]

Establishing a small hospital on the grounds of his residence, Sims invited several plantation owners to send their fistula cases to him. He operated on about eleven slave women in all, but three, Anarcha, Betsey, and Lucy, were with him for the entire three and a half years it took to perfect the procedure, each of them undergoing repeated experimental operations without anesthesia, about forty in all. The three women were young, Anarcha no more than seventeen, and each had been injured by complicated and protracted first births. Sims had actually been present at Anarcha's delivery, and her fistula was the first he had ever seen. Besides an enormous hole in her bladder, there was "an extensive destruction of the posterior wall of the vagina, opening in to the rectum." The poor woman was in constant pain, her urine running in a steady dribble, saturating bedding and clothing. Her pelvic region and thighs were acutely inflamed with sores "almost similar to confluent small-pox." Anarcha's life, Sims felt, "was one of suffering and disgust."[19]

Sims's initial attempts at repair were unavailing, but he was determined. If his account can be believed, so were Anarcha, Betsey, and Lucy, who nursed each other and like patients during recovery periods, assisted Sims at operations, and endured unspeakably painful surgery without protest. Unquestioning of the racial and class system that made these women available to him as human guinea pigs, Sims was nevertheless admiring of their endurance and grateful for their aid and support.[20] From our vantage point, it is impossible not to view these courageous slave women as making an emphatic contribution to the perfection of surgical techniques, not merely by the availability of their bodies, but by actively assisting and encouraging Sims in his work.

Sims solved three technical problems in the course of perfecting the operation for fistulae: First, he improved access to the operative field by using the knee-chest position. He then designed a vaginal speculum that greatly facilitated repair. Finally, he used silver sutures, which he believed to be far less likely to cause postoperative infection. In January 1852 he published his findings in the *American Journal of Medical Sciences*. A year later he moved to New York City. The Woman's Hospital he established there, one of the first of its kind in the country, gave him a public arena for demonstrating the new techniques to a wider medical audience. In ensuing years he made many trips abroad, garnering fame, fortune, and the admiration of the burgeoning international community of gynecological surgeons.[21]

Until the mid-1870s, practitioners operated primarily on ovarian cysts that were relatively easy to diagnose because of their size. In 1872, however, Robert Battey, a prominent southern surgeon from Rome, Georgia, removed a set of what he called "normal" ovaries for indications no more precise than acute menstrual difficulties and dysmenorrhoea (painful menstruation), publishing his results almost immediately.[22] Battey's description of the case indicates he believed his patient, a thirty-year-old woman without a uterus, who had first visited him at the age of twenty-three, to be in serious chronic distress. Indeed, she later reported that her suffering was so intense that she felt "there was no future for her in this life, and that death would be a relief."[23] After a seven-year course of internal applications and other palliative measures, Battey, encouraged by the success of ovariotomy for neoplasms, determined to removed her ovaries, bring on "the change of life," and thus reestablish general health.[24]

In effect, by the removal of what he insisted on calling "normal," as opposed to diseased, ovaries, what Battey did was to broaden considerably the indications for gynecological surgery and, in so doing, greatly expand the patient population to which such procedures could be applied. In addition, he was never adequately specific about symptoms that might require the procedure, offering only the statement that his operation was appropriate in "any grave disease which is either dangerous to life or destructive to health and happiness, which is incurable by other and less radical means."[25] In 1877, in an attempt at more clarity, he presented before the American Gynecological Society four indications for surgery: (1) when the absence of a uterus threatened a patient's life; (2) when it was impossible to restore an obliterated uterine cavity or vaginal canal by surgical means; (3) in cases of uterine or ovarian insanity or epilepsy; (4) in cases in which monthly periods produced prolonged mental and physical suffering.[26] A decade later, Battey refined these criteria even further, citing "oophoromania, oophoro-epilepsy, and oophoralgia," still indeterminate diagnoses of various types of nervous conditions, pelvic pain, and hysteria, conditions he presumed to be catalysed by the condition of the ovaries. This vagueness was in many respects an indication of the vast ignorance physicians of this period had of the structure and functions of the female reproductive system. Other surgical diseases, like appendicitis, were written about in this period using equally loose criteria of definition.[27] Unlike some of the younger gynecologists who began their careers in the 1880s, Battey did not use a microscope and attempted no pathological analysis of the organs he removed. He always contended that the ovaries he took from the bodies of his patients looked "normal" to the naked eye. But we shall see that this kind of gross pathology would increasingly become unacceptable.[28]

In the next chapter, we will take up the implications of such diagnoses as Battey's for the nineteenth-century medical construction of the female body. At present it is necessary only to note that Battey's stance virtually guaranteed his operation would be performed too frequently for a range of vague mental and physical symptoms. The consequent enthusiasm for the knife in doubtful cases of organic disease generated by his work eventually troubled not only hostile critics of surgery, but even leading practitioners of the new specialty. It has, of course, also provoked the disdain of a generation of feminist scholars and historians of nineteenth-century health care who took such procedures to be proof of the profound misogyny embedded in Victorian culture.

In 1872, the same year that Battey introduced his operation to the surgical world, Lawson Tait, a young British surgeon, removed a chronically abscessed ovary, expanding indications for ovariotomy in yet another direction. A few months later, he used bilateral ovariotomy to cure a case of bleeding fibroid tumors.[29] Also in 1872, the German surgeon Alfred Hegar lost a patient after an unsuccessful attempt at removing both ovaries for menstrual neuralgia. Though he waited five years before publishing these and other results, Hegar eventually became the leading ovariotomist in Germany, performing the procedure most frequently to control uterine hemorrhage from fibroids.[30] Further, between the 1850s, when surgeons were just beginning to use anesthesia, and the mid-1870s, when Tait, Battey, and Hegar established their reputations, others improved techniques for removing cysts and tumors as well. Mortality rates fell substantially, especially in the 1860s, after Joseph Lister developed a system of antisepsis based on Pasteur's early experiments in putrefaction and applied it to the operating theater in 1865. Though not all surgeons adopted Lister's methods, cleanliness became standard operating procedure. Spencer Wells, who completed his first successful ovariotomy in 1858, admitted a mortality rate of 34 percent in 1865. Only a decade later, that figure had dipped to 20 percent.[31]

SURGICAL GYNECOLOGY COMES OF AGE: 1880–1900

The rise of specialty hospitals like Sims's in the United States and England was an important chapter in the development of gynecology. These institutions played a such a unique role in advancing careers and perfecting technological skill that Sims once admitted to the English surgeon Protheroe Smith that without them, "you and I could not have done the work we have done."[32] Indeed, in 1888, Ely Van De Warker credited the women's hospitals and not the medical schools with teaching the new specialty. "We are living today," he wrote, "under a new dispensation in the matter of teaching gynecology. . . . Starting from the germ planted by our great master Sims in the Woman's Hospital of the State of New York, scarce a city of the land but has its hospital, great or small, public or private, where some faithful master, surrounded by a little band of followers, works and teaches."[33]

Despite these striking developments, die-hard critics continued to complain bitterly about the resort to surgery, even after 1880. In response, surgical pioneers repeatedly voiced resentment at the slow acceptance of surgical techniques, identifying themselves constantly with the advancement of science.[34] Generational and status rivalries nurtured this resentment.[35] The men who created the specialty of surgical gynecology, much like Sims, tended to be young and ambitious.[36] They challenged medical tradition in numerous ways, and the new surgical techniques for women's diseases offered them a secure place in the profession by allowing them to stake out uncharted territory.[37]

The relative openness of the field helps explain how a woman like Mary Dixon Jones managed to achieve professional prominence. It also offers a plausible hypothesis as to why American surgeons had the reputation of operating more often than British and European colleagues and appeared more tolerant of radical procedures of an experimental nature, especially as the specialty matured. Besides the much-touted American tendency to welcome and celebrate bold technological solutions to difficult problems, the lack of professional controls meant that virtually any general practitioner could attempt abdominal surgery with few professional sanctions. The only constraint seems to have been the growth of malpractice suits in the latter half of the century, though even this was apparently not enough to serve as an effective deterrent.[38] For all these reasons, practitioners of the new surgery saw themselves as persecuted pioneers, even as late as the 1880s.[39]

Larger developments in medicine may be evoked to explain some of this specific tension and hostility over the attraction of elite gynecological surgeons to pathology and laboratory science. The dramatic bacteriological discoveries in the last third of the century, coinciding with the consolidation of gynecological surgery, produced a new paradigm of experimental science. Whereas earlier in the century traditional medical belief systems still explained sickness as a condition affecting the entire organism, the new science dictated another approach. Researchers were beginning to isolate the pathogenic bacteria of epidemic diseases, and their successes promoted a new ideology of science consisting of an acceptance of the germ theory, the focus on specific diseases and body parts, specialization, and a growing enthusiasm for resorting to the evidence produced in the laboratory and the revitalization of cellular pathology. While older practitioners continued to emphasize clinical observation and the inevitability of individual differences in treatment, laboratory enthusiasts argued that the chemical and physiological principles derived from experimentation must inform therapeutics. Patient idiosyncrasies and environmental differences were gradually stripped of their significance, while reductionist and universalistic criteria for treatment took their place.[40]

The persistent skepticism of some American practitioners to the medical relevance of basic science, when tensions arose over what role laboratory physiology would play in treatment and practice, speaks directly to our exploration of surgical controversies. On one side were physicians trained in an older, Parisian tradition of empiricism who believed that, though basic science research might explain *why* things happened in the body in particular ways, clinical decisions could be informed only by direct observation of sick patients at the bedside, where the effects of therapy on uniquely different individuals could be critically monitored. Now at the end of their careers, these critics of laboratory science had not forgotten their own early intellectual rebellion in the 1830s and 1840s, when they had themselves rejected prevailing theories—the Enlightenment-inspired quest for laws, certainty, and systems—which were, by that time, producing such rigidity in medical treatment and practice that patients became alienated from regular physicians and doubters broke mainstream professional ranks. In response, they had emphasized the art embedded in the physician-patient encounter, and expressed the conviction that "medicine is, above all else, humane as well as human, that its beginning, middle and end is to relieve suffering, and that whatever is outside of this may indeed be science of some sort, but certainly is not medicine."[41]

Now, in the twilight of their careers, many of these same physicians looked askance at a younger generation of doctors, the latter trained in or oriented toward Germany in the 1870s and 1880s, where the prestige of the basic sciences was already secure. The older group believed their younger colleagues were duped by the questionable possibilities of rationalist systems, where the uniqueness of each patient could be lost. Being a good practitioner meant above all else exercising impeccable judgment, making careful choices at the bedside, highlighting not only the healing potential of the physician-patient relationship, but moral values as well.

While appearing to their detractors to be returning to the approach of a more benighted age, younger enthusiasts for laboratory medicine sought a newly constituted and experimentally based set of universal laws about how bodies functioned in health and disease, intending to transform medicine into an exact science. Unlike the traditional approach to care that often breached the wall between doctor and patient and depended on a body of shared, accessible information, the new scientific model mystified medical knowledge and furnished objectively agreed-upon criteria for setting standards in behavior, diagnosis, and treatment. For these young practitioners, many of them specialists in newly established fields of medicine, basic science was to foreshadow and shape future practice.[42]

Suspicions of and tensions over this new professional style were palpable in the latter third of the nineteenth century.[43] These were often channeled into hostility to radical gynecological surgery, which, in addition to reducing the whole patient to constituent body parts, embraced laboratory science, especially in the guise of pathology, with increasing enthusiasm.[44]

Also worth noting, especially for our exploration of the Dixon Jones affair, is the fact that different concepts of the good practitioner became gendered at the end of the nineteenth century. Some women physicians, whose most eloquent spokesperson was Elizabeth Blackwell, developed a carefully crafted articulation of female professionalism that, using the language of domesticity, valorized and gendered a newly emerging concept of empathic expertise. Empathy became intertwined with the public image of the woman doctor. Blackwell, for example, used motherhood as a central metaphor in her discussion of the ideal physician-patient relationship. Ironically, this ideology of female professionalism hearkened back to descriptions of the doctor's traditional role in bedside care prevalent earlier in the century, images dear to the conservative contingent of physicians I have just described, who were suspicious of the changes catalyzed by the new bacteriology and physiology. We shall see that Mary Dixon Jones, who embraced the new scientific style and did not necessarily follow the gender scripts provided by Blackwell, found herself denounced by both men and women in the profession, practitioners of both sexes loyal to a more traditional version of professional values and women who saw her assertiveness as inimical to their professional image and collegial status.[45]

Contemporaries may not have been aware of the fully ramified moral issues embedded in the struggle, but they certainly understood that medical knowledge was rapidly changing. According to the surgeon Howard Kelly, three crucial nineteenth-century developments turned the old gynecology "to seed," while creating a new specialty "full of life and vigor, sturdy, independent and aggressive." The first was anesthesia, which "robbed surgery of its horrors." Asepsis followed, which "robbed it of its dangers." Last, Kelly pointed to the important influence of "cellular pathology," which arose out of the researches of the Paris school and "came as a godsend to enable the operator to discriminate between malignant and non-malignant growths."[46]

Kelly's triumphant narrative is also interesting on other counts: Namely, it barely hints at the growing pains and controversies generated in the last decades of the nineteenth century, as gynecologists, old and new, struggled mightily to professionalize. A look at the nature of those controversies can tell us much about the interaction between structural developments, social ideology, and scientific and technological change in the making of the specialty, all factors that provided the crucial context for the Mary Dixon Jones affair.

FROM CONTROVERSY TO CONSENSUS: SURGEONS SHAPE THE SPECIALTY

Anesthesia certainly stimulated the use of the knife, and practitioner after practitioner commented on the obvious—that "surgery is the pivot around which is to revolve the gynecology of the future."[47] "A gynecologist of the future, without surgical attainments," argued T. Gaillard Thomas in 1879, "will be as impossible as an ophthamologist without them is today."[48] An Alabama physician detailing for his local medical journal a recent visit to New York to observe advances in gynecology concluded, "Operative gynecology is now sweeping the world."[49]

Surgeons experimented with new methods as they became more confident of success. By the 1880s, debates turned less than in the past on the legitimacy of the operation per se, though, as we will see, these disagreements did not disappear altogether. Instead, doctors discussed the efficacy of various techniques, including the use of the clamp or the ligature, vaginal versus abdominal routes to extirpation, the effectiveness and necessity of Listerism, especially the use of the controversial carbolic acid spray, the length of incisions, proper management of the pedicle (the stump of an organ left attached to the abdominal lining after excision), the validity of drainage, and various methods of cleansing the peritoneal cavity. Several approaches to plastic repair and treatment of uterine prolapse were devised and discarded during this period as well.[50]

In Great Britain, Lawson Tait's contributions to the technique of ovariotomy surpassed even those of Sir Spencer Wells. In terms of diagnosis, Tait distinguished his operation from Battey's and Hegar's by empasizing the connection between diseased ovaries and diseased tubes. In theory, at least, Tait was also extremely reluctant to operate for vague symptoms like neuralgia (nonspecific, but acute pain without demonstrable inflammation) and painful menstruation, although he did so occasionally.[51] In addition, "Tait's operation," as his version of the procedure came to be known, included the removal of the Fallopian tubes *and* the ovaries, and he argued that the appendages, and not the ovaries, were the most likely seat of disease. Unlike Wells, Tait eventually rejected Listerism in favor of what he always described as "soap and water." Also in contrast to Wells, whom he eventually came to view as a hostile rival, Tait emphasized the importance of pathological diagnosis and rejected the idea of operating when visible pathology was absent. Indeed, in 1879, he first introduced the radical idea of using exploratory surgery as an aid to diagnosis.[52] "The nearer we approach to Battey's principle in operating upon any case, the more unsatisfactory will be the result,'' he wrote in 1890. ''The nearer we approach to my principle in operating for gross and palpable disease, the more our patients will be benefitted.''[53]

Gradually, many operators began to distinguish the terms "ovariotomy" and "oöphorectomy" by the symptoms presented and the appearance of diagnosable pathology, the latter term most often used to refer to the extirpation of ovaries that *appeared* to be healthy. Tait aggressively identified himself with the former procedure, as did Mary Dixon Jones, who was a staunch supporter, and eventually distinctions between Tait's and Battey's operation rode on the presence of manifest pathology. In a letter to Dixon Jones in 1888, for example, Paul F. Mundé, the editor of the *American Journal of Obstetrics and Diseases of Women and Children*, clarified his own understanding of the differences in approach. Referring to Battey's operation as "oöphorectomy," he distinguished between this and Tait's version in part by drawing attention to Tait's list of indications: "diseased, even purulent tubes (chiefly) and ovaries." These guidelines for excision "are quite different from that for Battey's . . . when the disease of the uterine appendages is but problematical before and after the operation, which is performed often for merely reflex neurotic conditions." Mundé concluded that "in Tait's operation, there can be no question of the indication; in Battey's . . . the justifiability is still *sub judice*."[54]

It is clear from her many published articles that Dixon Jones preferred Tait's operation to the other versions of ovariotomy available, and both she and Tait exhibited a similar disingenuousness in their claim to be able to diagnose pathological conditions from symptoms only. Though Dixon Jones produced a sizable collection of professional articles on the pathology of the reproductive organs, her slides and specimens were made after, not before, her operations. In retrospect, one marvels at the slowness of surgeons to use pathological diagnosis before operating in cases other than cancer, but the adoption of new procedures could often be a gradual and complex process, and Dixon Jones and other practitioners were doing the best they could with the limited knowledge and methods available.[55]

Meanwhile, as leading gynecologists debated these questions, they continued through trial and error to improve technique. Success with ovariotomy for diseased ovaries and tubes emboldened many to attempt it for fibroid tumors of the uterus, as Tait had done early in 1872. As late as the 1870s, surgeons remained reluctant to perform abdominal surgery for these neoplasms, though myomectomy (removal of fibroids) through the vagina was attempted more often.[56] However, mortality rates from serious fibroid tumors, some of which weighed from six to twenty-two pounds, could be as high as 90 percent, and surgeons, who were interventionist by nature, were persuaded by such statistics to persist in a search for treatment.[57]

What operators feared most was a patient's bleeding to death; the vascularity of fibroid tumors and the uterine stump meant that new methods of hemostatis had to be devised. Tait's and Hegar's early success with fibroids was actually quite remarkable. In the United States, a period of trial and error ensued, in which operators experimented with myomectomy by devising various ways to arrest bleeding and avoid infection, using ligation in creative ways, designing various kinds of clamps, trying morcellation, or the cutting away by pieces, and concocting several new methods of drainage.[58]

The stubborn persistence of high mortality rates for myomectomy prompted the introduction in the 1880s and early 1890s of a new therapy—electricity— offered as an alternative to surgery.[59] Radical surgeons, like Dixon Jones and Joseph Price of Philadelphia, however, were skeptical. Price's contempt was particularly aggressive, and his instincts were on target: "When I am called finally to operate upon a patient who has been for weeks under the treatment of currents and counter-currents, and find her . . . not only no better, but worse, must I accept the reports of cures in identical cases simply on the affirmation of enthusiasts, often incapable of making a correct diagnosis?"[60] Within a few years, electricity proved less safe and effective than supporters claimed, and it gradually fell into disuse.

More successful than the use of galvanic current was the revival of an older procedure—hysterectomy—and its application to the treatment of fibroids. Although hysterectomies had been performed as early as the 1860s as a last resort for cancer, the results were unsatisfying, and the operation was considered too risky.[61] Surgeons suspected, however, that removing the entire uterus could aid in achieving hemostasis and help avoid infection.[62] In addition, since many believed that uterine fibroids could in some cases lead to cancer, employing the same technique for both conditions made logical sense. But it was only gradually that practitioners learned how to deal with the cervical stump.[63]

In 1888, Mary Dixon Jones performed the first total hysterectomy for fibroid tumors in the United States, offering a report of her first case to her colleagues at the New York Pathological Society. A year later, the general surgeon Louis A. Stimson of New York devised a successful method of ligating the ovarian and uterine arteries and "Presto!," according to Kelly, "the thing was solved." Dixon Jones's name thus became associated with the operation in some of the histories written by her contemporaries. LeRoy Broun, reviewing the development of surgical treatment for fibroids in 1906, praised her contribution but noted it was "strange that this was not suggested earlier." Eventually, abdominal hysterectomy for fibroids became the treatment of choice, and even ovariotomy declined in favor of the procedure.[64]

PATHOLOGY AND SURGICAL DIAGNOSIS

The question of whether one emphasized the more likely involvement of the ovaries or the tubes in diagnosing candidates for surgery, or preferred myomectomy to hysterectomy in cases of fibroids, was confounded in a world where the larger issues of clinical diagnosis still hung in the balance. Here is where Howard Kelly's retrospective observations regarding the three crucial turning points in the development of surgical gynecology, especially his remarks about the influence of cellular pathology, deserve renewed attention. In these matters, the years between 1880 and 1910 marked a transitional stage when, as Russell

Maulitz has observed, the pathological theory used in diagnosis and the role of the microscopist evolved in interaction with each other. Indeed, the decade of the 1870s, when Mary Dixon Jones returned to medical school for a second degree, was a critical juncture, when calls for the institutionalization of pathology in the United States gained momentum, resulting in the addition to many medical faculties of individuals who, if they had not studied in Germany themselves, were at least "attuned to the New German investigative model."[65]

The use of the microscope to diagnose and describe pathological organs needing surgical attention was far from routine, even when second-generation ovariotomists expanded the operating field in the 1880s. "In some instances," the British surgeon Thomas Savage confessed in 1883, "I feel sure there is nothing to be felt in the pelvis before operation, and we have nothing to guide us but the more or less constant pain and recurring attacks of inflammation."[66] This was not solely a question of lack of experience or familiarity with the new diagnostic techniques; more significant was the fact that the microscope was not accepted uncritically by all practitioners. Earlier in this chapter we noted the splits between individuals who welcomed and those who suspected laboratory science, highlighting older physicians' mistrust of general physiological laws, which they feared would interfere with clinical decision-making at the bedside. In many respects the microscope became for some a symbol of these larger tensions.

When advances in Parisian physiology discredited traditional heavy dosing at mid-century, the resulting therapeutic gloom stimulated a range of remedial approaches, including a movement toward what was called "physiological therapeutics."[67] This optimistic program pushed by youthful practitioners in touch with European developments proposed to link clinical practice with experimental science. Whereas older practitioners were quite content to use physiology merely to *explain* events at the bedside, emphasizing a strict clinical empiricism that underlined the importance of individual variation and direct observation, physiological therapeutists believed basic science should *direct* modes of practice. This meant studying the differences between the normal and the abnormal and systematically investigating the physiological effects of various treatments. It was here that the laboratory physician who sought, as we have already pointed out, reductionist and universalistic chemical and physiological principles, made a contribution. Inevitably, he focused less on the patient and more on the physiological process under investigation. The result was a competing definition of what constituted science in medicine and "a thoroughgoing rearrangement of the relationships among therapeutic practice, knowledge, and professional identity."[68] Debates between practitioners entailed not only how medical knowledge should be produced, evaluated, and applied, but also "divergent conceptions of professional identity and professional morality."[69]

Worry that the new regard for laboratory knowledge would turn physicians away from patients and "undermine the moral order of medicine" was particularly acute in the case of bacteriology, which focused a great deal of attention on microscopical pathology.[70] Indeed, these fears are best captured in the words of the German clinician Ottomar Rosenbach, whose polemic *Physician versus*

Bacteriologist was translated into English in 1904. "Nothing," he wrote, "has so injured the standing of the practitioner and of the medical profession as the eagerness of bacteriologists to transfer decisions from the bedside to the laboratory, and to regulate etiology, diagnosis and therapy . . . according to an artificial scheme, instead of making full allowance for the requirements of actual conditions which can only be judged by those who are present at the bedside and who are familiar with local conditions."[71]

These discussions raged among gynecologists. While Joseph Price's memorialist deplored the resistance of older practitioners to the "new pathology," he praised Price for his advocacy of advanced "scientific" ideas.[72] In an 1888 *Journal of the American Medical Association* editorial entitled "The Wave of Surgical Progress," the writer emphasized to readers that "the present ascendency of surgery" was in "large measure" due to recent advances in basic science, especially "the work that has been done in chemistry."[73] Even the British physician Sir John Burdon-Sanderson admitted in 1899 that surgery was more scientifically engaged than general medicine. "If a comparison be made of the two great branches of medical practice—surgical and medical," he remarked, "one of the most striking points of difference is that the influence of scientific discovery has been much greater in surgery than in medicine."[74] Others as well urged the relevance of the basic sciences—"anatomy, physiology, chemistry, pathology"—arguing that, for the surgeon, these were the only areas that could yield "positive knowledge."[75] Several cited the necessity of proper differential diagnosis, asserting quite cogently that knowledge of the normal, "healthy human ovary" was essential to accurately identifying true pathology. "A diagnosis," Richard Douglas, Professor of Gynecology at Vanderbilt University, reminded his colleagues, "is the capstone of the edifice whose foundation is pathology."[76]

Indeed, many of the most radical gynecological surgeons argued that pathological diagnosis shaped the scientific basis of their ideas and gave the specialty its well-deserved prestige. By the 1880s, they were affirming their superiority over physicians, arguing that surgery required *both* medical knowledge and careful technique. J. Ewing Mears boasted of the surgeon's transition from being "bleeder and barber" to "pathologist [and] diagnostician."[77] Moreover, gynecological surgeons deliberately cloaked their decisions in the mantle of the new science by invoking the microscope whenever possible. While older practitioners like Spencer Wells and A. J. C. Skene questioned the relevance of the laboratory to treatment, others rushed to revitalize pathological societies and found microscopical societies that gave the microscope a central role in diagnosis, even if, as Henry Clarke Coe pointed out regretfully, surgeons who embraced it as a tool too often conducted their laboratory analysis after the fact.[78]

Mary Dixon Jones participated actively in these debates. Though already in her late fifties when she began her surgical career, she embraced the use of pathological investigation in the clinical setting without any of the ambivalence of the older generation of practitioners. Working first with John Gibbons Hunt at the Women's Medical College of Pennsylvania, and then Charles Heitzman, a Hungarian immigrant and German-trained pathologist, she began publishing her pathological investigations in 1889, often producing slides and theories to accompany case reports and justify diagnoses. She regularly attended meetings of the New York Pathological Society, which met at the New York Academy of Medicine's new building on West 43rd street in Manhattan, and often presented specimens there herself.

In 1886, in a letter to George Shrady, the editor of the New York *Medical Record* and the individual who nominated her for membership in the Pathological Society, Dixon Jones obliquely chided the great ovariotomist Spencer Wells, who spoke disparagingly of Tait's operation (for the removal of uterine appendages) and claimed that he, Wells, had not perceived "one case among his one thousand ovariotomies" of "disease in the tubes." Dixon Jones blamed Wells's myopia on the lack of microscopical data: "All the cases I have had of Tait's operation" involved disease of the tubes even more so "than in the ovaries." "I must think," she concluded, "that in many of Sir Spencer Wells' cases there were diseased tubes. . . . Could his cases be reseen, and especially seen in the light of the modern microcopical science, I believe it would be found that many had diseased tubes."[79]

In a subsequent article, she took a similar swipe at her own nemesis among the Brooklyn "conservatives," A. J. C. Skene, who testified as an *Eagle* witness in court, calling into question her surgical judgment. When asked what aid the microscope was to the practicing gynecologist, Skene had replied "None whatever. . . . It is utterly useless in ovarian disease." Barely able to mask her contempt, Dixon Jones rejoined, "Yet all great surgeons the world over are earnestly looking to the teachings of the microscope to know more of the minute anatomy of each and every organ, the pathological changes that may occur, the nature of these changes, so that they may learn more of the etiology of the disease, how to prevent, cure, or check its ravages."[80]

Like other surgical colleagues, Dixon Jones deliberately spoke the language of the new science, which not only validated her work but attracted the attention of male colleagues. Her ability to "do" pathology subtly placed her among an elite group of men.[81] Indeed, by 1886, Dixon Jones was reading the medical journals with great gusto, corresponding with various colleagues in the field and frequently presenting specimens at sessions of the Pathological Society in New York City. At several of these meetings she no doubt met Henry Clarke Coe, former assistant to William Welch and a gynecological pathologist at the New York Woman's Hospital and Bellevue in the late 1870s. In 1886, Coe published an article that engaged the attention of his colleagues in an extended discussion of the uses of pathology in surgical decision-making.[82] It is plausible to speculate that this article, so wide-ranging in its willingness to address the difficult issues in the field, not only provided the inspiration Dixon Jones needed to continue her pathological investigations, but emboldened her to express her own views.[83]

Coe's remarks underscored an important moment in the self-critique of the new specialty and provided an opportunity to pause and reflect on what had been accomplished in the last decade. Much like his mentor, Welch, Coe made a cogent case for the relevance of pathological research to surgery. He began by affirming the phenomenal interest practitioners of the previous decade had in the removal of ovaries and tubes. He linked these developments to the growth of the specialty. But welcoming this attention did not free him from the worry that many of his colleagues had fallen into the habit of what he termed "a priori reasoning" in clinical decision-making. Surgeons alone were driving the resolution to operate, he complained, when such procedures also required the input of the pathologist. In malignancies, Coe admitted, pathologists were often called in to examine a piece of tumor or sample sarcomatous uterine tissue before surgery. "But the same gynecologist will remove the ovaries and tubes, and will afterward call upon the pathologist to justify the wisdom of the operation." This, Coe confessed, was "often extremely difficult to do." If pathological research had revealed anything in the last decade, it was the onerousness of the researcher's task and the widespread ignorance of ovarian inflammation and its sequelae. "It should be remembered," he told his readers, "that within the ovary there is ceaseless activity, changes as subtle and eluding as the vital principle itself. . . . Under these circumstances, how difficult is it to affirm where the normal ends and the pathological begins!"[84]

In view of this still hesitant relationship of pathology to surgery and other clinical specialties, it took courage for Coe to say what he did, especially in the widely read *American Journal of Obstetrics and Diseases of Women and Children.*[85] But Coe was eager to stake out important claims for the relevance of pathology to gynecology. This was his most important point; the second, very much related to the first, was an oblique and gentle attempt to give shape to the amorphous debates regarding "too much surgery" that were agitating gynecologists in the 1880s.

There is no question but that the dramatic advances achieved in the last decade and a half stimulated what even contemporaries promptly identified as a *furor operandi*, or operative mania, a moment in the history of the specialty that at least one historian has aptly characterized as the "hysterical adolescence" of gynecology.[86] Once bold, but careful practitioners like Tait, Mundé, Sims, Battey, Price, and Thomas solved many of the technical problems of hemostasis and reduced infection, lowering the mortality rates for a variety of procedures, gynecological surgery became deceptively easy and accessible to a company of less experienced and imperfectly trained practitioners. These were likely to be generalists and surgeons living in the more remote towns and regions of the Midwest, West, and South. Others who entered the field were simply young and inexperienced. Indeed, as S. C. Gordon of Portland, Maine, recalled, a " 'craze for operating' " took "possession of the surgical world and every young man ambitious for renown in this fascinating department of medicine, 'fleshed' his maiden knife in the abdomen of some confiding victim to inexperience and immature judgment."[87] In the midst of these developments, Rufus B. Hall of Cincinnati offered the same diagnosis. "Abdominal and pelvic surgery today," he admitted, "is practiced by as restless and ambitious a throng as ever fought for fame upon the battlefield. There is probably no state in the Union," he guessed, "which cannot produce at least one man from each county who has made one or more abdominal sections in the past few years."[88]

Many complained that colleagues were being driven by the basest of motives: professional ambition or outright greed.[89] When "we see the records of countless exploits with the laparotomists' knife," Malcolm McLean confessed in an orgy of self-criticism,

> we are easily persuaded that, to be modern, we must be bold and dexterous. We must not fall behind in records, if we do in the aggregate number of our cases. A little reading, a little breathing of the laparotomist's atmosphere, whether we be in the operating room or in the halls of scientific societies, and we are converts to the new faith and boldly enter in. A few short months roll on and we are ready with our "year's record in laparotomy." With pride we point to our scores of successful cases, and we feel convinced that we have at last struck the panacea for most of woman's ills.[90]

But the craze for surgical solutions was driven not solely by practitioners. Individual commentators understood that pressure from patients also played a role in their sense of what was acceptable treatment. "Pelvic operations on women," admitted one practitioner, "has become a fad. It is fashionable, and the woman who cannot show an abdominotomy line is looked upon as not in the style, nor belonging to the correct set. It is a mark of favor and considered as pretty as the dimple on the cheek of sweet sixteen."[91] And, indeed, although this opponent of ovariotomy characterized such patient attitudes as frivolous, patients' desires and their complex attitudes toward their own bodies did play a part in the overall decision to operate. In the late 1880s, some doctors even noted that their patients left them to seek operations from more radical practitioners. Albert Brinkman, for example, the secretary of the Brooklyn Pathological Society, confessed to his colleagues at a case presentation to the King's County Medical Society in 1889 that he had recently succumbed to such pressure from a patient. Consulting with both Dr. Buckmaster and Dr. Skene on behalf of a woman who had complained of severe painful menstruation, painful intercourse, anemia, and hysterical symptoms, he was advised by both colleagues to try everything else before operating. But before he could complete a course of palliative measures, "the insufferable anguish caused the patient to tell me that if I refused to operate she would go to New York to have it done." In revealing his decision to operate, Brinkman inadvertently revealed the existence of a New York City–Brooklyn professional rivalry. "Although a physician should not be influenced by his patient," he admitted, "still it is the duty of Brooklyn physicians to keep their cases and operations in Brooklyn, and I concluded to operate. I saw nothing else to be done."[92] This became a major issue in the Dixon Jones controversy, and patients' wishes proved to be a persuasive element in her defense. When he testified against Mary Dixon Jones during the libel trial, A. J. C. Skene complained of her willingness to operate on at least two of his patients without his approval.[93] Perhaps he also resented her strong identification with radical New York surgeons, who may have appeared more eager to satisfy patients' wishes than his more moderate local colleagues.

Those wishes obviously played a significant role in the physician-patient encounter. Indeed, therapeutic decisions resulted from the confluence of a number of different "voices" contributing to a complex process of diagnosis and treatment. Women's self-reported symptoms always initiated the physician-patient relationship, after all, and produced the basic data for doctors' medical theorizing.[94]

This confluence of voices and professional pressures prompted a full-scale debate at the end of the 1880s over the role of pelvic surgery in women's health. Splits between practitioners gave rise to three identifiable gynecological camps, labeled by contemporaries as radicals, moderates, and conservatives, according to their willingness to opt readily for surgery.[95] The medical journals brimmed over with position papers as, one by one, indications for each specific operation, from ovariotomy to hysterectomy, were revisited, rethought, and reevaluated. It is no accident that, in the midst of this acrimonious debate, Mary Dixon Jones became embroiled with the Brooklyn *Eagle* over the nature and frequency of her surgical procedures. Controversy was in the air, and the public was not oblivious to it, though public scrutiny made many practitioners uncomfortable.

For example, the Brooklyn surgeon Edwin A. Lewis complained bitterly to his colleagues of a clientele both "over-educated and badly educated on matters medical and surgical." His patients had no aversion to giving suggestions to their physicians on how to proceed. Lewis blamed the press. "The secular press and some of the better magazines have taken up medical matters," he grumbled, "and almost daily one may read descriptions of wonderful surgery and marvellous cures." But the literature on medical topics was "so unscientific, if not positively untrue," that it was "harmful, rather than of use." The result was that "the simplest cases are often magnified by the fears of the family into grave disorders."[96]

We have already reviewed some of the explanations for the increased criticism of laparotomy from within the specialty. Cultural pressures also motivated certain practitioners, who nursed an idealistic notion of women's child-bearing capacity and deplored various procedures because they rendered women sterile. We must remember that the late 1880s and 1890s marked the maturation of racial and sexual science, where biological explanations replaced religious and ontological ones for sexual differences and helped bolster belief in the superiority of Anglo-American, indeed, Western European civilization. Imperialism, and the attendant scientific explanations for the desirability of civilizing primitive peoples by force, became the stuff of political and social discourse in complex ways.[97] Embedded in this larger cultural moment, indeed partially responsible for it, medical journals filled their pages with ruminations on the importance of maternity, tightly linking "woman" to "her function of procreation" and the treatment of "the organs connected herewith." Cries of women being "spayed, unsexed, mutilated" were common, and many conservative practitioners, some of them female, drew parallels between gynecological surgery and vivisection.[98] Other practitioners were convinced that the operation of ovariotomy placed "the marriage relation distinctly on a lower plane," believing that it was impossible "for a husband to love his wife as is her due knowing that she is physically incapable of becoming the mother of his children."[99]

No doubt these feelings influenced Thomas Addis Emmet's discomfort with the revival of hysterectomy. His views were typical of those of the older generations of surgeons. At the annual meeting of the American Gynecological Society in 1897 he observed that the perfection of the operation actually "stands as a terror to me," for he was "often tempted to do it when I would not think of it if the result of the operation was not so successful. The danger of the procedure is the least obstacle to our progress to-day, for its execution has become too easy."[100] The fullest expression of these morally driven views, however, came from Ely Van De Warker, who linked laparotomy to fears of race suicide. Calculating the loss of population in unborn children to be in the millions since operative surgery commenced, Van De Warker declared categorically that "a woman's ovaries belong to the commonwealth; she is simply their custodian."[101]

Many women physicians subscribed to these maternalist anxieties. Elizabeth Blackwell, for example, was outspoken in her opposition to ovariotomy and vivisection. She proposed several times to rally female physicians against the wholesale sterilization of women, prompting Mary Putnam Jacobi, one of Dixon Jones's mentors, to reply in a fit of pique that "there is not such special sanctity to the ovary!"[102] But Blackwell was not isolated in her resistance. An annoyed Mary Spink responded to a colleague's ridicule of women doctors with a string of accusations against male physicians' quick resort to the knife:

> As for the removal of the ovaries, the fact is that women physicians object to the wholesale onslaught upon those innocent organs, which originated with so-called reputable physicians and has been continued by men mountebanks to that degree that nearly every city in the land has several "private homes" or sanitariums" for the purpose of removing those organs. . . . [103]

Amidst these emotional outbursts most practitioners stood fast, mocking the cries of "Unsexing women!" "Preventing their bearing children!" "Enemies to posterity!" and so on in favor of the claim that these unfortunate sufferers were "unsexed by disease." "All the capabilities of maternity," asserted Mary Dixon Jones, "all the physiological functions of the generative organs were as completely destroyed as if she had not had the organs." Performing the operation, indeed, "makes the sick woman a more perfect woman, makes her capable of performing life's duties and meeting life's responsibilities."[104]

Moral qualms may have produced the most dramatic of the critiques of over-operating, and doubts about the relevance of basic science to clinical practice prompted others, but there were by the end of the century a set of thoughtful misgivings of a new professional and scientific nature forcing practitioners to reevaluate their approach in more serious ways—ways, ironically, that supported the increasing role of laboratory science. Because of ongoing attempts to explore the chemical, physiological, and pathological processes of the female reproductive system, information gleaned by surgeons gradually began to indicate that these organs secreted fluids significant to female body chemistry.

Technological improvements stimulated the new course. Changes in fixing and staining techniques in the last three decades of the nineteenth century, for example, simplified microscopical investigation, while new lenses provided better, less clouded images. Knowledge of the endocrinology of reproduction was still in the future, and doctors only imperfectly understood the role of the ovaries, tubes, and uterus in ovulation, but these new technical developments encouraged more detailed study of the morphology of cells and cellular processes.[105] Physicians became increasingly more aware of how little they really knew, and some responded by finding new reasons for a more precise pathology and greater attention to differential diagnosis. By the end of the century there emerged out of these developments a fresh reluctance to extirpate organs.

Henry Clarke Coe had underscored the necessity of this approach in his 1886 article on the frequency of diseases of the uterine appendages. Barely thirty years old, he had risked incurring the wrath of Lawson Tait and other powerful practitioners at home and abroad. Undaunted, he continued throughout his career to urge more precise histological distinctions between the normal and the pathological, and, eventually, others joined their voices to his.[106]

In 1894, for example, the British gynecologist C. H. F. Routh published a three-part article in the *Medical Press and Circular* in which he exhaustively investigated the pathological conditions of extirpated ovaries, concluding that organ secretions were important to body chemistry and excision should be exercised with caution. Referring to the researches of Brown-Séquard, who was then studying the testicular extract of animals, Routh suggested that practitioners would do well to pay more attention to the "symptoms in after life" of the "castrated woman."[107] Likewise William Goodell of Philadelphia aptly titled an article "What I Have Learned to Unlearn in Gynecology," in which he noted his gradual understanding that the "womb, like the nose, has its own secretions." A study of those had led him to exercise greater caution in the decision to operate.[108] Indeed, even the radical surgeon S. C. Gordon, who was in principle so adamantly opposed to the move away from total extirpation that he once called the uterus a "useless bag," indicting surgeons' reluctance to remove it as "purely sentimental," admitted that "retaining the ovary or ovaries" conceivably supplied "something in the human economy which tends to limit . . . nervous disturbance."[109]

For a time radicals and conservatives hurled epithets at each other, the former accusing the latter of endangering life by refusing to confront disease boldly and thoroughly, the latter convinced that impatient operators with dubious diagnoses risked women's lives unnecessarily.[110] The issue of specialization was also a factor in the debates, as both sides condemned general practitioners for performing gynecological operations, and turf battles over whether general surgeons should be doing pelvic operations ruffled feathers and exacerbated already existing professional tensions. Indeed, some specialists, like L. S. McMurtry of Louisville, the sixth president of the American Association of Obstetricians and

Gynecologists, blamed general surgeons for the "reckless" operating of the 1880s, claiming they undertook operations "upon inadequate and erroneous conceptions of pathological conditions, and often, indeed, without any definite pathological data whatever."[111]

By the mid-1890s, conservative surgery took on new meaning, as the majority of gynecologists conceded that the excesses of the 1880s should not be repeated. Perhaps the fullest expression of the new attitude came from Charles P. Noble, a Philadelphia surgeon and a friend and colleague of Howard Kelly's before the latter left Philadelphia for Johns Hopkins. Not long ago, he began, conservatism meant "non-operative or medicinal therapeutics." He proposed instead to use the term in its "entymological sense." For Noble and an increasing number of his colleagues, this meant that "all methods of treatment which promote the best interests of the patient must be considered conservative. . . . Conservative treatment may embrace the most radical measures, the essential point being that they promote the best interests of the patient."

In addition, Noble continued, "the term . . . is also applied to surgical operations which have for their purpose the preservation of organs or tissues, and in this sense it is used as opposed to exsective [sic, meaning to cut out] surgical operations." Beginning in the 1890s, then, the trend among younger surgeons was to resect (cut away parts) of organs wherever possible in order "to cure the patient of her disease while retaining her sexual organs with their functions of menstruation and procreation." Many practitioners also began to leave small fibroid tumors alone, as they discovered that some stabilized in size. Myomectomy (removal of the fibroid only) in place of hysterectomy or removal of the ovaries and appendages was once again chosen as the optimum treatment for about 20 percent of larger growths.[112] Still, Noble did not shrink from hysterectomy when it was indicated. It was, he urged, still "true conservatism" in the majority of cases, when the danger from the tumors themselves far outweighed the risks of operation.[113]

Radical surgeons, such as Price, Tait, Dixon Jones, Charles L. Reed, and S. C. Gordon, remained suspicious of these new attitudes for several reasons. Resection in unskilled hands could be an invitation to reoperation if diseased tissue was inadvertently left in the pelvic region. True conservatism in the sense that Noble had meant it, they felt, cured disease quickly and permanently. They urged early and total extirpation. In addition, myomectomy was a more difficult procedure than hysterectomy in most cases, given the technical advances of the 1880s, and could be extremely dangerous.[114] Thus, the "new conservatism" did not silence debates between radicals and conservatives in the 1890s, though one might argue that they became more muted, as practitioners agreed that some sort of operation was usually necessary.

A. J. C. Skene, always conciliatory, described the new situation in 1891:

On the one side, we find those who insist that if there is a suspicion of disease . . . the abdomen should at once be opened and the diseased parts removed. . . . On the other side there are many who (while just as competent diagnosticians) favor waiting and trying less heroic treatment, or until the evidence shows plainly that surgical treatment alone is capable of giving relief. For convenience we might denominate the two classes radicals and conservatives. In thus contrasting the experience of the two parties, it should be understood that the one . . . is as skilled in operating and in diagnosis as the other.[115]

Once again we recall that Dixon Jones's libel trial occurred in the midst of these discussions, and it is clear that these professional debates provided an important context in public deliberations of the case. It is worth noting before leaving the subject of Skene that his performance in testifying against Dixon Jones, of whom he emphatically disapproved, was not nearly as generous as the statement he offered here, made at a meeting of the King's County Medical Society a year before the libel trial took place.

By the end of the decade of the 1890s, gynecological surgeons could look back on three decades of positive accomplishment. They had created a specialty now boasting of skilled experts in the field, two prestigious national societies, the American Association of Obstetricians and Gynecologists and the American Gynecological Society, dozens of state and local organizations, a Section on Gynecology and Obstetrics of the American Medical Association, three or four specialty journals devoted exclusively to the diseases of women, a respectable body of pathological work on diseases of the female reproductive system, and the beginnings of specialty training in medical schools and hospitals. In addition, thousands upon thousands of women with serious, life-threatening illnesses had been helped by the surgical procedures perfected during these years of experimentation.

Gynecologists themselves, of course, were much inclined to be forgiving of their own excesses. They understood that experimentation was essential to progress. "Innovations of pronounced value usually arouse enthusiasm, and enthusiasm, especially that of youth, generally goes to extreme," observed Carlton C. Frederick to his colleagues in the American Association of Obstetricians and Gynecologists in 1890.[116] L. Coyteux Prevost of Ottawa, Canada, agreed. "If a certain number of patients have been wrongly operated upon by surgeons in too great a hurry to resort to the knife, how much more numerous," he estimated, "are not the women whom an untimely reserve on the part of the surgeon allows to die or to lead a miserable existence!"[117]

Certainly gynecologists were entitled to give themselves credit for alleviating the suffering of many sick women. Female patients also deserve recognition for their persistence in seeking out medical solutions and refusing to accept their ailments with stoic resignation. However, attention to the language physicians used to describe female patients—for example, references to "castrated women" or descriptions of the uterus as a "useless bag"—reminds us that these surgical innovators often stepped beyond their medical roles. They participated in the construction of a dominant cultural image of the female body as fragile and full of difficult, incomprehensible working parts, and they deployed a powerfully effective conception of femininity that constrained women in a variety of ways and sanctioned their confinement within the separate, private sphere of family life. Though they likely demonstrated caring and concern to individual patients, their language also encouraged a relationship to women's bodies in the abstract that possibly mitigated against undue sympathy with patients' real physical distress. Doctors were not alone in this effort; it was, after all, the age of Darwin, when intellectuals of all stripes sought justification "in nature" for social arrangements. Many, including Skene, were proud to claim cultural authority for themselves and their colleagues. "The differentiation of sex was receiving due attention," Skene wrote of the last third of the nineteenth century,

> and the characteristics of woman in all her infinite variety of structure and functions, and their relation to health and disease, were well outlined in the minds of the foremost gynecologists. The relation of the reproductive system to the general organization had received liberal consideration. The scientific discoveries at this time paved the way for the emancipation of woman in her social, ethical, and political life about which philosophers and philanthropists have had much to say. . . . [118]

Skene's comments remind us, as does the complexity of this brief history of gynecology, that the libel trial of Dixon Jones was an event that stood for considerably more than contemporaries, who perhaps saw it primarily as a story of ethical and gender transgression, may have understood. The trial brought together important and weighty questions in medicine, professionalization, and the role of science in society, marking Dixon Jones as an important transitional figure in the movement toward modern medical standards of appropriate surgical intervention to treat female pathology of the reproductive system. Thus, her story must be located not only, as has just been done, within the recent historiography of medicine, but also within more modern debates about the role of the medical profession in managing women's health. Today, doctors are still guilty of over-medicalizing the normal reproductive events of women's lives, and, next to Caesarean section, hysterectomy is the second most common surgical procedure in the United States. Roughly 550,000 women receive the operation every year, and predictions are that, when baby boom women reach the likely age, the present number will increase to 802,000 annually. Some 90 percent of hysterectomies are performed for nonmalignant conditions similar to those experienced by the nineteenth-century patients we have described. Moreover, some contemporary gynecologists advocate the operation as a cancer-prevention measure for women who have completed child-bearing. Their arguments, perhaps somewhat overzealously summed up by R. C. Wright in the journal *Obstetrics and Gynecology,* have a familiar ring: "The uterus has but one function: reproduction. After the last planned pregnancy, the uterus becomes a useless, bleeding, symptom-producing, potentially cancer-bearing organ and therefore should be removed."[119]

The problem, of course, is not inherent in the technology itself, and doctors are only partially to blame for its overuse. Much of the evidence offered in this chapter has suggested that, like the present, nineteenth-century physicians functioned within a larger health care system where women's voices were not heard equally, as either patients or practitioners. Social conceptions of femininity guaranteed that to be the case, while constructions of masculinity, coupled with a masculine professional ethos so integral to medicine, indeed to the entire sex/gender system, gave doctors, most of whom were men, the authority to dominate in discussions about female illness. But this is not to say that they always used their power irresponsibly. Many women welcomed the relief medical technology made possible. Certainly some wanted to be operated on, as do many today who suffer the ill effects of bleeding fibroids and premenstrual and perimenopausal pain. Thus, it is wrong to see female patients as passive victims, either then or now. Surgical procedures often improve health. In the end, it seems, we must return to questions of power: who has it when invasive medical procedures are being invoked and to what ends are such techniques used.

If we consider the role of power in the history just sketched out, we see that Dixon Jones's identity as a woman clearly affected the manner in which she went about her work, the motivations behind her surgical radicalism, and how she was judged. Crucial to this discussion are the implications of Ely Van De Warker's claim that a woman's ovaries belong to the nation. Such a statement reminds us that the Dixon Jones libel trial also opens a window onto structures of authority and larger public discourses about the body, the nation, and the place of women as perpetuators of the race. These questions were as deeply embedded in the schisms within the medical profession and the rapid changes in techniques and attitudes occurring within surgery as were the more mundane problems of what kind of incision best avoids infection and how a practitioner could say for sure that painful ovaries were infected. In the following chapter, we will take up some of these weightier topics, when we examine gynecology's specific perceptions of the female body.

5

Gynecology
CONSTRUCTS
the Female Body
and a Woman Doctor Responds

We have learned that although female aspirations to a career in surgical gynecology at the end of the nineteenth century were comparatively circumscribed, a woman with Mary Dixon Jones's boldness and sensitivity to effective strategies of self-advancement could achieve a respectable, though not stellar place in this masculine world. Dixon Jones not only supported but pioneered radical approaches to surgery. She helped make pathological diagnosis an important aspect of evaluation and treatment. She promoted gynecology by using and validating controversial procedures that more conservative practitioners were still reluctant to accept. In all these ways she deserves recognition as a staunch advocate of more modern surgical methods. Yet, given the powerful critiques of surgical gynecology that have emerged in our own time, what may have appeared only a generation ago as a remarkable achievement now seems tainted. New understandings of the unequal power relationships between doctors and female patients in the clinical decision-making process have changed our perspective. We are particularly uncomfortable with the use of invasive procedures no longer considered necessary to effect a cure. These reservations generate doubts about Dixon Jones's motives and lead us to require a better understanding of the intricate intellectual and social context in which she did her therapeutic thinking.

Moreover, our contemporary suspicion of doctors has been fueled in the last two decades by a rich literature on the oppression of women by the medical profession, much of it concentrating on the second half of the nineteenth century.[1] Some of this work has been insightful and convincing, prompting pointed questions about Mary Dixon Jones. For example, if, in craving male colleagiality, she purposely kept her distance from female professional networks, embracing medical procedures that contributed to cultural definitions of women as weak and sickly, are we not obligated to judge her harshly? Or was she simply a male-identified woman suffering from a bad case of false consciousness? How can we approach her career with a greater sense of balance, avoiding the oversimplication of these extremes? Additionally, how can an understanding of her medical theories bring us closer to making sense of her involvement in a public imbroglio like the libel trial?

In this chapter, I want to explore what happened when nineteenth-century women physicians authorized themselves to speak on the subject of their own bodies. Their willingness to claim a place in heated contemporary discussions on female health and disease is surely one of the developments that foreshadowed the Dixon Jones affair. Did women doctors speak in one voice, and were they able to alter the terms of the debate? Admittedly, all gynecologists' scientific decisions were variously influenced by social ideology. How did this predisposition play out when the gynecologist was a woman? By what methods did Mary Dixon Jones, an active proponent of gynecological surgery and a leading expert in the field, empower herself to speak? How was her surgical training implicated in her point of view? Did she passively tolerate "received" professional wisdom, or, in constructing and constituting the female body, did she balance scientific training with her subjective knowledge as a woman? What sort of therapeutic decisions could such a reconciliation produce, and did these interventions accomplish anything on behalf of women physicians as a group or benefit the patients she treated?

NATURAL FACTS: MEDICAL SCIENCE CONSTRUCTS WOMAN

Doctors accepted as a law of nature that the determining factor from which all other male-female differences derived was motherhood. Actual and potential maternity accounted not just for obvious visual differences in bodily structure, but for psychological dissimilarities, also assumed to be natural. Thus the sexual division of labor, which assigned women to the private sphere of the family and men to strive in the public and political world, merely carried out what Nature had intended. Physicians added that the female reproductive system governed psychological and physical health in women. Misuse or neglect of its dictates caused illness and disease.

Moreover, sickness and health emerged as ubiquitous concerns of Victorian culture, and a rising faith in medical science among the middle-class prompted women increasingly to seek medical treatment. Their illnesses appeared to confirm physicians' emphasis on woman's reproductive apparatus as the driving physiological force of her being.[2] We have seen in our discussion of gynecology as a specialty that women complained of a variety of ailments, such as ovarian cysts; uterine infections; displacements and lacerations following childbirth; menstrual derangements, including profuse bleeding or the absence of periods; tumors; fibroids; and various forms of cancer. All of these diseases were painful and debilitating; all involved the reproductive organs.

No wonder physicians perceived that one hallmark of being a woman in the nineteenth century was to experience ''the pathology of femininity.''[3] They believed female ill-health to be widespread, and that reproduction was fraught with danger. The English obstetrician William Tyler Smith, for example, characterized parturition as an event that stood ''at the boundary between physiology and pathology; being attended by more pain, and being liable to a greater number of accidents, than any other act of the economy.'' When historian Wendy Mitchinson examined the patient records of a Canadian hospital from the year 1892, she found that the sex organs were implicated in disease causation by practitioners even when the patient's illness was something ostensibly unconnected, like gastritis or tuberculosis.[4] No severe constitutional disorder, observed the American gynecologist Dr. Arthur Edis, ''can long continue in a woman during the predominance of the ovarian function without entailing disturbance. . . . And the converse is also true, that disorder of the sexual organs cannot long continue without entailing constitutional disorder, or injuriously affecting the condition of other organs.''[5] Even medical advertising in the popular press reinforced such views, suggesting that female patients probably shared them.[6] As the surgeon George Rohé acknowledged, ''Among the general public and the medical profession the influence of abnormalities of the sexual organs in producing mental aberrations is . . . believed in to a considerable extent. Indeed, some of the highest authorities in mental diseases, as Esquirol and Guislain, emphasize the overwhelming influence of the genital organs, especially in women, in the production of insanity.''[7]

Though all practitioners indicted the reproductive system, the component parts on which physicians focused their therapeutic efforts shifted according to medical fashion. In the mid-1850s, for example, practitioners highlighted the womb as the site of most disorders. In the second half of the century, first the ovaries and then the fallopian tubes became the objects of clinicians' attention. By the 1880s and 1890s, reflex theory, which had actually been proposed earlier in the century, shifted the interest of some practitioners from the organs of reproduction themselves to the interaction between the reproductive system and the brain, a process some theorists believed was governed by the vascular system, though others highlighted the nerves.

The theory of reflex irritation posited that nervous connections running along the spine joined all the organs of the body together, including the brain, and that in this way irritations in one part could cause derangements even in distant sites. These disease states could occur quite independently of human volition. Thus the blood, the sensory arcs, and the sympathetic nervous system worked together, and a change in the brain's vital energy or, conversely, a local ailment in a particularly sensitive organ could have disastrous sympathetic consequences elsewhere in the body.[8]

Also significant was the belief that the body functioned as a closed system, possessing a finite amount of vital energy. Using up too much in one particular activity could leave inadequate resources for other important physiological tasks. In the case of women, this theory spoke directly to their child-bearing responsibilites. Any physical strain that potentially compromised their capacity to reproduce was suspect. For physicians like E. H. Clarke of Harvard, whom we shall meet again later in this chapter, or Ely Van de Warker, this included, in particular, advanced educational studies, and a number of practitioners opposed the higher education of women on these grounds.[9] While the concept of reflex irritation could theoretically be applied to males and females, women's nervous systems were characterized as more sensitive, and so they were considered more vulnerable to diseases of nervous origin. Indeed, the theory of reflex irritation enabled gynecological surgeons to operate for a range of indeterminate mental disturbances, prompting a heated debate among gynecologists, neurologists, and alienists (early psychiatrists), with female physicians often pitting themselves against gynecological surgeons as well.[10]

Presuppositions about female virtue, which generally had to do with sexuality, also governed dominant medical presumptions about women. Indeed, feminist historians have written quite ingeniously about the various ways nineteenth-century theories of female sexuality were deployed for what feminist scholar Mary Poovey has called "the ideological work of gender." The Victorian period was a time when the bourgeois family was naturalized, and the model of separate spheres helped inscribe a host of new institutions and social relations, from the shaping of policies toward the poor, regulating prostitution, and rethinking divorce law, to new forms of literary expression and the development of social, political, and economic theory. Indeed, Poovey shows how images of women and constructions of female desire were indispensable to a model of male capitalist social identity and to the English national character more generally. Especially significant was the way in which traditional Enlightenment renderings of virtue, which had previously emphasized class-bound definitions of male disinterestedness and civic benevolence, were gradually relocated, articulating a new discourse about gender that was embedded in the language of domesticity. Virtue became identified with sympathy, altruism, and social benevolence, qualities decidedly feminine and safely ensconced in the private realm of family life. This new morality was crucial to the consolidation of bourgeois power because it linked ethical and empathetic behavior to a figure (woman) rhetorically "immune to the self-interest and competition integral to economic success" and "preserved virtue without inhibiting productivity." Social order and confidence in a humane and stable society depended on believing that the images of home-oriented, generous, nurturant, and maternal women represented reality. Indeed, social well-being was powerfully connected to economic and political developments that appeared best to bolster middle-class familial relationships. It followed that sexually misbehaving women perceived as flaunting their virtue became metaphors of social disorder.[11]

In their role as clinicians, doctors thus had something to say about virtue in their discussions of female sexuality, but the messages were truly mixed. Persisting from earlier religious constructions were images of Eve the temptress, which represented women not only as libidinous, but perversely so. Superimposed on these were newer notions of female passionlessness, modesty, and purity, fundamentally connected to shifting definitions of virtue.[12] Nineteenth-century medical therapeutics reflected both points of view. Self-styled guardians of female purity, many physicians hesitated to do needed pelvic examinations or propose other treatments that might give offense. Not surprisingly, patients who exhibited any kind of blatant sexuality were labeled deviant and/or diseased and occasionally subjected to mutilating procedures, the rarest and most grave of which was cliterodectomy, performed occasionally for frequent masturbation or promiscuous sexuality diagnosed as nymphomania.[13]

Taken as a whole, medical discourse about the female body exercised a powerful role in shaping late-nineteenth-century definitions of femininity that constrained women and limited their opportunities in a variety of ways. For example, historians have cited a host of invasive medical procedures allegedly animated by these ideas. They have dwelt most forcefully on the orgy of gynecological surgery that took place in the last two decades of the century, arguing that conceptions of female biology sanctioned "transgressive" surgical procedures—operations that endangered lives even as they provided opportunities to try out a range of new therapeutic modalities and techniques.[14]

That surgeons boldly explored the internal body cavity, experimenting with a variety of surgical treatments on their female patients, is an established fact. There were countervailing developments as well, however, which also require attention. While it was primarily *men* who first used the authoritative language of science to speak and write about the female body, the absence of women's voices in medical practice was less stark in the United States than in England or on the continent. Women did learn to speak for themselves in America, first as physiological lecturers in the health reform movement, then as sectarian medical practitioners, and, finally, after mid-century, as regularly trained and professionally licensed physicians.[15]

Moreover, even the dominant discourse was never as unified as some scholars have claimed. All language, even scientific, is inherently unstable, and in the nineteenth century it contradicted itself on the issue of woman's place in several ways. Not only did individuals experience scientific knowledge differently, depending on their position in the social order, but what constituted knowledge itself was articulated in dissimilar ways by various institutions and groups. In the case of gynecology, a range of factors converged to color doctors' theoretical and therapeutic decisions, including the entrance of women into medicine, professional and class rivalries, diverging constructions of gender, disagreements over therapeutics and the role of the good practitioner, the desires of the patient and her own perceptions of disease, and the politics of medical specialization. As a result, medical science and gynecological theory in particular was the site of competing definitions of both gender *and* science.[16]

In what follows, I will revisit the emerging specialty of surgical gynecology, this time testing the gender ideology gynecologists produced against the constellation of theories I have just summarized. Did the surgical gaze modify or alter conceptions of the female body in significant ways? How did clinical experience, the act of invading the bodily cavities and removing diseased organs, the attention to cellular pathology and differential diagnosis, affect understandings of femininity and masculinity? When women began the practice of gynecological surgery, did their personal experiences of their own bodies color their perception of the biological theories generated in their specialty? Were tensions apparent? Did they resist some of the more extreme constructions of female frailty? If so, in what manner was this resistance framed? Once again we can address some of these larger questions by exploring aspects of Mary Dixon Jones's medical career.

GYNECOLOGICAL SURGERY AND FEMALE HEALTH

Discussions of female health and disease in the gynecologial literature from the late 1870s through the turn of the century gradually altered in content and narrowed in focus. Perhaps the change can be best characterized as moving away from material that drew conclusions from biology about proper female roles and behavior and reaching toward approaches characteristic of the increasingly narrow and reductionist gaze of the new medical science. This meant that doctors slowly paid less attention to offering social commentary in the medical literature and expanded their consideration of technique, diagnosis, and treatment. This orientation was welcomed, indeed even catalyzed by surgeons, and it highlighted diseased tissue and inflamed organs more often than it pondered the social role of these body parts.

Given the complex nature of the changes in medicine that I described in Chapter 4, in terms of both the content of scientific practice as well as the fashioning of new images of science and scientific authority, it should not be surprising to find generational differences in gynecological writings about femininity as well. Some of these shifts mark the influence of the new science, while others exhibit evidence of the acceptance of women physicians' voices and the integration of their point of view into discussions of female health and disease.

How closely did gynecologists subscribe to the depictions of nineteenth-century femininity that I have just cited? Did those with a surgical orientation offer a different perspective? What altered in the wake of changing visions of science and practice? The careers and ideas of a few representative figures, recognized leaders in the field, can stand as emblematic of some interesting disjunctions in the specialty.

Thomas Addis Emmet (1828–1919), a New York surgeon admired by Mary Dixon Jones, has been described as "one of the great founders of modern gynecology." The son of a University of Virginia professor of natural history, chemistry, and *materia medica*, Emmet hesitated as a youth before committing himself to medicine but, with the encouragement of several of his father's friends, eventually received a diploma in 1850 from Jefferson Medical College in Philadelphia. He immediately took a position as resident physician at the Emigrant Refuge Hospital on Ward's Island in New York City, where he gained five years' experience in general medicine, treating a large number of patients, performing over 1000 postmortem examinations, and opening a private practice. In 1855, he met J. Marion Sims, who appointed him assistant surgeon at the newly established New York Woman's Hospital, the first of its kind in the United States. Emmet remained Sims's assistant until 1861, when the latter resigned as chief surgeon and Emmet assumed full responsibility for the surgical work and the management of the hospital. In 1872, he surrendered managerial responsibility, but remained a visiting surgeon there for the next thirty years. Coming to Sims with a broad experience in general medicine, Emmet learned state-of-the-art surgical techniques, and soon invented many of his own. Like Sims, he became a brilliant operator for vesico-vaginal fistula, developing new instruments as he progressed, and invented an operation for repair of cervical tears known as trachelorraphy, which had brief currency among his colleagues.[17]

In 1879, Emmet published a textbook, *The Principles and Practice of Gynecology,* which Howard Kelly held to be the "first thoroughly scientific, comprehensive book on the subject in English." True to the principles of Parisian empiricism, it boasted of extensive statistical tables, for which, according to Kelly, Emmet "rightly" claimed no parallel "to be found in the whole range of gynecological literature."[18] Emmet also demonstrated an awareness of pathology and its importance to diagnosis and treatment, especially in his chapters on diseases of the ovary, where he was able to coherently summarize prevailing European notions regarding the origins of tumors.[19]

When it came to issues of women's health, however, Emmet's ideas and opinions are representative of conservative views typical of his day. Outlined in the first chapter of his 1879 text, entitled "The Relations of Climate, Education, and Social Conditions to Development," and expanded for the third edition, published five years later, were a series of familiar assertions on the topic of male-female differences, including assumptions about women's more delicate constitution, the social obligations of maternity, and the necessity of preserving female sexual purity and innocence.

Ideas about the incommensurability of male and female first gathered momentum in the eighteenth century and were carried into the next with increasing force. Scholars have explored the power of such concepts, locating their origins and logics within the scientific community, and then tracing the ways they were inscribed in institutional practices, social organization, and daily life. Medical theories were deeply influenced by culture and social structure. They also shaped society in complicated ways. Occasionally they were contested, as we shall see in Dixon Jones's case, but not always in the most obvious or straightforward manner.[20]

For Emmet, puberty marked the fault line of sexual incommensurability, because before then, "the progress of development is equal in the two sexes." After the eleventh or twelfth year, however, "until old age," there was "wide divergence." At puberty "the nervous system becomes dominant in the female organization" and girls became "as susceptible to external influences as the barometer is to atmospheric changes." The moment of puberty was determinative, because "an impression for good or evil once made upon the nervous system, especially while in the adolescent period, is permanent."[21]

Emmet's belief in the hypersensitivity of pubertal development led him to support the theories of E. H. Clarke on female education; indeed, he admitted, "my own experience leads me to believe that the evil is even more serious than he has represented."[22] In 1873, Clarke, a professor at Harvard Medical School, published *Sex in Education: A Fair Chance for Girls,* a bestseller when it appeared. Clarke argued a version of the closed energy theory. He contended that higher education was sapping the reproductive development of especially talented girls. The result was "monstrous brains and puny bodies; abnormally active cerebration and abnormally weak digestion; flowing thought and constipated bowels."[23] Emmet, too, believed that the energy needed for physiological functioning was finite. "The young girl commences life with an inheritance of a certain amount of nerve force," he cautioned, "which, if squandered in mental culture, will leave the physical growth defective at some point."[24] With a touch of class defensiveness, he declared himself not necessarily opposed to the "highest grade of education for woman as befits her station," but felt that females should not be schooled beyond the primary grades until adolescent development was over and the reproductive system had matured, at which time a girl would "be better fitted to become a wife." If custom "would allow some approximation to this plan," Emmet concluded, "I believe the women of our country would bear more children, would be better able to discharge their maternal duties, and would preserve their youth and vigor many years longer." For Emmet, who harbored fears of race suicide, these facts were paramount. Though education was pleasant in a woman, it was not necessary. "It is woman's mission to populate the earth, and it is a most noble one, carrying, as it does, God's blessing upon her in proportion as she is able to fulfill her trust," he concluded.[25]

Emmet was a passionate believer in reflex theory, and in tandem with an up-to-date recognition of the significance of ovarian pathology, he maintained a strong commitment to reflex action as the ultimate, if not proximate, cause of women's diseases. "The various symptoms of ovarian disorders are but an evidence that nature's laws have been put at defiance, and that the nervous system has been overtaxed," he wrote. "Who are the sufferers . . . ? The young girl who has had her brain development out of season; the woman disappointed or crossed in love by a man not worthy of her; those who have been ill-mated, and, often, the unmated—she who has sold her person, under the guise of marriage, for money or position; the prostitute; and she who degrades herself and sacrifices her womanhood by resorting to means to prevent conception. In all of these, the nervous system has been first abused."[26]

Emmet's reverent construction of the female body, which carved out a safe and subordinate place for women in the home, was shared by other leading lights among the first generation of gynecologists. Alexander J. C. Skene (1838–1900) is of particular interest to us, because Skene dominated the medical scene in Brooklyn, testified at Mary Dixon Jones's libel trial, and demonstrated open contempt for her style of practice. Along with Emmet, Skene was one of the founders of the American Gynecological Society. When he died in 1900, his eulogist called him "one of the last" of gynecology's "great pioneers." Skene received his medical diploma in 1863, and in his early years assisted Austin Flint of New York City, a participant in the American Medical Association (AMA) Code of Ethics controversy and a clinician whose views represented the old guard generalists who were suspicious of laboratory medicine.[27] Like Flint, Skene did not use a microscope in practice, and his suspicions of the over-use of both ovariotomy and hysterectomy earned him a reputation as a surgical conservative.[28]

Skene published his first textbook on women's diseases in 1888. A year later, he produced a little volume called *Education and Culture as Related to the Health and Diseases of Women*. The ideas in this work were reprinted in his magnum opus, *Medical Gynecology: A Treatise on the Diseases of Women from the Standpoint of the Physician* (1895). While the first text is almost free of editorializing about the nature of women, *Education and Culture* proved Skene to be in perfect agreement with Emmet on the subject of male-female differences.[29]

For Skene, like Emmet, women's primary duty was to children and the home. "Owing to the general complexity of their sexual organs, both in structure and function," women were more frail than men.[30] While "in mind" (intelligence) Skene noted little divergence in the sexes "save in degree," he believed the psychological differences were stark. Skene also joined Emmet in subscribing to a theory of reflex action, focusing on the ovaries as the organs "peculiarly prone to disturbances."[31] Deranged sexual organs, he argued, often produced insanity, although how this occurred was still "in many cases a mooted question."[32] In contrast to Emmet, however, Skene held no brief against female education; for him female ill health was due to environmental causes—mental or physical overtaxation of a variety of kinds or unfortunate heredity. In terms of his sexual construction of women, he cherished their innate purity, which he called the "monogamous instinct." Woman's superiority over man "from the ethical point of view," he noted, "makes the desire of equality of the sexes far more necessary for man's advancement than for her own."[33]

Many gynecologists of Skene's and Emmet's generation shared a version of the ideas about femininity laid out in the writings of these men. However, two important developments, one external to gynecological surgery, the other embedded within its growth as a specialty, worked to modify a rigid construction of womanhood, at least for some practitioners.

The first was the gradual participation of women physicians trained at regular medical schools in discussions about female health. In Chapter 4, I suggested that some women physicians were gendering and reconstituting an older, more holistic approach to physician-patient relationships. Even at the beginning of their campaign to enter the profession at mid-century, they represented themselves as able to fill a special place in the profession because of their special skills at nurturing. In addition, they complained about the male perspective, convinced that they would "supply a deficiency" to medical theory and practice in regard to the diseases of women. If they had pursued medicine earlier, Anna Longshore-Potts wrote in 1897, "today women would have more healthy bodies."[34]

Women physicians, most of whom specialized by default in the treatment of women and children, used science to "talk back" to their most conservative male colleagues. For example, taking up positions as resident physicians at the newly established women's colleges of Smith, Vassar, and Mt. Holyoke, they monitored the health of college girls and began to publish statistics that contradicted the Clarke thesis about the injurious effects of higher education. In 1881, graduates of the New England Female Medical College, Emily and Augusta Pope, teamed up with Emma Call, an early alumna of the University of Michigan Medical School, which had opened its doors to women in 1870, to publish a ground-breaking survey on women physicians sponsored by the American Social Science Association. All three were staff physicians at the New England Hospital for Women and Children, a female-run institution. Examining the health of 430 women doctors, they concluded that "some unnecessary anxiety has been wasted" on the issue of higher education and the health of women. "We do not think," they concluded, "it would be easy to find a better record of health among an equal number of women, taken at random, from all over the country.[35]

Nevertheless, dominant ideas had substantial explanatory power, and whether a woman physician trained at an all-female or coeducational institution, she most likely received an up-to-date medical education. This meant learning the same prevailing medical theory as her male peers. Still, women physicians, just like their male colleagues, exhibited a diversity of opinion on the subject of female health. Several subscribed to conservative assumptions about the sexual division of labor and believed in the delicacy of the female constitution.[36] Some women doctors viewed puberty as a worrisome time for young girls. "For a year or two," Margaret E. Colby told the Iowa Society of Medical Women, "we as physicians, should urge the necessity of fewer studies, or shorter study hours . . . and instruction in regard to the physical changes, their significance and value."[37] Even M. Carey Thomas, the indominatable president of Bryn Mawr College and a fierce supporter of higher education for women, was uncertain of what rigors the female body could endure: "We did not know when we began whether women's health could stand the strain of education. We were haunted in those days by the clanging chains of that gloomy little specter Dr. Edward H. Clarke's *Sex in Education*."[38] But whatever their views on female health, what they had in common was the desire to emancipate women from the confines of a narrow role dictated solely by biology. Thus, even women physicians who subscribed to a conservative understanding of the female body and worried overmuch about female endurance had a stake in drawing different conclusions than male peers on the implications of certain cultural truths.

There is clear evidence that these women doctors' voices had an impact on the professional company of gynecologists in interesting and revealing ways. Indeed, many male physicians conceded female colleagues a certain expertise where female health was concerned, while others felt it necessary to cite women doctors' opinions on the subject to bolster their own authority. Surgeon Charles A. L. Reed, a decided liberal on the subject of women's health, who enthusiastically supported higher education for women and believed civilized women to be no more sickly than their primitive sisters, invoked Mary Dixon Jones on the subject of brain differences between men and women. Agreeing with her that higher education improved women's bodies as well as their minds, he characterized her as a "successful practitioner with an extensive *clientele* among women."[39] Even a conservative such as Thomas Addis Emmet, for example, felt obliged to invoke the authority of both Elizabeth Blackwell and Mary J. Studley, a physician at the State Normal School for Girls in South Framingham, Massachusetts, to make a point about the importance of strong physical development for pubescent girls.[40]

For their own part, women doctors participated enthusiastically in expanding gynecologists' role as monitors of female health. Indeed, they helped in numerous ways to broaden the specialty's authority among the lay public. After Anna Fullerton, resident physician and surgeon at the Woman's Hospital in Philadelphia, gave a paper on her gynecological practice to the Section on Obstetrics and Diseases of Women at the Annual AMA meeting in Philadelphia in 1897, Howard Kelly, by then a towering figure at the new Johns Hopkins Medical School, was quick to affirm in the ensuing discussion that "it was in the hands of physicians to model very largely the future generation, to carry out those plans which we know will result in the prevention of disease, and in producing better women and a better race in the next decade." He confessed that this subject "had for a long time been prominently before his mind in connection with gynecologic work." Other male physicians in attendance were intensely curious to elicit Fullerton's opinion of bicycling for women, a new and controversial sport in the 1890s. Skeptical questioners raised the possibility of bladder damage and the danger of weakening certain muscles, with more extreme objections, such as fears that women would receive masturbatory pleasure from the bicycle seat, making the rounds in the medical journals. At this session, it was Fullerton who was deferred to as the expert, and, as an experienced woman gynecological surgeon, her support for the bicycle as a form of exercise carried weight.[41]

In other examples, Charlotte Blake Brown, founder of the Women's and Children's Hospital in San Francisco, delivered a paper entitled "The Health of Our Girls" before the California State Medical Society in 1896. Brown's point was that lack of exercise and sleep, not puberty per se, accounted for female adolescent ill health, and that boys suffered from similar bad habits. Her audience did not contest her conclusions, but more interesting was the respect afforded Brown and her subject matter by her male colleagues. Similarly, the Johns Hopkins Hospital *Bulletin* reviewed Anna Galbraith's *Four Epochs of a Woman's Life*, a volume on female health written primarily for lay women, not once, but twice, ruminating with great seriousness on its "good sense," "clear and simple" style, and "successful use of technical terms without confusion to the uninitiated."[42]

Women physicians wielded a measure of authority, despite some male physicians' expectations that they would advocate conventionally gendered positions on various controversies in the field. An intriguing demonstration of the latter, and of the spectrum of male attitudes, is a heated exchange that took place in 1892 between Anna Fullerton and G. Betton Massey, a well-known proponent of the use of electricity in treating gynecological ailments. Fullerton had delivered a paper before the Philadelphia County Medical Society on abdominal surgery at the Woman's Hospital of Philadelphia, in which she acknowledged the importance of early operations in many cases, and strongly supported the idea that only trained surgeons and not generalists (general practitioners or all gynecologists) should operate. Though the presentation was a highly professional, middle-of-the-road position on the usefulness of surgical solutions, during the discussion Massey pressed her hard, asking why the "conservative side of gynecology" was not represented in her paper. "It seems to me," he continued revealingly, "that with women who enter the practice of medicine there would be the strongest incentive to at least test what could be accomplished by non-operative gynecology. I regret that so little has been done in this connection at the Woman's Hospital." Dr. Joseph Hoffman immediately came to Fullerton's defense, retorting that "Dr. Fullerton can tell Dr. Massey a great deal about conservative gynecology. She can tell him about electricity, about poultices, about iodine, about hot water, about rest, and about all the other tomfoolery which tries to get pus out of the pelvis. . . . There should have been enough . . . to convince everyone that we do not want to operate on everything."

But Massey pressed the issue, and eventually Fullerton herself, visibly annoyed, responded. "My paper presented the principles on which we work at our hospital," she stated. "Perhaps it will answer Dr. Massey better if I state that during the time that I have been connected with the Woman's Hospital we have had 18,000 gynecological cases . . . only 179 on whom abdominal operations have been done." This exchange, worth dwelling on to capture the flavor of the interaction, demonstrates, of course, that many male physicians *expected* women to take a conservative approach to the issues, and were occasionally sorely disappointed. Judging from Fullerton's published articles, she *was* a relatively cautious operator; indeed, much more conservative in her clinical judgments than Mary Dixon Jones.[43]

All doctors exhibited a variety of approaches to the question of female health and disease. In making decisions to operate for hysterical symptoms, most women surgeons did appear to exercise extreme caution, as did many of the more conservative gynecological surgeons, including Thomas Addis Emmet and A. J. C. Skene. Certainly women surgeons were aware of the opprobrium these operations provoked in certain quarters and were cognizant as well of the debate in their own ranks regarding gynecological surgery. But the handful of women who chose to specialize in gynecological surgery and managed by the end of the 1890s to perform hundreds of laparotomies were also highly trained professionals who, like all surgeons at the time, struggled to balance scientific, social, and subjective knowledge. As Anna Fullerton made perfectly clear in her response to G. Betton Massey: When deemed necessary, none would hesitate to remove ovaries for hysterical symptoms.[44]

MARY DIXON JONES AND THE FEMALE BODY

When speaking of female health and disease, Mary Dixon Jones was remarkably unsentimental about the female body and stubbornly resistant to traditional ideas of feminine weakness and ill health. Ironically, it was very much this cast of mind that drew criticism when she took her place on the witness stand at the libel trial. But while such an intellectual approach got her into trouble in 1892, it generated a remarkable creativity that allowed her to intelligently ponder the origins of female reproductive disease in spite of the constraints placed on medical knowledge by time and place. Indeed, she consistently and emphatically rejected any hypothesis holding women inherently prone to illness. For example, she sharply criticized clinicians like Emmet, who feared that excessive mental exertion among adolescent girls hampered the development of their reproductive organs, contemptuously dismissing closed energy theories in any guise. She vigorously assailed the claim that sterility and undeveloped uteri were proportionately more frequent among educated women. She offered her own experience, first as a student and then as a teacher in "the largest and most advanced college for women in this country" as evidence for these assertions. "Over three thousand young ladies came under my observation," she wrote,

> who, during the period allotted to sexual development were subject to continuous "severe and laborious intellectual labor"; yet in all this number, and in all these years, I do not recollect a single one giving any indication that "the reproductive organs were not naturally and promptly developed, and that their functions were not normally performed." . . . The young ladies who were subjected to these severe intellectual tasks grew healthier and stronger.

Nor did she put much stock in biologically based concepts of male-female difference. "If study prevents development, by diverting the vital forces from the sexual organs at the very time when their exercise is most needed," then excessive "brain-work" threatened boys as much as it threatened girls. "Where is the difference?" she demanded. "Woman is subject to the same laws of growth and health as is man, and like him she is capable of high mental cultivation, and, at the same time of retaining the full power of her procreative functions."[45] Demanding the right "to call a halt" to false claims that college "indisposes to matrimony and unfits for maternity," she insisted that college-educated women made better, more devoted, and more enthusiastic mothers. They welcomed children "more lovingly" and gave them a stronger "mental inheritance."[46] Pursuing the matter in an article on insanity, she wrote, "It is not the 'sex' that causes insanity, but the disease of the brain in either sex."[47] Morever, while several of her colleagues worried that the negative reproductive effects of higher education even led to race suicide, she denied women's responsibility for lower birth rates among the middle class, insisting that "small families do not come from the higher education of women."[48]

Nor was Dixon Jones prone to the bathos some male and female physicians displayed when they discussed the inevitable sterility resulting from ovariotomy. Better to save lives than wring hands, she advised. She disliked the notion that women who lost their ovaries were in some way unfeminine, and she contradicted the belief of many practitioners that the operation rendered them less sexual or desirable. "Removing diseased uterine appendages," she insisted, "is not unsexing a woman, it is restoring her from helpless invalidism to all the possibilities and opportunities of life and labor. It is not taking away the possibility of her having children—that has already been done by disease—it is only removing the cause of suffering."[49]

When it came to treating hysteria, Dixon Jones's clinical reporting demonstrated probably more faith in surgical solutions than even many of her male colleagues, although her writings on the subject do display an awareness of the cultural sensitivity of such operations. Though her clinical case records are riddled with protestations of caution, the careful reader discerns unmistakably that she removed ovaries and tubes for reflex symptoms quickly and repeatedly. Indeed, one notes a certain disingenuousness in her published work, causing us to ask if it was not this same element of equivocation that the jury noted in her behavior at the libel trial. Her very first case report, for example, was a diagnosis of "hystero-epilepsy due to reflex irritation," and she performed many operations for similar symptoms in the next several years, even as her published work continued to contain disclaimers.[50]

By 1888, the specialty was entering a period of collective self-criticism, and Dixon Jones may well have felt on the defensive. One incident, of which she was fully aware, referring to it several times in her own articles, was the "Imlach Affair," which rocked gynecologists in England in 1886. Francis Imlach, a surgeon at the Woman's Hospital in Liverpool, was accused by several colleagues at the Liverpool Medical Institute of performing unecessary ovariotomies for reflex symptoms. Disturbed by the high percentage of patients undergoing ovariotomy at the hospital, critics were even more troubled to hear that Imlach had himself performed over 80 percent of them, many more than the other attending physicians. An investigation was launched that drew in some of Britain's most renowned surgical gynecologists: Spencer Wells, Thomas Keith, Lawson Tait, Granville Bantock, and Thomas Savage. The committee interviewed patients and practitioners alike, reassessing the indications for ovariotomy and expressing ethical and clinical reservations about this type of surgery. The report condemned Imlach's decision to operate in several cases. Imlach's reputation was further damaged by a sudden lawsuit brought against him by a patient in the summer of 1886. Though the suit ended in acquittal, the hospital investigation dragged on and eventually catalyzed a vitriolic public debate over sexual surgery between Lawson Tait, who defended Imlach, and Spencer Wells, who condemned his overeager scalpel. As a result of the inquiry, Imlach was not reappointed to the hospital staff. Eventually he had to give up gynecological practice. As a result of the affair, the rift between Spencer Wells, representing conservative surgeons, and Lawson Tait, the enfant terrible of radical surgical gynecology in England, became irreparable.[51]

Dixon Jones visited England in 1886, at the height of the affair, and even spent a day in court as a witness at Imlach's trial. He was accused of removing healthy ovaries without consent. Dixon Jones's written notes of this experience, published a decade later, express her adamant conviction that Imlach was being charged without cause by an ignorant and venal patient. She was relieved when he was exonerated and attributed his acquittal in part to the "great surgeons"— Tait, Thomas Savage, James Aveling, J. Greig Smith—who defended "their persecuted brother" "so nobly and well."[52]

Perhaps because of Imlach's trial, she felt compelled to appear cautious when reporting operations for reflex symptoms to her colleagues. Contrasting herself to Battey, she wrote in an article published that year that she would never remove *"healthy"* ovaries if she thought the lesion was elsewhere. "I have never operated on a case, but I had full and substantial reason to diagnose incurable diseases of the appendages. . . . I would not remove them for mental or neurotic diseases, even if I had failed in long trials of tentative measures, and had the cordial, full, and deliberate sanction of experienced practitioners, *unless* I believed the *appendages were diseased.*"[53] And yet one cannot help but feel that Dixon Jones was traveling a slippery slope. Elsewhere in the same article, for example, she admits that microscopical examination is often necessary to diagnose disease. "We cannot always tell from the naked-eye appearances whether the ovaries are diseased or not."[54] But neither she nor her colleagues were at this time using the microscope for preoperative biopsies. It was only after organs were removed that sections were taken and slides made. Admitting, as she had, that visual diagnoses were not always accurate, how, then, could she be sure that her conclusions were always correct? Repeatedly Dixon Jones fell back on self-proclaimed diagnostic acumen: "Before its removal," she remarked about one case, "I knew well from the history and examination that it was diseased."[55] About another she wrote: "Though at the time of the operation the ovaries did not show such manifest appearance of disease, still I *knew there was as much necessity for their removal as if they had been tubes full of pus.*"[56]

Thus, in her overall approach to controversial issues regarding female health, Dixon Jones undoubtedly shared with other radicals a willingness to promote surgical solutions as the best and quickest cure. As we have already seen, she identified with this group and greatly admired Lawson Tait, whose work was often cited in her own publications. She disdained the delaying tactics of many practitioners and rejected palliative methods when surgical ones were available. Indeed, she blamed many deaths on hesitant practitioners who warned of the consequences of acting precipitously. Like Tait, she even supported exploratory surgery for diagnostic purposes. How can we understand these views? Was Dixon Jones simply an anomaly, an early example of a male-identified woman whose lack of womanist consciousness made her the exception that proves the rule?

We have already learned that there was no perfect fit between a practitioner's social views and therapeutic choices. Conservative physicians who were suspicious of gynecological surgery—a therapeutic stance toward treatment admired by many scholars of women's history—could maintain rigid opinions about sex roles. Some, uncompromising regarding expanded roles for women, were also resisting surgeons' focus on localist concepts of disease and clung to holism, ostensibly on women's behalf. The conservative Boston gynecologist George W. Kaan, for example, might be speaking for some feminists today when he chastised radical surgeons for doing women a disservice because they failed "to appreciate that the whole organism of a woman is closely related to her function of procreation" and that removal of ovaries could jeopardize a patient's general health. Meanwhile, others, who welcomed the turn toward the new science, used it to underscore the need for confining women to the home.[57] As I have tried to show, we cannot easily or neatly correlate therapeutic approaches with either enlightened or repressive views toward women.

This said, the majority of women doctors were indeed more cautious about surgery than most of their male colleagues, and they frequently deplored tampering with women's child-bearing capabilities, though rarely in the language of race suicide. Though few male physicians spoke of the subject in as unadorned a manner as Van Der Warker—who, we remember, asserted a woman's ovaries belonged to the nation—many referred to the subject obliquely. Their language was coded, but the point taken nevertheless. Once again Skene is exemplary. He does not address the issue of race suicide directly, but he is uncompromising in his commitment to the sexual division of labor. Men and women were made for different purposes in life and "each is best and ablest in the position designed to be occupied by each respectively." The home was "woman's kingdom," and "to be a wife and mother" the "chief end and object of a woman's life." Indeed, "the fulfillment of the injunction 'to multiply' is the highest earthly function of woman," he wrote. Failure to do so might not unsex women, exactly, but it did them grave damage, frequently leading to insanity."[58] On this subject Skene sided with Emmet, who argued that "functional inaction or sterility, is a potent cause of disease."[59]

For many scholars who have written about nineteenth-century gynecological surgery, the sympathetic approach for a woman doctor would have required more skepticism toward ovariotomy and other invasive procedures then Dixon Jones evinced. Her obvious enthusiasm for the knife seemed out of place to many contemporaries as well, and would lead some to conclude that she was motivated more by the aggressive and exuberant desire to deploy and improve on new techniques than by a concern for what was actually best for her patients. Certainly there were male and female colleagues at the libel trial who believed this. But her work in pathology once again confounds any quick identification of one therapeutic modality with men and another with women, just as it cautions us not to oversimplify our correlations between choice of therapy and social ideology. Gender operated in complicated ways when practitioners chose a particular treatment, and often the messenger—whether it was a male or female—could be just as important as the content of the message itself.

DIXON JONES AND THE PATHOLOGY OF THE FEMALE REPRODUCTIVE SYSTEM

Dixon Jones was particularly proud of her writings in cellular pathology, which substantiated malignant cell formations and identified new forms of disease. Like many of her colleagues, eagerness to cloak surgical decisions in the patina of the new science of the laboratory prompted this work, in which she depicted herself as a clinician who brought the laboratory to the bedside. During the last decade of her life, between 1892 and 1903, the articles she published were almost exclusively on gynecological pathology.

A glance at these writings reveals a powerful surgical cast of mind, not surprising in an individual who intended to be counted among the premier gynecological surgeons in Europe and America. However, I also want to suggest that they reveal Dixon Jones responding in a gendered fashion to pathology's intellectual and theoretical problems regarding disease description and causation. I will argue that both her subjective experience as a woman and her connections, however tenuous later in life, with the women's medical movement colored her approach to pathology, and that gender identity and specialized surgical knowledge acted together to shape her thought and her therapeutics in specific ways.

Because Dixon Jones did not write a textbook, we have only an incomplete record of her ideas. We must piece together her opinions from her published articles. In the last two decades of the nineteenth century, doctors saw plenty of sick patients who came to them complaining of acute or chronic pain in the pelvic region. It was an axiom of diagnosis at the time that pain was most often an indication of disease, and probably of inflammation. Surgeons badly needed guidelines to help them decide when to operate for generalized symptoms. The more academically oriented of them used pathology—studying excised organs under the microscope—to develop an approach to diagnosis and treatment. Thus, many of Dixon Jones's pathology reports are interspersed with case studies in which she demonstrates over and over again that the decision to operate was justified by subsequent pathological findings. This is the surgeon in her speaking. Also speaking is the rebellious woman whose character would be called into question when her career became the subject of public discussion. More than any other aspect of her career, her writings in pathology demonstrate her continued insistence on her right to be engaged on masculine territory, fighting battles on male terrain, in particular the very frontiers of medical science.

Clinicians like Dixon Jones did not seek merely to justify their surgery, however. They speculated about where infections came from, how they developed, and what organs, tissues, and cells were being transformed into what. Among academic pathologists located primarily in Germany, France, and England, there was a great deal of debate over simple questions like the formation of pus, cancer, and scar tissue. What, pathologists consistently asked, was a particular inflammation's tissue of origin? Additionally, were inflammations the result of local abscess, or did infected cells migrate into the pelvic region from elsewhere in the body? Surgeons tended to think locally, while physicians thought systemically.[60] Thus it was altogether possible for the pathological interpretations of surgeons to differ from those of physicians in part because of their specialty's intellectual/clinical orientation. Some of the tension in the specialty at this time can be accounted for by this dichotomy. Some gynecologists thought systemically, like physicians, while most gynecological surgeons took a localist perspective. Indeed, the idea of infection from without tended to privilege surgical solutions, for removing inflamed tissue at the first signs of disease could easily appear simple and effective. Although 100 years later modern medical science has learned that an either/or approach is not productive, thinking locally was relatively new and revolutionary, and, in the late nineteenth century, moderation was not the order of the day.

As one works through her pathology, one discerns in Dixon Jones's discussions a consistent localist stance on the origin of inflammation. This approach should not surprise us, for if the origin of disease is local and not systemic, surgery can be easily justified. But if this were all that Dixon Jones had to say, we might conclude that her opinions differed in no discernible way from those of her male colleagues who preached surgical removal as a panacea. But there are other themes in her writings that suggest that Dixon Jones was also engaging in debates regarding the putative health and disease of the female body, even as she made contributions to pathological theory.

In a series of articles on the origin and formation of fibroid tumors, she addressed a school of pathological thought that attributed fibroid tumors to the degeneration of unused ova in the ovaries. The primary proponent of this theory was the German pathologist Julius Cohnheim (1839–84), whose studies on suppuration (discharge of pus) and inflammation revolutionized the field. Cohnheim argued that the growth and structure of tumors could be explained by their origin from embryonal cells when, at that earliest stage in fetal growth, more cells than were actually needed for the development of a particular body part were produced. He hypothesized that not only did embryonal cells have greater reproductive capacity, but that a "quantum" of unused cells remained in the body. It was from this residual embryonal tissue, he explained, that tumors arose.[61]

Dixon Jones adamantly criticized this theory. She opposed Cohnheim's hypothesis using an older, design-based argument centered on the belief in a supreme and rational Creator. Although she was perfectly willing to accept the suggestion that tumors develop out of embryonic material, she emphatically rejected the notion that groups of unutilized cells remained present with no function other than to randomly metamorphose into disease. Such a theory implied some "serious mismanagement" in the workings of human physiology, which, she reminded her readers, "was made in perfect wisdom. There were no defects, no arrested development to tissues remaining in a latent condition, certainly no arrangement beforehand for the formation of abnormal growths or fibroid tumors.'' Tumors, she concluded, come from ''some changing pathological state, and can only be formed by the tissues being diseased. . . .''[62]

At first glance, we are struck by the quasi-religious nature of this argument, and the somewhat uncomfortable juxtaposition of perfectionist theories of divine creation with the more mechanistic approaches of laboratory science. In 1902, when the article was published, such arguments were rapidly going out of style among her medical and scientific peers. But Dixon Jones was a transitional figure, and while invoking creationism, she was also joining forces with the bacteriologists, who believed that all diseases, even cancer, were caused by infections brought in from outside the body.

Her ideas have implications for understandings of the female body as well, and although it is impossible to know whether the religious language was sincere or used as a mode of entry into the debate, the subtext of much of her discussion revolved around her refusal to define any female bodily function as inherently abnormal. For example, later in the same piece, engaging once again with the argument that normal cells at a later date can give rise to distinctly abnormal neoplasms, she asks, ''Are we justified on technical or scientific grounds in pronouncing any function of the body or the time of its appearance abnormal? Infinite Wisdom,'' she continues, ''has made the human body and there are no imperfections.''[63]

Cohnheim, in contrast, specifically implicated the female body by suggesting that ''the history of the genitals offers . . . a striking example of abnormal growth, depending on inherent disposition in *the enlargement of the uterus during pregnancy.*'' This is abnormal? she responds with rhetorical sarcasm. ''This most important and frequent function of one-half of the human race? If abnormal, would there not be continued departures, irregularities, and unexpected variations, and even, at times, grotesque presentations? Instead of that, there is not a departure from the exact standard except from acquired disease, or some recognized pathological condition.'' The uterus is a marvelous organ, adaptable to all of its functions, she continued, ''which are equally normal, namely of carrying, nourishing and supporting for nine months the young foetus. . . . How, we do not know; *but we do know that these functions are not pathological.*''[64]

Dixon Jones was applying the new germ theory to diseases of the female reproductive organs. ''I hold,'' she continues, ''that a fibroid tumor of the uterus . . . is a new growth, resulting from the tissues of the uterus being, by some infection or microbic excuse, reduced to inflammatory or medullary tissue.'' Fibroid tumors, she continued, are the cause of great suffering, ill health, and even death among women. Cohnheim would have people believe that such conditions are ''divine gifts''—that the Creator in his wisdom, ''after saying, 'Let there be light,' may have added, 'and let there be placed in the womb of women germinal material to develop into tumors; and then all things can be pronounced very good.' ''[65]

Of course, Dixon Jones's insistence on the inherent health of the female body was not meant to suggest that women were not vulnerable to disabling illness. Indeed, as a surgeon who believed that in many instances an operation should be the first, not the last resort, she had much to say about infected tubes, suppurating ovaries, life-threatening tumors, and the ravages of cancer. Yet, again and again, in her case reports as well as in her pathological theories, Dixon Jones repeated her conviction that diseases of the female reproductive system were brought in from the outside. Poor diet and improper hygienic habits among female adolescents often caused microbial infection, as did venereal disease passed to unsuspecting wives by imprudent husbands. The most common cause among married women who had already borne children was infection stemming from the poor management of parturition by obstetricians.

Dixon Jones did not invent the microbial explanation for female disease, nor was she the only one to be attracted to it. Many male pathologists favored it as well. Rather, the marketplace of medical ideas on the subject of disease causation circulated actively in this period around two antipodes: disease from within versus disease from without. The microbial, though not strictly speaking the newer of the two theories, since it was actually resurrected from the past in new guise, seemed the most fresh and exciting, but it was only one of many available theories in this rapidly agitating eddy of ideas. The Cohnheim theory was another. My argument is not that this approach was necessarily female, but, rather, from Dixon Jones's perspective, it was logical to be drawn to the theory that most freed the female body from its association with inherent pathology. Nor is it surprising that as a surgeon she would gravitate to a theory that readily authorized surgical solutions to cure.

SURGERY AND THE NEW LANGUAGE OF SCIENCE

In identifying Dixon Jones with a surgical cast of mind, one that embraced the use of pathology and the contributions laboratory science was making to clinical practice, I want to link her with a younger group of gynecological surgeons, a cohort that stands in marked contrast to the generation of gynecologists represented by Thomas Addis Emmet and A. J. C. Skene. I do so less because of her actual age than because of her approach to science. I argue that two factors worked to alter gynecology's image of the female body in the late nineteenth century: the entrance of women physicians into discussions about female health and the practice of health care, and certain changes in approach catalyzed by the new science itself. Emmet and Skene represented those practitioners who clung to more traditonal views of women and were transitional figures where the development of the new scientific language was concerned, especially in the way their social commentaries were interspersed with scientific data in their textbooks on gynecology and surgery.

Indeed, the marked shift in language in the gynecology textbooks by the turn of the century is part of my argument. Standing in noticeable contrast to the earlier works of Skene and Emmet was the publication of a huge and definitive volume edited by Howard A. Kelly and Charles P. Noble, two very active gynecological surgeons in mid-career at the turn of the century, who helped refine and solidify developments in the specialty in their early careers and gradually became dominant figures in surgery and surgical gynecology in the years after 1890. Their textbook, *Gynecology and Abdominal Surgery*, published in 1907, opens a broad window onto the changes of the previous three decades. Clearly technique and diagnosis have made great strides. But what is most instructive about the volume is that it is absolutely devoid of the philosophical theorizing endemic to most gynecology texts only two decades before. Skene himself contributed an essay on "ovariotomy," and, though his death before the work was published evokes a kind of symbolic passage, even *his* language had changed. His chapter, like the other twenty-four, including the two penned by women physicians, is stark in its utter concentration on scientific data and surgical technique.[66]

Certainly the more traditional treatises were still being produced. Indeed, many mourned what they feared was the passing of gynecologists' active role as social engineers. Henry Parker Newman, for example, a Professor of Clinical Gynecology at the Chicago Post-Graduate Medical School and Vice President of the Chicago Gynaecological Society, complained in 1896 that surgical specialization had separated "the surgeon from the diagnostician." He viewed gynecology's affiliation with surgery as a deplorable "narrowing" of the gynecologist's "opportunities and a belittling of the esteem in which he aims to be held." Indicting his colleagues for retreating from their former willingness to comment extensively on ways to handle the health problems of female adolescents, he pleaded, "Our interest in her constitution must not be centered alone in its pathology, but must extend to the developmental period when evil influences exist to determine later suffering and disease." In Parker's view "the work of advancing the concrete advantages of the specialty," which included the details of treatment, still needed to be combined with the equally important task of "forwarding the abstract good of humanity as it is bound up in the welfare of woman."[67]

In Kelly and Noble's volume, however, there are no passages prescribing women's social role. The emphasis is on cellular pathology, diseased organs, and optimum surgical technique. The language of medical science had changed, and it was nowhere more visible than among surgeons, who always tended to take a localist view of disease. Dixon Jones's two trials, both the one for manslaughter as well as the libel suit, were also devoid of the social editorializing that might have occurred a decade and a half earlier in a public discussion of gynecological surgery. This is not to say that complex assumptions about gender and women's proper roles were not operating on the level of subtext; but what is *equally* noticeable in the courtroom proceedings is the language of the new science, powerfully embodied in the jars of specimens preserved in alcohol on display as exhibits to the jury and the public.

Kelly and Noble's textbook suggests that, by the first decade of the twentieth century, as knowledge and expertise became more differentiated, sociological discussions of femininity and sex roles passed out of the vocabulary of surgery and gynecology. Probably other institutions and professionals—namely, sociologists, psychiatrists and psychologists, journalists, magazine editors, and advertising agents—took up the slack.[68] Nevertheless, nineteenth-century surgeons' localist perspectives, concentrating on specific diseased organs rather than holistic views of the body, could and did provide opportunities for gender to become a less salient aspect of medical treatment. Operative techniques, first used on female reproductive organs, were eventually transferred elswhere within the body. For example, James Murphy boasted at the first conference of the British Gynaecological Society in 1891 that ovariotomy had "opened up a whole field of abdominal surgery, so that many men who started as gynaecologists are now our most brilliant surgeons, successfully attacking the uterus, the spleen, the liver, and all the organs contained in the abdomen."[69] The surgical treatment of appendicitis, for example, gained a great deal from improved techniques in surgery and asepsis, including experimentation with various incisions, the use of the clamps or ligature, and notions of proper drainage first pioneered by gynecological surgeons like Mary Dixon Jones. Cancer research was also stimulated by the postoperative researches in pathology made available by the removal of diseased female reproductive organs. It can be argued that dealing with cancer on the cellular level might have allowed researchers to forget about male-female differences and return to a more gender-neutral model of disease.[70]

There were other significant possibilities embedded in the changes in science and scientific language in this period as well. For blacks and Jews responding to scientific racism and anti-Semitism, the shift in language was a crucial one. It allowed them to operate within the ostensibly neutral discourse of science, with scientific empiricism setting the terms of the debate. Gradually science could be used to critique its own excesses, which, in the case of nineteenth-century scientific racism, included highlighting faulty data and questionable logic. Embracing the language of objectivity, African Americans and Jews *did* find ways to represent themselves "in alternative yet 'scientific' terms." Becoming scientists and intellectuals themselves, even on a "separate but equal" basis, allowed them to "keep open and contested arenas of knowledge that otherwise might have become completely 'naturalized.' "[71]

Like other marginalized groups, women physicians also used science to critique biological constructions of femininity that buttressed woman's confinement to the private sphere, seeking an alternative epistemology of the body. Mary Dixon Jones's work in pathology was part of this effort, and her career needs to be placed within these broader social and intellectual changes, offering further proof that her story is embedded in the wider context of historical changes in science and professionalization taking place at the end of the century. In spite of her feelings of hesitancy regarding the efficacy of connection to the female professional community in advancing her research and surgical career, she counted herself a member of the small group of women physicians who struggled to develop more emancipatory theories of women's health and worked to find a place for themselves in a male profession. Unlike many of her male peers, she advocated the surgical removal of the sex organs without subscribing to a disease theory of the female body. But her obvious desire to succeed in a man's world did not deter her from disagreeing with male practitioners over what treatment she believed was right for her female patients. She doubted neither the positive effects of surgery nor her theoretical justifications for it. Surely she was women's advocate in her insistence that they should not be judged inferior to men on the grounds of biology. Her own ideology of gender, namely, that woman must not be reduced to her ovaries or uterus, allowed diseased organs to be removed without fanfare. Doing so, she argued, did *not* make her patient less of a woman. Gender considerations colored her surgical decisions just as they did the opinions of other women doctors who may not have approved of them. Her alternative construction of the female body joined with the voices of other women physicians to provide political, psychological, and intellectual support to those committed to changing the material conditions of women's lives.[72]

It is also true that her clinical decisions differed little from those of many male colleagues. Indeed, *they* used *her* to authorize their own gynecological practices, and this was at the expense of approaches being advocated by other women physicians such as Elizabeth Blackwell, Eliza Mosher, and a group of women physicians in Brooklyn who disapproved of her methods. Not surprisingly, Lawson Tait and Henry McNaughton-Jones, two world-renowned radical surgeons in Great Britain, were delighted to have a woman surgeon on their side. They lauded Dixon Jones's accomplishments in several published articles and welcomed her as a bridge both to female patients and skeptical colleagues.[73]

The possibility that Dixon Jones was aiding and abetting the surgery of men like Robert Battey and Lawson Tait, whose procedures some feminist scholars have condemned, returns us finally to questions historians have raised regarding physicians' participation as ideological protagonists in the painstaking social transformation of gender roles that took place in the latter half of the nineteenth century. Taking their cues from the assumption that language *produces* the meaning of bodies, rather than simply reflects it, some scholars have argued cogently that sickness and health, though passionate concerns of the Victorians for their own sake, also served as metaphors for other social conditions. Thus, late nineteenth century literary and medical narratives of disease accomplished several different goals. One of the most significant was to displace cultural issues, especially anxieties about order and disorder, onto bodies, especially female ones. Commentators have often framed these developments as a narrative of power relations, a story about the strong oppressing the weak.[74]

At its best, this scholarly work has made a significant contribution to our understanding of how gender ideology was produced and sustained, offering an acute analysis of one of its many possible social effects. But Mary Dixon Jones's story cautions us against collapsing medical theory into a coherency that ignores both changes over time and sites of possible contradiction and inconsistency, namely, professional disputes, specialty tensions, and gendered and generational differences among practitioners. It encourages us instead to consider the therapeutic results of specific therapies on specific individuals in specific medical contexts. Ideas about male-female differences certainly structured gynecologists' assumptions about the female body. But to posit a direct and causal relationship between ideology on the one hand and therapeutics and technological developments on the other is too simplistic. Unless we decline to take the lives of physicians seriously, we must also incorporate into their decision-making process the influence of new technology and the increasing prestige of modern scientific ideals, two developments that exercised a powerful effect on Mary Dixon Jones's career. It is important to remember that, after almost a decade in practice, she returned to medical school to begin a career in surgery.

How do we explain the odd combination of her identification with masculine professional networks and her willingness to counter accepted theories of female pathology? One answer is to try to avoid presentism. Dixon Jones's strong connections to the woman's movement early in life validated her aspirations in medicine even as she found only limited use for the professional community of women doctors. Her interest in science strengthened her ability to question. So too did her subjective knowledge, her lived experience as a woman. Yet, rather than use this knowledge to oppose the practice of her male colleagues, she found a way to ratify gynecological surgery in the interests of women and give herself the status within the specialty she craved. The female patient suffering from pain and tenderness in the pelvic region, accompanied by systemic disability and perhaps even hysterical fits, would have just as likely lost her ovaries and tubes to Mary Dixon Jones's probing scalpel as she would have to one of Dixon Jones's male colleagues in New York City, Boston, or Philadelphia. But the meaning of that experience was surely different to patient and practitioner, and warrants our careful attention. In the next chapter we will learn more about Dixon Jones's relationship with her patients, perhaps further complicating the too-easy assumption that her professional ambitions overshadowed her ability to demonstrate concern for their needs.

6

"The Lured, THE ILLITERATE, the Credulous AND THE Self-Defenseless": Mary Dixon Jones AND HER PATIENTS

In the previous chapter we examined how Dixon Jones's perspective as a woman helped shape her response to scientific debates over the origins of female reproductive pathology. I argued that the patient's experience with a female physician like her could be an extremely complex one. Many factors influenced diagnosis and treatment, and, in spite of Dixon Jones's refusal to accept prevailing theories emphasizing the sickly nature of women's bodies, she chose aggressive surgery for a variety of ailments, just as a male colleague who believed in women's inherent physical weakness but preferred operating might have done. Here the question of doctors and their patients will again be taken up, more specifically, the relationship between Dixon Jones and the women she attended. The voluminous testimony given at the two trials, combined with newspaper reports and Dixon Jones's own case records afford us a rare opportunity to peer through the door of the late nineteenth century consulting room. We learn how female patients regarded their bodies and their illnesses, and how Dixon Jones behaved with her clients. We note as well their expectations from doctors and patterns of patronage. Indeed, the sources are rich enough to allow us to speculate in some detail about the vexing question of doctor-patient relations at the end of the nineteenth century, and what follows is offered not just as a significant component to the narrative of this historical episode, but also as a contribution to the emerging historical literature on patienthood.

FINDING A DOCTOR

In much of the literature on male physicians and their female patients in the nineteenth century, there is an implicit assumption that sick women were brought to the doctor primarily by husbands, family members, or friends. Carroll Smith-Rosenberg's insightful study of hysteria, for example, presents us with the image of a woman ceasing to function within the family, taking to her bed, while forcing others to assume the role of wife, mother, or daughter. "Worry and concern bowed the husband's shoulders," we are told. "His home had suddenly become a hospital and he a nurse." Presumably it was the husband who summoned the doctor to the patient's bedside. In Joan Brumberg's *Fasting Girls*, parents, most often the mother, sought medical advice and treatment for recalcitrant daughters. Finally, Mary Poovey's exploration of the "silenced female body" and its relationship to professional struggles in mid-century England represents female patients as passive participants. Doctors "enter" the birthing room; they "attend" the hysteric. Just exactly how they get there remains a mystery. What seems lacking in Poovey's account is the possibility that physicians might actually have been *invited* to deliver treatment by the sufferers themselves.[1]

Though these narratives may indeed be accurate, they do not tell the whole story. Evidence from Mary Dixon Jones's career offers a stark corrective to these prevailing assumptions about patient care. One of the first things we learn is the degree to which women were actively managing their own medical affairs.[2] The material allowing us to draw this conclusion is striking in its abundance. In Brooklyn in the 1880s, it appears, female patients' bodies were far from being silenced; on the contrary, sick women attended carefully to physical signs and symptoms and monitored their illness experiences with self-assertive determination.[3] Few of them needed a physician to tell them they were not well. Moreover, women sought the advice of numerous practitioners to mollify their enduring pain and chronic discomfort. When dissatisfied with a particular physician's therapy, they moved on, demonstrating no enduring loyalty to a specific doctor or a particular mode of treatment.

Activating patient discontent was the fact that consensus on how to treat gynecological ailments, even among specialists in the field, did not exist. Patients could always seek—and find—another opinion. For example, a typical patient had undergone a variety of treatments before she sought out Dixon Jones, including:

> fly-blisters to be repeatedly placed over the lower part of the abdomen, and leeching at intervals; some [doctors] used pessaries which she said "always made her worse"; for nine months she was treated for "inflammation and misplacement," with no relief; a year later she was treated for "ulceration," no better results; for five years she was treated for "uterine congestion." The next physician, after attending her for some time, said he could do nothing more, and relieved by [sic] hypodermatic injections of morphia. Her last physician treated her for valvular disease of the heart; said the uterus was misplaced and bound down by adhesions. He also attempted to introduce pessaries, which, as before, "gave great distress."[4]

Most patients moved from doctor to doctor, passionately hoping to mitigate disabling symptoms and restore functionality and competence to their lives. The testimony at Dixon Jones's trial reveals that in some cases women consulted with over twenty physicians before knocking at her office door. It perhaps should not surprise us that the dictates of a consumer culture were exercised by many in their quest for effective medical care. It was, after all, primarily women who comprised the clientele of department stores in this period, and shopping was coded feminine in the late nineteenth century. Becoming the primary purchasing agents for their families aided women in viewing themselves as responsible household managers, and they took pride in their ability to shop around. Why should not the same rules of consumption apply to medical care? Whatever the causes, there existed a lively medical marketplace in Brooklyn and New York City, and the business of gynecology was apparently booming.

Mrs. Alfred Strome, for example, told both the Brooklyn *Eagle* and the *Citizen* in 1889 that she had been sick for fourteen years before she consulted Dixon Jones. She sought the opinion of Dr. Westbrook, who had advised against surgery on the grounds that it would kill her. "Not satisfied with this," Strome recalled, "I went to several other physicians in the city and elswhere, but with the same negative result." "Having abandoned all hope of a radical and permanent cure," she was eventually convinced by a friend to visit Dixon Jones. The doctor removed Strome's abdominal tumors and cured her.[5] Another patient Dixon Jones treated in 1884, about whom she published a case report, had already tried twenty-one doctors, and a third, whose discomfort was so acute she threatened suicide, confessed to having appealed to "thirty different physicians."[6]

Some of the best specialists in New York City and Brooklyn had examined Mrs. A. E. Scholtz, including "Dr. Skene, Dr. Thomas, Dr. Fowler and others." None had suggested surgery. After a talk with her friends, Scholtz sought out Dixon Jones, who successfully operated on her for a tumor.[7] Victoria James, an African American patient, confessed to seeing "six doctors before I went to . . . [Dixon Jones's] hospital and none of them did me any good."[8] Mary Vibert had fourteen doctors in as many months come to her house.[9] When Mary Gearon was asked on the witness stand what Dixon Jones had told her about the nature of her surgery, she replied, "Well, I can't remember, I have been through so many doctors since."[10] Similarly, Mrs. Frances Stroble came to Dixon Jones's Madison Avenue dispensary in 1887, after being ill for twenty years. "She had been to all the doctors she could get at," the *Eagle* reported her as saying, "but they did her no good."[11]

Perhaps as intriguing as the idea that female patients exercised a considerable amount of initiative in finding a physician is the evidence that their referral networks were more likely to be comprised of other women, rather than male doctors. Indeed, the latter were only one route among many in the search for a physician, and their suggestions carried no more authority than did recommendations from other trusted or even casual sources. Stories of exactly how patients wound up on Dixon Jones's therapeutic doorstep are a fascinating study in female community, telling us much about the degree to which women, not only close friends but casual acquaintances, shared concerns about body and health matters. Indeed, the inordinate interest displayed by the crowds of respectable women who sat faithfully in the courtroom throughout the trial, attentively listening to the libel proceedings, can be taken as additional evidence of this generalized concern that communities of middle-class women shared for matters gynecological.[12]

The women involved here seemed implicitly to understand the nature of each other's suffering; they reported their movements from one doctor to another in matter-of-fact tones. Their decisions appear to have been taken on their own, or in the presence of female friends; there were apparently very few husbands involved at the initial stages of choosing a physician. Mrs. Steinfeldt, for example, was recommended to Dixon Jones by her sister, Mrs. Gerry, while Mr. Bruggeman testified that his wife sought out the doctor on the advice of a friend, Mrs. Sophie Smith. Although he accompanied her on her first visit to the doctor, it was she who "did all the talking."[13] Mrs. Euphemia Tweeddale's referral also came from a friend, Mrs. French, who had been similarly afflicted since the birth of her little boy and was about to undergo an operation.[14] Mrs. French's source of information was Mrs. Mason of Greenpoint. Ida Hunt was recommended to Dixon Jones by the same Mrs. Mason, whose husband, John, a bricklayer, was doing some work at the Hunt household. Hunt gave the man lunch one day, and, when she complained of pain, he boasted that Dixon Jones had cured his wife of similar symptoms.[15] Likewise, Mrs. McCormick came to Dixon Jones's dispensary because of the recommendation "of a lady with whom I became acquainted," while Mrs. Strome, who had already consulted Dr. Westbrook and had been advised by him against surgery, was induced by her friend Mrs. Hulten to seek out Dixon Jones. Henry Gunther's wife came to the dispensary on the advice of a female neighbor, while Augusta Offeldt was urged to see Dixon Jones by a woman physician who had treated her in New Jersey. Like Offeldt, Mrs. Miller preferred a woman doctor. Miller's family physician, Dr. Wheeler, sent her to Dixon Jones, explaining to the *Eagle* that Miller had used a woman doctor while living in New Jersey and wanted another. Although he knew Dixon Jones only through her published work, he was impressed enough by it to recommend her.[16] Mrs. Gale told a reporter that Sarah Bates also wanted a woman doctor.[17] Kunigunde Rettinger came into contact with Dixon Jones when she brought a sick friend to the dispensary. Both women were German, and although there was an interpreter present, she reported that "Dr. Mary Jones understands some words of German." While examining the friend, however, Dixon Jones told Rettinger that she, too, was sick and needed treatment.[19] Some female advice-givers had already undergone successful operations, and reports of being cured were most certainly influential. Others undoubtedly chose Dixon Jones because they hoped a woman physician would charge a little less.

NARRATIVES OF ILLNESS

Most of these women suffered chronic pain or experienced occasional bouts of acute distress. Many were literally "worn out with suffering."[20] Dixon Jones's published case records, as well as testimony on the witness stand, frequently speak of years of misery. Often ill feelings were accompanied by patient frustration with physicians, who seemed unable to relieve their torment. Pain could be exacerbated by a more generalized depression and anxiety, making clear how difficult was patient experience. When one reads these tales of lives shattered by acute invalidism, it is easy to understand why women might have aggressively sought out a potentially dangerous procedure. One such patient, "a teacher by profession," was brought to the hospital "in her husband's arms." She "took no interest in life," and her nervousness prompted Dixon Jones to liken her to "a frightened deer."[21] Mrs. Scholtz confessed that Dr. George Fowler had diagnosed a tumor and had urged her to go to the Woman's Hospital in New York for an operation. She "did not like the idea and spoke of my dislike to several of my friends." But one of them told her "that Dr. Mary Jones had operated upon her and done her good. Then I made up my mind and went."[22] Mina Emerich, a fifty-year-old washerwoman, endured constant soreness in her lower abdomen. Dixon Jones diagnosed her case as cancer of the uterus and recommended surgery, warning that the operation was a difficult one and might not be successful. But Emerich told the *Citizen* that she wanted the operation. "I wanted anything that would relieve me, either by cure or death."[23] Similarly, the Reverend Baldwin, a friend of Mrs. Sarah Bates, one of several women who eventually died from her surgery, told the *Citizen* that "the patient herself begged to have the operation performed as her only hope."[24] Dixon Jones claimed that Ida Hunt also came to her "determined upon getting relief," complaining that she had "not drawn a well breath in ten years."[25]

The evidence suggests that often Dixon Jones was sought out specifically because she had a reputation for radical measures, and that many of her patients came to her with the determination to have surgery even before she offered a diagnosis. This fact may also explain why Dixon Jones performed more surgeries than many others in Brooklyn; it is always possible, though the available evidence cannot tell us, that she had an atypical clientele. Nevertheless, the attitudes these women bore toward their ill and malfunctioning bodies—including their willingness to risk the dangers of radical surgery—can be teased out of her case records. Such evidence serves to remind us that the patient experienced her body *both* as a physical entity *and* a culturally constructed one. In other words, how her body felt to her, and how she and her doctor flagged her symptoms, interpreted her illness experience, and decided on a course of action was mediated by cultural expectations surrounding motherhood, sexuality, and wifely responsibility, just as surely as it was dictated by organic disease and physical pain. These interviews between physician and patient helped define Victorian society's boundary between health and disease.[26]

There are numerous examples of women asking for surgery, nervous at any delay, and, in some instances, "begging" to be admitted to the hospital. Mrs. T., who saw Dixon Jones in 1888, informed the doctor that she wanted to be relieved "even if it were necessary to perform an operation," asking if "the ovaries might be removed." One of Dixon Jones's earliest cases, a young woman from Maine, who "urged it and urged it very strongly, [and] almost grew angry when I put it off, said:—'She wanted the operation if she died under it.' "[27] So, too, did H. J., "a frail little woman, aged twenty three years," who was so anxious and impatient to have "her ovaries taken out" that "many times when other patients were to undergo operations she would wish it was her."[28] Some patients objectified their diseased organs so vividly that they envisioned them as invading foreign bodies. One twenty-five-year-old, for example, a young woman who allegedly begged for surgery, lay in bed and "often marked from the outside of her clothing the boundaries of the blood cyst, saying 'There it is, and I want to get clear of it.' " Another, a mother confined to her bed since the birth of her last child, dramatically laid her hands on her pelvis and gripped herself, exclaiming, "Such a misery!"[29] It seems extremely unlikely, given the corroboration of patient testimony, that Dixon Jones was guilty of misrepresenting these facts. She was careful to describe her role in such instances as wholly professional—which meant displaying an unwillingness to be unduly influenced by patient demands without appearing unsympathetic. When Dixon Jones operated, her case records make clear, it was always because the doctor, not the patient, deemed it necessary.[30]

It is not unreasonable to conclude that the desperation many women felt at being chronically unwell led to unconventional and often bizarre forms of behavior, and some of Dixon Jones's patients reported a variety of what she labeled hysterical symptoms, responses that were terrifying not only to friends and family, but to themselves. One such case, Miss L. M., had her first attack fifteen years before she saw Dixon Jones, enduring pain so sharp that she often "had to scream with the agony." Unmarried, she was "extremely nervous, hysterical, and her mental condition was somewhat disturbed." Her friends who accompanied her said that "she was not exactly right in her mind." Dixon Jones diagnosed ovarian disease.[31] Mrs. Alice M. C., aged twenty-five and married, had her first attack a few months before her wedding, at age eighteen. Afterward, her health grew worse, and she began having spasms and fainting spells, sometimes ten to twelve a night, appearing with regularity during her menses. "In these convulsions," Dixon Jones recounted, presumably sifting through the patient's narrative, "she was at times unconscious, 'acted strangely,' twisting and throwing herself into all conceivable attitudes and positions . . . neck swelling out enormously; then she would spring straight up in bed, showing almost superhuman strength, or she would be all doubled up in agonizing pain." "So frightful were her convulsions," Dixon Jones continued, "that her excellent husband once said, 'He would rather she would never come out of ether than be as she had been.' " The patient felt just as strongly as he that she would try anything, even at the risk of death. In another of these cases in which the husband was involved, Dixon Jones remarked sympathetically, "I know the mild-mannered man had groaned under her tantrums and felt that he could not live with her and her two ovaries, too."[32] For similar reasons did Mrs. Margaret Gunther beg "again and again to be relieved by an operation," appearing "grieved and dissatisfied at every delay."[33]

Though many women were forceful in opting for operations that would render them sterile, Dixon Jones occasionally delayed such a procedure to allow a last opportunity to become pregnant, even at the risk of patient dissatisfaction. "Still I hesitated," she recalled of one such case, "put off from time to time even against the wishes of the patient and her friends, and thereby incurring their displeasure."[34] In contrast, other patients sought her out because they were unable to conceive.[35] Dixon Jones and her male colleagues were often approached to deal with problems of infertility, sometimes a side effect of infection.[36] One such young wife, whose "cry was that of Hannah's," came to the doctor in 1887 accompanied by her mother. An ovariotomy performed on her relieved the young woman's symptoms. Though the doctor insisted that it was disease and not the surgery that had rendered her sterile, the patient was understandably distraught. Not all was lost, however, because Dixon Jones could at least assert with confidence that the procedure had not destroyed this wife's sexual desires, an example of Dixon Jones's unwavering insistence that childless women could still be loving wives. "So far from it, this patient assured me to the contrary."[37] Another patient, also a woman who had yet been unable to have children, came to see Jones because "marital relations" were "so painful she could not endure them. She, too, suffered so much that she was anxious to have the operation."[38]

While patients understood their pain and emaciation to be abnormal, they still worried about not being able to fulfill their roles as wives, sexual partners, mothers, and wage-earners. Mrs. L., for example, was a nervous wreck. Married seven years, she was "as incapable of being a wife as a mother."[39] An important aspect of patients' constellation of reported symptoms was culturally determined by their acceptance of nineteenth-century sex roles. The inability to manage household responsibilities caused women and their families considerable anxiety, and a significant sign of improvement always included the observation that the patient was managing to do her work once more.[40] One patient, whom Dixon Jones operated on in 1887, a woman with seven children, felt better after the operation than she had "for fifteen years." Her husband reported that she had gained weight and strength, looked well, and "commenced at once her heavy labors, doing the household work and washing for a family of eight persons."[41] But, as Nancy Theriot has so insightfully observed, enriching Carroll Smith-Rosenberg's early argument regarding the possible advantages of the sick role for hysterics, these case studies demonstrate how patients used their bodies to gain a certain measure of legitimation. For women who could not easily fulfill their duties, or whose symptoms led to unladylike or hysterical behavior, doctors' diagnoses of disease could play an important psychological role. At least for a time it evoked sympathy from friends and family, even as it served to temporarily relax cultural expectations for the individual sufferer. The patient with seven children, for example, could be forgiven for not doing her housework; and, as was true for the woman to whom sexual intercourse was repellent, the "medicalized body" allowed women a significant form of breathing space conveniently sanctioned by the scientific authority of the physician.[42]

THE PHYSICIAN–PATIENT ENCOUNTER

The case records reveal that the support her confused and ill patients received from Dixon Jones was appreciated. Perhaps historians' assumptions about power relations between physicians and patients need to be rethought, weighing more carefully the influence of patient desire and intention. We have already shown that in the meetings between Dixon Jones and her patients, as in all such conversations, both doctor and client had notions of what was normal and abnormal. Patients sought out medical advice when they understood their bodies to be ailing, and Dixon Jones, with great confidence, shaped their symptoms, legitimizing their discomfort by validating the urgency of medical treatment and sometimes also by naming its source. Both attributed the origins of female ailments primarily to disorders of the reproductive system. From patient histories, mediated through Dixon Jones's voice, or given in their own voices on the witness stand or to a reporter, what is first apparent is that many women already had a coherent sense of "why" they were ill and what should be done about it. They did not have to be told that surgery was a possible treatment; they already knew, and some were quite anxious to have it.

In an interesting twist, though Dixon Jones corroborated her patients' experiences, *they* underscored and legitimated *her* therapeutics as well. Offering the possibility of a cure gave Dixon Jones confidence in herself as a clinician, serving to reinforce her belief that she was doing the right thing. This was especially important because, as we have seen, her treatment methods were controversial. Certainly Dixon Jones and her radical surgical colleagues were able to push with relative safety against the boundaries of the specialty's diagnostic and treatment norms in part because they always pictured themselves working in the patient's best interest; their procedures were invariably represented as life-saving. Dixon Jones offered additional comfort in her stubborn refusal to see her patients' bodies as inherently to blame. She was convinced these women suffered not because their bodies were weak, but because disease had been inadvertently introduced from the outside—by dishonest husbands who concealed venereal infections from innocent wives, by inept (male) clinicians who practiced insufficient antisepsis during parturition, or by the contaminations, tears, and organ displacements that too often accompanied difficult deliveries. Moreover, the psychological and physical state of her patients gave Dixon Jones the cultural and medical incitement to try radical solutions. Though doctors generally urged caution in the treatment of female ailments, an increasing impatience with illness and disease also emerged in the social discourse of the late nineteenth century, standing in tension with more familiar themes valorizing the frailty, pale countenances, and vaunted delicacy of middle-class women. Patients willing to risk their lives proved a perfect constituency for Dixon Jones's bold surgical and diagnostic approach. We do not necessarily have to view female patients as passive victims to concede that Dixon Jones needed her patients— and perhaps in some way used them—just as much, if not more, than they needed her.

If we recognize the complexity of this negotiated relationship, or the role of choice in the circuitous paths patients trod to her doorstep, it is not so surprising that instances of gratitude and good feelings abound when treatment proved successful. The newspapers printed some of these testimonials, and Dixon Jones's published articles are also full of accounts of patient gratitude. Mrs. Augusta Offeldt averred that Dixon Jones was "very kind and treated me nicely." A former lady manager of Dixon Jones's first hospital, writing from California, told the *Citizen* that "she never left my bedside for three days and nights and brought me safely through." Miss Elizabeth Carter, interviewed by the *Citizen* while a patient at the Woman's Hospital, enthused, "the longer I am here the more I learn to love Mrs. Jones." Another hospital patient, Nora Kelly, said of Jones that "I never saw her equal in kindness." Mrs. Steinfeldt admitted that "she talked very nicely." Mrs. Mary Bibbert, who could not lift a chair or a broom before the doctor's surgery cured her, stated, "Dr. Jones was always kind to me. She treated me like a mother. I love Dr. Jones." Likewise Mrs. Alice Moore, the daughter of Mrs. Mason, the woman who recommended Dixon Jones to Ida Hunt, cured after a six-week stay in the hospital, claimed, "I couldn't have had better care from my mother than Dr. Mary gave me." "No Doctor," according to Clara Schaeckla, another satisfied patient, "ever treated [me] so well as Dr. Mary Dixon Jones did." Clara Hartisch "had tumors filled with pus . . . two of them, on each side, . . . about the size and shape of a goose egg." Mary Dixon Jones removed them "and cured me entirely. She was very good to me, as she was to all patients." Finally, Mrs. Helen Nash called Dixon Jones an "angel." "If you go down to Hudson Avenue and take a pencil and paper with you," she told the *Citizen*'s reporter, "you will find hundreds of people, blacks and whites, to speak of the goodness of the doctors."[43]

Some of these women were clearly desperate. Others were likely less ill but flattered and buoyed up by the attention they received, both as private and as hospital patients. Indeed, when patients liked Dixon Jones, they praised not only her own skill but the institutional setting of her hospital. Clara Hartisch, for example, told the *Citizen* that the place was clean, the food good, and that all nine of her fellow inmates were content. Margaret Walsh had three operations and received solicitous attention. "Dr. Charley Jones sat up with me for six nights and has made me broth and oatmeal himself to be sure it was right," she reported. Walsh paid nothing for her surgery, though she was asked to help care for Mrs. Fisher, which she was happy to do.[44] Mrs. Alfred Strome had a similar experience with Dixon Jones. "For three days and nights she sat at my bedside," Strome remembered. "Whenever I opened my eyes, my gaze met hers. 'Anything you want, my dear?' she would say. Of course I cared only for water, and she used to bring it to me herself."[45]

Dixon Jones believed that her interest in her patients inspired their trust. She reported that in the hospital dispensary she "over and over again . . . taught poor women . . . how to care for their health, the health of their children, and even many times discussed household hygiene." While treating a primarily German population in 1887, she frequently had "forty, fifty, or more patients a day," and worked mainly alone. "Many times I would enter, women sitting all around, the room full of patients, I, in my broken German, would give them first a little lecture on health, tell them about ventilation, pure air, and the care of their children." It was in this particular dispensary that she "found the greater portion of the tubal disease that went to the Women's Hospital."[46]

Naturally, Dixon Jones's case studies emphasized positive outcomes and even miraculous cures. She described patients with countenances "beaming with happiness" after surgery, and quoted letters from former clients that spoke of "rapid" recoveries and "perfect health after fifteen years of suffering."[47] But not all reports of Dixon Jones's treatment were positive, of course, and the Brooklyn *Eagle* took advantage of the patient dissatisfaction unearthed by its reporters to publish pointed complaints about her in their 1889 articles. Some of these are confirmed quite emphatically in court in 1892. A few accounts describe an imperious clinician who exercised a good deal of authority and power, using fear tactics to manipulate women into submission, and not always thoroughly informing them of the nature of therapies and outcomes. One recurring theme in these negative reports is Dixon Jones's insistence that a particular diagnosis was life-threatening, and that an immediate operation was imperative. Given what has been said about the importance to Dixon Jones of the belief that such a diagnosis was accurate, we can understand the complex meaning of this forcefulness on her part. But the doctor's own need to be emphatic in her diagnosis did not always sit well with her patients. Dixon Jones told Kunigunde Rettinger, for example, that she would "drop dead" if not treated, and when the patient voiced reluctance to undergo surgery, she added that "an operation is nothing." When the court later asked Rettinger why she did not seek a second opinion, she explained that "I didn't think it necessary, as she said I was so sick and would not live three months. I believed what she said."[48] The example of Rettinger reminds us that some women did not have the sense of worldly competence to question physicians' diagnoses. The fact that Rettinger was working-class, German, and spoke broken English may have been relevant in this case, but there is not enough evidence to move beyond speculation about the role of ethnicity and class.

Sophia Sass went to see Mary Dixon Jones in 1888. She thought she had catarrh and rheumatism. At her second appointment the doctor informed her that she suffered from a tumor and would live only five or six months unless she submitted to an operation at the hospital. But Sass wanted to be treated at home. Dixon Jones refused, promising instead that she would be cured in three weeks' time. "You are very sick. You must have treatment. You are diseased," she added. When Sass heard the word "diseased," she confessed that she "got kind of scared." Eventually agreeing to go to the hospital, Sass was not informed what kind of surgery she would undergo, nor that it would render her sterile. Moreover, her hospital stay stretched from three weeks to five. Kate Thompson averred that after she had hurt her back lifting a stove, she consulted Charles Jones, who sent her to the hospital to see his mother, whereupon an operation quickly followed. Thompson had not understood herself as giving consent to this surgery, telling the court, "I cannot write, and did not make my mark for anybody." A couple of nights later she woke up "in a terrible condition. My stomach was cut open." It was three weeks after the event before Charles Jones explained exactly what had been done.[49] Several other patients, including Emma Memmen, Mrs. McCormick, Mrs. Scholtz, Mrs. Schaeckla, and Mrs. Elizabeth Hartman, testified that they were told they would die or go insane if they were not immediately operated upon.[50]

In addition, some patients and their families, confirming one of the critical themes in the 1892 libel trial, complained that Dixon Jones did not tell them the whole truth regarding their illnesses, or demonstrated noticeable insensitivity to emotionally difficult situations. Mary Corning's father claimed that Dixon Jones minimized his daughter's discomfort after surgery and discouraged the family from seeking a consult from physicians at the Cumberland Street hospital. Even he could see that his daughter was very sick. Thomas Cassin testified that when he tried to visit his wife several times at the hospital after her surgery he was denied access. Eventually she died without his having seen her. Henry Gunther also complained of poor communication from Dixon Jones, who told him his wife needed an operation, but used such technical terminology that "[he] didn't understand what the words meant exactly. They were too heavy for [him]. . . ."[51] Mrs. Gale, Sarah Bates's sister, went to visit her at the hospital after her surgery and reported that Bates looked terrible. When Gale asked whether a second physician could consult on the case, Dixon Jones mentioned two doctors in New York, adding that "They don't know as much about this case as I do." Mrs. Gale was tending her sister the night Bates died, and re-marked to Dixon Jones that she feared Sarah was doing poorly. Gale claimed the doctor contradicted her, saying, "Oh, she is doing very well." Only later in the evening did Dixon Jones admit that Bates was dying, and began filling out the death certificate. When Gale declared angrily that "she isn't dead yet," Dixon Jones answered, "Oh, she can't live much longer."[52] Hannah Hennessey rued the day she let her daughter, Lizzie, a starcher in a Troy, New York, steam laundry, become a patient at Jones's hospital. When released, Lizzie had to be put in an insane asylum, where she died. On the other hand, Nurse Olsen of the Woman's Hospital testified that Lizzie Hennessey was addicted to whisky, perhaps an attempt to mitigate Dixon Jones's culpability, since the received wisdom was that drunks often ended up insane.[53]

Yet, as we already have seen, many positive reports of Dixon Jones's treatment contradicted these claims of disregard for patient rights. Theodore Eisenhut told the *Citizen* that when his wife went to the hospital for surgery, Dixon Jones explained to him that his consent was necessary, and he gave it. Similarly, Mrs. Nellie Dorsey testified that when she was ill in 1886, she saw Charles Jones, who told her she had a tumor and sent her to the hospital. She and her husband were told of the operation in advance, an operation she had requested. Before it was done Jones took her to Dr. Gill Wylie in New York for a consultation. Moreover, her hospital stay stretched to six months and she paid not a cent.[54]

Occasionally Dixon Jones's kindnesses appeared disingenuous. Some patients described the doctor as "too friendly" or suspiciously adept at manipulating them. Mrs. Gale reported that the doctor "was so plausible and smiling and talked so strongly of the dreadful contagion" that for a while she agreed not to try to visit her sister. While Mrs. Tweeddale admitted that Dixon Jones "spoke very lovingly as if she pitied me excessively," she disliked the valency of Dixon Jones's words. She "succeeded in making me very nervous about myself." Meanwhile, Tweeddale accused Charles Jones of intimidation. When she complained to him about her operation, "he got very white and raved at me until I was frightened and took back all I had said. I was all alone in the house and he looked very fierce."[55]

Just as the doctors' supporters extended their praise to the hospital care they received, complaints about the Joneses' bedside manner were also translated into a critique of care in their hospital, suggesting that pre- and postoperative management at the institution was typically uneven, with resources often scarce. Two-thirds of the patients were usually treated for free, while one-third paid various sums for their keep. Like other hospitals, sometimes convalescent patients helped out, especially if they were nonpaying, by doing light housework or sitting through the night with sicker inmates.[56] Mary Johnson, for example, was asked to "wait upon two other patients there who were helpless." She also testified that she knew of at least one woman, a Mrs. Williams, who ran away from the hospital after surgery because they were going to require her to work. Emma Memmen complained that Dixon Jones asked her to help around the hospital while her wound was still open. She did dishes, mostly, until she moved to Dixon Jones's house. There she cooked, washed, and scrubbed. She had paid the Joneses $16 for her operation, and received $8 a month for working at the house.[57]

Although paying patients had a better experience, some of them were decidedly hostile. Mary Johnson testified that when she came in for her surgery, the hospital was crowded. Dixon Jones told her that she would have to sleep in the basement. "I objected to this, as I was a pay patient. I told her I would go home sooner than sleep down there." She was given the nurse's room. Another paying patient, Mrs. A. E. Scholtz, who had nothing but praise for Dixon Jones as a surgeon, deplored the general conditions at the hospital, noting an over-burdened nurse responsible for eighteen patients; the bad food; and the lack of cleanliness. She had initially requested that her surgery take place at home. Dixon Jones demurred, arguing that the "simplicity and asepsis of a hospital can rarely be established in a private residence." Described by the *Eagle* as of a higher class than some of the other patients, she was promised her own room by Dixon Jones, who testified in 1892 that it was normal procedure to treat private patients in the hospital, rather than at home, especially if they required a lot of care. Scholtz admitted that she was prepared to "make all due allow-ances for such conditions in such places."[58] Kate Thompson remembered a day or two during her stay when there was no nurse at all, and the patients were left to care for themselves.[59] Many complained of not being given enough food, though it is likely that the hospital put patients on special diets both before and after surgery, and some of these complaints may have been prompted by poor communication rather than poor care.[60]

It is difficult to interpret these multivalent patient reports, partly because few hospitals were felicitous institutions in this period. In a small and financially marginal institution such as this one, it is plausible to assume that patient care remained uneven. Though one must surely inquire whether class was a factor in differential treatment, the evidence in this regard is inconclusive. Certainly it is true that gynecological surgeons in general factored in the class of their pa-tients when deciding on a course of treatment. They did not always wish to admit that this was so, of course. A. P. Dudley liked to remind his colleagues that "the wife of the millionaire and of the poor man should be treated alike, and both receive the advantage of an operation when called for."[61] But most practitioners felt that the compassionate course was to operate on working-class women as soon as possible, because the exigencies of their family economies demanded a return to work as soon as possible. "The greater the poverty of the patient, and the greater duties which she is called upon to perform," argued Dixon Jones's colleague Charles Noble, "the sooner, in my judgment, is radical treatment called for." Middle- and upper-class women, in contrast, had more resources, and the rhythms and obligations of their lives could support a length-ier regimen of palliative treatment before turning to surgical solutions. In con-trast, Dixon Jones appeared to believe in surgery for everyone.[62]

Additional support for the conclusion that class was not necessarily an influential factor in the differential treatment Dixon Jones offered her patients was gleaned by an attempt to break down patient satisfaction by class, an inquiry that yielded inconclusive results. Patients, physicians, and other professionals who testified at the 1892 libel trial and for whom residential information was available, including 38 physicians, 45 patients, and 46 other witnesses, were located by residence on a large Brooklyn map. Using a variety of sources, neighborhoods were coded into three types—monied, including old and new wealth (Brooklyn Heights and the "Hill" communities, Prospect Park, and Park Slope); mixed-class areas, comprising Bedford, the immigrant-dominated East-ern District, and the areas east and south of City Hall; and lower-class districts,

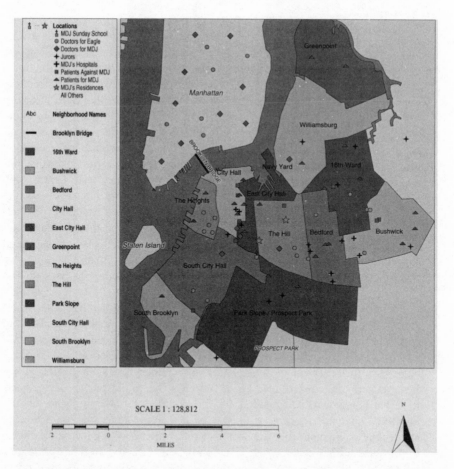

Brooklyn, 1892, with resident locations of trial participants. The author is grateful for the technical assistance of Fourth Dimension Interactive.

primarily located around City Hall and extending along Brooklyn's Sixteenth Ward and north toward Greenpoint. Combining the testimony of all groups together revealed what one might expect: that the bulk of Dixon Jones's support in the 1892 trial came from her surviving patients, most of whom lived in lower-class communities where all three of her dispensaries were located, or in the mixed-class sections adjacent to them. Moreover, her opposition came primarily from physicians, with mixed testimony from others living in wealthy and sometimes mixed neighborhoods, where not only Brooklyn's doctors but also businessmen and other professionals tended to reside. If we concentrate solely on the residences of patients, the evidence does not indicate clear-cut class discrimination in Dixon Jones's care—many free patients felt they were treated well, while clearly some paying patients were mishandled. The sample of wealthy patients from whom there is oral evidence is small—only a handful of individuals—too sparse to allow confident generalizations beyond the speculative assertion that class did not appear to be a significant factor.[63] Though one might expect an ambitious and upwardly mobile woman like Dixon Jones to give special treatment to the better sort of patient, direct evidence to back up this claim does not exist.

Complaints from some patients, however, do suggest that her behavior regarding the payment of fees could appear offensive and might be expected to make the Brooklyn community of physicians and other respectable professionals uncomfortable. A handful told the *Eagle* that Dixon Jones displayed an inappropriate concern for money. Mary Corning's father, for example, alleged that Dixon Jones offered to reduce his $1100 fee if he would procure her patients from his hometown, Bridgeport. Mrs. Tweeddale informed an *Eagle* reporter that when Dixon Jones came to operate on her at her home, she was undressed and feeling vulnerable when the doctor suddenly attempted to procure the money to pay the anesthetist, Dr. King. King, on the other hand, told the court that he did not need his money at that moment, and that he charged less for his services than the amount Dixon Jones had requested. Theodore Goodman alleged that immediately after operating on his wife at home, Dixon Jones asked him for $25 to cover the removal of the tumor. But his wife had already paid her the $25, and he was clearly annoyed that she sought an additional sum from him.[64] The significance of this testimony, even if true, is inconclusive. One of Lawson Tait's nurses admitted that he often overcharged his paying patients in order to give poor women free care, just as hospitals do today. It is possible that this practice was common among many surgeons.[65]

Other patients testified that Dixon Jones brazenly sought testimonial letters from them. After Mrs. Eisenhut's operations, she was approached by Dixon Jones on two different occasions to write letters of good report. One time she simply signed a statement that was already prepared for her, at another she was dictated a letter that she wrote in her own hand, in spite of feeling "too ill." She spoke only German, could not write in English, and gave her testimony in court through an interpreter. Emma Memmen was also apparently asked to write two letters, one before her operation stating that she had been sick. The second letter, full of technical language, was dictated to her by Mary Dixon Jones.

Emma claimed she did not know the words she was writing down, and that the request came before she was paid her wages. Her sister, Annie Heisenbuttel, who was also a patient, wrote a letter in German similarly dictated to her by Jones.[66]

Indeed, these incidents are hard to interpret. Dixon Jones admitted encouraging the Memmen girls to write testimonials, but denied dictating them. Certainly the canons of professionalism by the end of the century demanded a quiet dignity around the payment of fees. In addition to excessive venality, self-advertisement was emphatically frowned upon, not only in medicine, but in other fields as well. On the other hand, women physicians were generally paid less, with every indication that patients expected as much, if not more from them then they did from male clinicians. They may have been driven to seek patients and payment more actively. But an open and aggressive approach to money was not just unprofessional, it was unladylike. Dixon Jones's apparent avarice, coupled with the unrestrained self-promotion revealed in her requests for letters of praise, clearly disconcerted the conventions of middle-class gentility. That such qualities would be displayed apparently unself-consciously by a woman served to render Dixon Jones the negative other, the "woman out-of-bounds" who blatantly disregarded the ethical niceties of respectability. As we have shown in Chapter 1, the *Eagle* certainly picked up on this theme in its descriptions of her, and played to its audience relentlessly. In this sense the newspaper policed the boundaries of behavior between doctor and patient, reading Dixon Jones's character in a fashion that spoke to the larger issues of "gentlemanly" conduct in medicine.

POWER, THE BODY, AND THE PHYSICIAN–PATIENT ENCOUNTER

How, in the end, does one reconcile these two contradictory images of Dixon Jones—the one a physician sought after and implored to perform surgery, whose bedside manner was kindness itself and whose technical skill gave countless women a second chance at life, the other a darker and more ominous characterization of a greedy practitioner deficient at honest communication and insensitive to patient needs? For some insight it may be helpful to return to the structure of the physician–patient encounter and the context in which it occurred.

Contemporary studies of patient compliance recognize that the concept itself is ideological and historically determined, part of the structure and discourse of a particular medical system.[67] Indeed, modern assumptions about the proper relationship between doctor and patient require a delicate balance of kindness and authoritarianism in the caregiver and a modicum of acceptance and pliability in the client. These conventions emerged after 1900, with the development of contemporary modes of treatment and care. Researchers recognize that even today a number of factors influence patient acquiescence, including prior experience with health care practitioners, financial situation, acceptance of or discomfort with the patient role, a preference for illness or health, rejection of or respect for medical intervention, familial attitudes to therapy, and personality conflict between patient and caregiver. During the latter third of the nineteenth century, a new, more authoritarian version of scientific medicine arose, riding on the coattails of the culture's faith in the validity and power of science, and the status of physicians markedly improved. Habits of patient compliance were also inevitably in transition at this time, and at least some of the conflicting stories about Dixon Jones reflected the uncertainty of this change. We can surmise, for example, that the behavior and response of patients to the authority of physicians varied more at the end of the century than decades later, because twentieth-century expectations for acceptable interaction between surgeon and patient were not wholly formed, and the triumphalism of surgery as a specialty yielding dramatic cures had not yet occurred. In a medical world like the one we have described, in which patients shopped around for an agreeable practitioner and often had a great deal of prior experience with treatment, the conflicting stories of Dixon Jones's bedside manner make some logical sense. Dixon Jones was probably not consistent in her behavior toward her clients. It is surely possible that she was an emotionally volatile individual, whose erratic interaction with patients reflected changes in mood. But it is perhaps more plausible to note that, in the changing world of late nineteenth-century medicine, Dixon Jones, perhaps even more because she was a woman, tried out various approaches to patients, combining manipulation and a degree of disingenuousness with authority and the appearance of erudition. For some women this affect worked, for others it clearly did not. Moreover, the descriptions of Dixon Jones's manner reveal as much about patient expectations and cultural context as they do about her. The imagery evoked recalls the familiar angel-witch dichotomy conjured up at the trial, suggesting that patients' perceptions of a woman practitioner mirrored larger cultural themes.[68]

The case studies and court testimony combined help us locate within concrete, specific historical narratives the theoretical assertion that women's bodies were both a fabrication of scientific and medical discourses *and* a biologically grounded organism. Medical, moral, and commercial discourses structured the search for relief from pain for most of these patients, but the tumors, the bleeding, the infections, the inability to conceive caused enormous physical distress. Ironically, physical suffering, which clearly involved the cycle of reproduction, coupled with cultural constructions of femininity, converged in the Victorian period to underscore assumptions that could easily be used by conservative social commentators to reinforce prevailing notions of sexual order and hierarchy. Thus female patients and their practitioners, who together accounted for their protracted suffering by reference to women's reproductive system, underscored women's difference from men and reinforced the notion of separate spheres.

In this determining of social roles, the medicalization of the female body can be viewed as a function of the secularization of culture in general. Besides strengthening the ideology of separate spheres, surgical gynecology's disciplining of the female body also contributed to the rationalization of *female* household labor, just as factory life restructured the labor of men. For Dixon Jones, as well as for most of her patients, an important goal was the restoration of the patient's ability to perform household tasks. Over and over again, satisfied women measured their recovery by their ability to sustain long hours completing chores, either for their own families or as servants in the families of others.[69]

And yet, as constrained by gender as the lives of these female patients were, we also learn from this material that the power relationships it describes were imprecise and indeterminate. These accounts paint a complex portrait of both patient autonomy and dependence. Though the doctor-patient relationship often appears imbalanced, these women are never completely without agency. In the nineteenth century, they were able to convert a set of available resources into a measure of control over their own illnesses. One form of resistance involved using the dominant medical culture's tendency to construct women as weak for purposes not originally intended. Thus, women who needed validation for their inability to function as competent wives and mothers could use diagnosis and treatment to achieve respite from too much responsibility.[70]

In addition, although the self-direction patients displayed in seeking out a health care practitioner certainly did not guarantee quality of care, the availability of female networks that aided women in finding medical consultants remind us that doctors were at least in part dependent on patients for cooperation, income, and reputation, just as patients needed physicians who could display skill, integrity, and genuine concern. Nineteenth-century doctors were certainly in a position to use their privileged position as experts to exploit patients through the performance of unnecessary procedures or by giving less than quality care. Many sought to reinforce the emerging status hierarchy the profession collectively craved. But it is also possible to assume that physicians usually tried to act in the best interests of their patients. Surely their choices in this instance were mediated by culture, but it is also important to note that "the exploitative aspects of medicine are exerted through the useful ones." Even when the balance of power remained with the doctor, control was not inherently bad; it could enable as well as constrain.[71]

The evidence suggests that Dixon Jones took a kind, but decisively authoritative stance with her patients. It also seems clear, however, especially from the eloquent testimonies on her behalf, that some of these women benefited enormously from the fact that she was a woman physician. While timid patients might have overly trusted her because of her sex, being treated by a woman who embodied the dictates of the new masculine professional ethos, but who refused to acknowledge that women's bodies were either inherently diseased or vulnerable to the alleged strains of higher education and "brain work," offered an alternative to the most narrow conception of female roles. We will never know definitively how the majority of Dixon Jones's patients experienced her as a practitioner. The evidence presented here, however, fleshes out the nineteenth century physician-patient encounter in new ways, reminding us once again that women practitioners like Dixon Jones could be both embedded in as well as critical of the medical culture of their time.[72] The remaining chapters will assess the price Dixon Jones paid for her efforts.

7

Prologue:
Gynecology
ON TRIAL FOR
MANSLAUGHTER

We left Mary Dixon Jones and her son
Charles in acute professional crisis at
the end of Chapter 1. The Brooklyn
Eagle had run a successful smear campaign that cast grave doubt on their
personal integrity, suggesting that they
took advantage of patients and practiced inferior, indeed irresponsible
medicine. Though they attempted to
defend themselves to *Eagle* reporters
by giving their own version of events,
they were unable to alter the negative
public image the newspaper had so
carefully crafted. The *Eagle* twisted
their words, cast doubt on the veracity
of their explanations, and cited their
testimony as further proof of wrongdoing. Not even the Brooklyn *Citizen*'s willingness to take their side
could mitigate the worst effects of the
Eagle's sensational revelations. At the

end of May 1889, the two physicians were indicted for second-degree murder in the death of Sarah Bates, and manslaughter in the case of Ida Hunt. They were arraigned, arrested, and held in jail until a wealthy widow who admired their work put up bail. As if this were not humiliating enough, over the next several months, no fewer than eight former patients, emboldened by events, sued Dixon Jones for malpractice.

In the preceding chapters, we explored the social and historical context of these events, suggesting that the story brings out into the open a variety of anxieties troubling late nineteenth-century Americans. These include emerging models of professional identity and new forms of practice within medicine, as gynecological surgeons developed innovative approaches to the female body in health and disease. Though some historians have characterized these pioneers as biased toward surgical solutions and all too willing to perform unnecessary operations, the more accurate explanation is more complex. The very real suffering of nineteenth-century women, the perceived lack of alternatives to surgery for doctor and patients, the exciting advances in surgical techniques arising out of trial and error, and the extraordinary courage of ordinary women, who chose an often dangerous procedure as an alternative to chronic, debilitating pain, contributed substantially to the growth of the field. Among the few female practitioners of gynecological surgery was Mary Dixon Jones.

We have also noted the changing role of the press in American life, and have speculated as to why the *Eagle* might want to take advantage of the suspicion the general public harbored of hospitals, doctors, and the new science of medicine by running a campaign. We have tried to show that questions about the philanthropic role and obligations of Brooklyn's respectable middle classes to medical charities was also at issue, as was the larger question of Brooklyn's image as an independent city geographically and economically linked to New York. Now we must turn to the court cases themselves, which in many respects remain the dramatic centerpiece of this story. In these court proceedings, Dixon Jones would be called to account for her medical therapeutics, while her career and character would be relentlessly assessed. As we shall see, the manslaughter trial proved to be a dress rehearsal for the main event.

BLIND JUSTICE

Unfortunately for Mary Dixon Jones, the wheels of justice moved slowly. For purely bureaucratic reasons, it took almost eight months for the Hunt case to come to trial. Again and again she and her son pleaded with the District Attorney to try the matter "forthwith" or dismiss. They had good reason to lament their fate. Seven court terms passed between their indictment in May 1889 and the trial in February 1990. In the meantime, they suffered egregiously, experiencing a sharp curtailment of what was once a "large and lucrative practice." Given the fact that they earned their living as physicians, and that they were charged with "having, by unskillful practice and neglect, caused the death of patients," it is no wonder they petitioned the court repeatedly for speedy resolution, fearing their "sole means of support" was slowly slipping away.[1]

On February 17, 1890, the case of the *People vs. Mary A. Dixon Jones and Charles Dixon Jones, Physicians*, was called before Judge Bartlett, in the Oyer and Terminer Division of the state supreme court. Ironically, the first ten individuals examined as prospective jurors confessed to prejudice against women physicians, so it took two days to assemble the required twelve men. Indeed, an astonished Judge Bartlett took note of the "general feeling against female physicians" in court, and the *Citizen* devoted an eloquent editorial to the defense of women doctors the following day.[2] The Joneses had assembled a team of lawyers led by Richard S. Newcombe, a partner at Donohue, Newcombe and Cardoza, but also including George G. Reynolds, Stephen C. Baldwin, assistant to Newcombe, and Charles A. Jackson. All, with the exception of Newcombe, would return in 1892 to conduct her libel trial. Much rested on the case for both sides, because District Attorney Ridgway had already announced publicly that if this prosecution was not successful, he would drop the indictment in the case of Sarah Bates. A victory for the Joneses, in other words, would amount to an exoneration.[3]

Compared with the libel trial that occurred two years later, the Hunt manslaughter case was relatively simple and straightforward. Though it, too, attracted enough public attention to crowd the courtroom, it was tried in only six days, and the arguments were not complicated. Soon into the trial it was determined that there was no incriminating evidence against Charles Dixon Jones, and the judge agreed to instruct the jury to acquit him. Ridgway then presented the relevant evidence gathered by the grand jury, and little that had not already been printed by the *Eagle* in 1889 came out at the trial. He attempted to show that the treatment Dixon Jones gave Hunt after the operation was "brutal." In addition, he claimed, she contradicted herself regarding the tumor she removed, first claiming that it had "burst" and then, when Hunt's father asked to see it, that it had been sent to Paris. The substance of the District Attorney's accusation was twofold: First, that the abdominal wound was improperly dressed, impugning Dixon Jones's surgical skill, and second, that removing Hunt so soon after an operation either caused or hastened her demise.[4]

Ida's parents, the DeVoes, and her husband took the stand, all testifying that Dixon Jones insisted that Ida be removed to her home the night before she died. Mary Gearon, a patient in the hospital at the time, stated she saw Ida cast off the ether cap and struggle in protest immediately preceding the surgery.[5]

In addition to these witnesses, Ridgway called up several physicians, asking all of them whether removing a laparotomy patient from the hospital with an abdominal wound like Hunt's "might accelerate her death." None gave testimony that proved decisive. Herbert E. Williams felt the trip did hasten death, but his testimony was discredited when he admitted he had never performed a laparotomy and had little surgical experience. Glentworth Butler agreed with Williams, though his surgical experience was also minimal. More weighty were the opinions of George R. Fowler, surgeon to both Seney and St. Mary's hospitals, and A. J. C. Skene, Brooklyn's most distinguished gynecologist and professor at Long Island Hospital Medical School. Each agreed the midnight ride hurried the demise of poor Ida Hunt. [6]

But Newcombe presented a more convincing defense. He announced at the outset that he would bring in expert witnesses who could testify to Dixon Jones's outstanding surgical expertise. Even before he turned to the question of skill, however, he tried to show that Ida Hunt's ovarian troubles were the result of venereal disease acquired from her husband, from which pains she suffered for a long time. After the operation, Newcombe contended, she knew she was dying and wished to go home; her family complied with this request against the wishes of the doctors.[7]

Newcombe began building his case during the cross-examination of prosecution witnesses, at which he proved quite skilled. He discredited much of George DeVoe's testimony, pointing out how it ran counter to statements he had made to the grand jury. Even the *Eagle* was forced to admit that Ida's father "made a poor witness," one who "contradicted himself frequently, forgot the things he had said in his direct testimony and then pleaded deafness as an excuse."[8] When Ridgway put James Hunt on the stand, Newcombe succeeded in getting him to admit that before he married Ida "he had been obliged to call in a physician for himself personally." Hunt declined to state the nature of his complaint "on the ground that it would disgrace him," but everyone in the audience understood that it was venereal disease.[9]

Newcombe then summoned a number of witnesses who knew Ida Hunt and testified that she was eager to have the operation. For example, the Reverend A. Z. Conrad of the Ainslie Street Presbyterian Church had visited her in the hospital a few days before surgery and "she seemed in good spirits." The Reverend Charles E. Miller of Greenpoint Methodist Church also spoke to her there and "she seemed hopeful." A fellow patient, Mrs. Boodi, a determined witness despite harassment from the district attorney, added that Ida was "fearful of the result" because "she had a sickness that might cause blood-poisoning." Ida named the disease herself, Boodi alleged, and added that if she died, "she would blame her husband."[10]

Nurse Olsen, Mary Dixon Jones, and Charles all contradicted the DeVoes' story. It was Ida's family, not Dixon Jones, who decided that she should be brought home to die. Indeed, Charles claimed to have told his mother to convey emphatically to the DeVoes that if they insisted on taking Ida home, the doctors would retire from the case. Charles gave details of the operation at great length, pointing out that the wound had been only partially stitched up to leave room for drainage, and that it would "naturally" gape a little, "a frequent occurrence in operations of that sort." Indeed, on cross-examination he had little difficulty allowing that the carriage ride might indeed have hastened Hunt's death. He also admitted to suspecting within twenty-four hours after surgery that the patient had developed septicemia, but he "had hoped to save her."[11]

Mary Dixon Jones added that when Ida Hunt first presented herself as a patient, she had said, "I have not drawn a well breath in ten years."[12] During her testimony, Dixon Jones's lawyer introduced into evidence a signed "postal card,'' allegedly in Ida's hand and addressed to her husband, with a note scribbled on it saying, "If ovaries diseased will have them removed." Dixon Jones claimed Ida had given it to her before the operation took place. According to the *Eagle*, the doctor admitted that she never explained to Hunt "the exact method of the operation," nor did she tell her that "an incision would be made in her abdomen." Her excuse was that she assumed Hunt understood what would happen to her because she had conversed with "other patients who had undergone a similar operation and were convalescing." She concluded emphatically that she would not have operated had not Hunt asked her to do so, though she considered the operation imperative.[13] She added that Mary Gearon was not in the operating room and could not have seen signs of struggle during the administration of ether to Hunt, but that patients undergoing anesthesia had been known "to kick about a good deal when intoxicated . . . and not fully under its influence."[14]

Both sides used medical testimony, but Dixon Jones's lawyers enticed many of gynecological surgery's most eminent practitioners to court to give testimonials to her medical competence. Dr. George Everson, a Brooklyn gynecologist who had been called in to examine the nature of the wound when Ida Hunt's body was exhumed, averred that the operation had been "skillfully performed." He also denied rumors that, on seeing the body, he had exclaimed, "This is murder, gentlemen."[15] But more impressive were the statements of New York and Philadelphia physicians who, to a man, told of Dixon Jones's surgical skill. William M. Polk, for twenty years an attending physician at Bellevue, where he helped create the gynecological service, had read the medical articles published by the Dixon Joneses and "judged them competent . . . as far as he knew." He had known Mary Dixon Jones by reputation for two or three years and had visited the hospital once. He was somewhat critical of what in his view was inadequate communication with patients, emphasizing that he always sought additional consent for surgery from parents, husbands, and natural guardians, and "never performed such an operation on a patient without informing her and her friends of every detail and danger." However, he believed that in the case of Hunt "every care had been taken and the work properly done." Nor did he think Dixon Jones's overall mortality rate for laparotomy excessive. After examining the specimens removed from Hunt's body, he pronounced them "badly diseased," stating that "it was right that they were removed." Moving the patient after surgery, however, was a different question, and something he always believed was extremely dangerous.[16]

Henry Clarke Coe, physician to the New York Cancer Hospital and editor of the *American Journal of Medical Sciences*, followed Polk. Coe first addressed the issue of whether nurses could be trained to give ether, in response to the aggressive questioning District Attorney Ridgway directed at Nurse Olsen calculated to raise doubts about the professionalism of the Joneses, who had allowed a former chambermaid to administer the anesthesia. At his hospital, Coe averred, a nurse always gave ether. Moreover, "he had had nurses who had been chambermaids, and considered that they made as good if not better nurses than women from other walks in life."[17] He, too, knew Dixon Jones and had visited the Woman's Hospital and seen her complete "one of the most difficult of surgical operations." He considered the preparations for Hunt's operation as described by the Joneses to be skillful and, after examining the organs removed, pronounced them badly diseased and justifiably removed.[18]

Next came the pathologist Charles Heitzman, president of the Brooklyn Microscopical Society, who had known Dixon Jones for twelve years and considered her "a very assiduous, hard-working student." For the last eight years she was a constant attendant in his laboratory, and "he could speak of her only with praise."[19] Heitzman corroborated her pathological diagnosis after examining specimens from Hunt's body. Then Robert Tuttle Morris, instructor in surgery at the Post-Graduate Medical School in New York City, endorsed the surgical abilities of both Joneses, which he had witnessed at several operations. Dr. Mary Jones's "skill and technique were unusually good. She had exhibited all the nerve necessary." In the case of Hunt, the operation was particularly "well performed." On the issue of informed consent, he would operate on a twenty-six-year-old patient with her permission even if the family didn't display "proper understanding." As for the DeVoes' wish to take Ida home, "it was a common occurrence for relatives . . . to demand the patient's removal immediately after an operation." He himself would object to it, but if relatives proved stubborn and insistent, he would allow it. "If a doctor accompanied a patient home after the relatives had emphatically insisted upon removal, it would indicate that he was unusually solicitous about the patient's welfare."[20]

Dr. Joseph Price, a hugely successful and widely published gynecological surgeon often spoken of as "The American Tait," founder and physician in charge of the Preston Retreat, a hospital for women in Philadelphia, and W. Gill Wylie of New York, Professor of Gynecology at the Post-Graduate Medical School and, like Polk, an attending physician at Bellevue, were the last medical witnesses on Jones's behalf. Price affirmed Dixon Jones's professional reputation and had read her published articles. He felt perfectly comfortable operating on the consent of the patient alone, and judged the surgery on Ida Hunt to have been "skillfully performed."[21] He claimed it was quite common for physicians to bring their private patients to hospitals to be operated on. He himself had often contended with relatives demanding the removal of a patient too soon. Although he usually gave them their way, he always made it clear he would not be responsible. He did not think the removal in Hunt's case accelerated her death.[22] Gill Wylie had known Dixon Jones for six years, had seen her operate several times, and had consulted with her in about "eight or ten cases." "She was," he insisted, "a very careful and cautious operator."[23]

Following the expert medical testimony, a few character witnesses were called by both sides, and the defense and prosecution rested.[24] In his summation, Reynolds, taking over from Newcombe, reiterated charges of an *Eagle* conspiracy against the Joneses, alleging that the manslaughter indictment would never have come up without a purposeful effort at defamation of character. He reminded the jury that Ida Hunt was a strong-willed woman who had suffered for a decade from the side effects of venereal disease, and that her intentions to have an operation and, when peritonitis set in, to be brought home to die were irrefutable. He reviewed the confused testimony of the DeVoes, and reminded the jury of the overwhelming evidence that Dixon Jones was an experienced and knowledgeable surgeon.

For his part, the District Attorney denied emphatically that he was the mouthpiece of any newspaper, continued to question Dixon Jones's expertise and decision-making abilities in the case of Hunt, emphasized her cavalier notion of informed consent, and warned the jury that if they did not do their duty and convict, the public would find "no safety from an unskillful or careless operator armed with a license to cut people up." Finally, Judge Bartlett charged the jury to "brush aside" all medical evidence, stating that the case rested simply on whether Dixon Jones had been guilty of criminal negligence. It was not enough, he explained, to believe the snow ride accelerated Ida Hunt's death; they must also assume Dixon Jones's culpable negligence in bringing the ride about. The jury retired for four hours before returning a finding of not guilty.[25]

The Brooklyn *Citizen* felt vindicated and celebrated the verdict, which it held to be as much against the Brooklyn *Eagle* as it was in favor of Dixon Jones. That newspaper had called her "nearly every foul name that foul minds could suggest," but when push came to shove, could offer little proof of wrongdoing other than the fact that Dixon Jones may have erred in judgment by allowing Ida Hunt to leave the hospital and go home. Luckily, the jury was not deceived by the *Eagle*'s maliciousness any more than was Judge Bartlett, whose charge to the jury during his summing up made the poverty of the accusations clear. Meanwhile, the *Eagle* had come close to shattering the public confidence in "honest and manly" journalists. In the end, however, the *Citizen*'s efforts had prevailed. It had managed to defend the honor of a worthy "Brooklyn matron, whose hair has grown gray in the service of Brooklyn people, and whose achievements in the world of science are among the high honors of the female intellect of the Nineteenth Century."[26]

The *Eagle*, of course, was not so sanguine that justice had been done, arguing that what had prejudiced the case was Judge Bartlett's restriction of the indictment to the second count, setting aside the question of Dixon Jones's medical judgment and skill in the performance of ovariotomy and concentrating only on whether it was wise to send a patient home after an operation. The acquittal under these circumstances proved nothing other than the jury's reluctance to send a woman to prison for an instance of bad judgment. The larger issues still remained, especially the question of the "management of hospitals sustained by public money" and the "wholesale recourse" to ovariotomy when it is often unnecessary. In these matters, the *Eagle* concluded, "there is need of reform," and "it is to be hoped that out of the trial will grow a greater vigilance."[27]

The people of Brooklyn seemed ready to exonerate the Dixon Joneses. Certainly those "thousands of persons" who attended the trial appeared by the end to be on her side, and dozens of people interviewed afterward expressed satisfaction with the verdict. Dixon Jones praised Judge Bartlett for his "clearness of insight" and impartiality. Many speculated that the *Eagle* would now be obliged to settle the pending libel trial out of court.[28]

For the most part, Brooklyn's medical community was silent. Some consternation regarding the controversy was displayed at the New York Pathological Society, however, an extremely important specialty organization for an ambitious gynecological surgeon like Dixon Jones. Sponsored by no fewer than three distinguished New York practitioners, she had been admitted to membership in 1887 and had delivered several papers to that body in the previous two years. When the *Eagle* articles started to appear, the Society's Committee on Ethics appointed an investigatory body to look into the possibility that Dixon Jones had acted unprofessionally. The members of this committee worked hard, writing to principals in Brooklyn, taking notes on the Minutes of the Woman's Hospital Board of Trustees that Dixon Jones remanded to their care, and carefully sifting through the newspaper articles of both the *Eagle* and the *Citizen*. They concluded that there were severe irregularities, indeed, perhaps even fraud, perpetrated in conjunction with the incorporation of the hospital, but a decision on whether to expel Dixon Jones was tabled. She remained a member in good standing until her death in 1907. This outcome most certainly reflects the fact that Dixon Jones had powerful friends in the organization, but a note to the chairman of the investigating committee from the society's treasurer is also telling, revealing that gender hostility was alive and well among its members. "Dear Doctor," John H. Hinton wrote to J. C. Peters in May of 1889. "Jones's dues are fully paid up—You don't get Mary on the hip in that way—Women Doctors are a nuisance—."[29]

In contrast to Hinton's annoyance, the *Medical Record*, New York's premiere medical journal with a national circulation of over 10,000, expressed great relief at the trial results in a full-page editorial published soon after the affair came to a close. The original indictment, it explained, was built on "a series of baseless charges" brought to bear by a "Brooklyn journal of large circulation." As "absurd" as these were, their persistent reiteration "inflamed the public mind against the doctor, almost ruining a hitherto untarnished reputation." But throughout the ordeal, Dixon Jones "not only showed herself to be a skilful surgeon, but an admirable witness for the profession, in proving its resources, emphasizing its achievements, and upholding its dignity."

The lessons of the case were significant, according to the journal. The first was the unsettling vulnerability of reputable physicians to the "anonymous and unfounded charges" of a "daily paper." The second was the risk of public discussion of "the medico-legal points in this remarkable case," which came close to establishing a dangerous precedent. Had the verdict been against the defendant, insisted the *Medical Record*, "a death-blow would have been aimed at progressive surgery":

> If the surgeon, assuming, as he necessarily does, grave responsibilities, should be held accountable for errors of professional judgment, thousands of operations which are now undertaken for the saving of human lives would be abandoned. The desperate cases, which would require desperate remedies, would necessarily die unrelieved, in fear of suits for malpractice, if not for actual manslaughter. Even the com-

moner injuries would be hesitatingly treated, in fear of legal consequences; and the maimed, the halt, and the blind would be present
everywhere to mock the high and noble resources of our art. As it is,
we congratulate Dr. Jones, and the profession at large, that we again
touch solid ground, and are enabled to vindicate our rights for protection in the freest possible use of individual judgment in the treatment
of our cases.[30]

For many, the story of Mary Dixon Jones and the Brooklyn *Eagle* had
come to a close. But not, it seems, for the principals involved. In 1891, a new
Woman's Hospital of Brooklyn was established when the state supreme court,
on charges stemming from the original grand jury indictment, dissolved the old
hospital on the grounds that it was never legally incorporated.[31] Moreover, the
Brooklyn *Eagle* refused to settle the pending libel suit out of court. Nor, even
more surprising, did Mary Dixon Jones, probably encouraged by her recent
vindication in court, drop the charges. Two years later, Brooklyn was treated to
yet another public spectacle in the form of a major trial, this time a sensationalist
extravaganza that rendered the measly manslaughter case a paltry nonevent. We
will explore the libel trial in detail in the next chapter.

8

SPECTACLE
IN BROOKLYN

For the citizens of Brooklyn in February and March of 1892, the courtroom became a stage. Commencing three years after the *Eagle* began its exposé, the libel trial might well be likened to the public enactment of a popular, serialized mystery novel, now come to life as a morality play. Throngs of well-dressed men and women, "very different from an ordinary courtroom crowd," and many of the principals involved faithfully attended the proceedings. Judging from the "remarks caught in the corridor as the crowd is dispersing," the *Eagle* observed, the "cumulative effect" the testimony had on these observers was "considerable."[1] The manner in which onlookers followed events "reminded one of the time when all Brooklyn was discussing the astounding revelations as to the management of the Woman's Hospital.'' With public interest hardly abating "since the matter was first brought to the attention of the city," the *Eagle* pronounced the "courtroom craze" a "mania that is incurable." The same people came, "day in and day out, rain and shine, regardless of the nature of the case or the technicality and monotony of the testimony given."[2]

The crowd's loyalty was to be marveled at, especially because of the sheer physical discomfort of the site. Located in an old downtown building, the huge courtroom was dotted with "antiquated gas fixtures" that shed a "dreary light," especially in the late afternoons. Windows could not be completely shut, and "chilling blasts" of cold air steadily swept across the tables and desks of the participants. During the proceedings, one juryman actually "wrapped his feet up in his overcoat."[3]

Moreover, the *Eagle* observed, the Jones affair had "begun to exert a morbid fascination upon the women of the city." As the court case dragged on, their numbers steadily increased, such that soon "the back part of the courtroom was pretty well filled with alert, feminine faces, eagerly stretched upward and forward as the women on the witness stand told the pitiful story of their sufferings." In view of what we have learned about women's interest in gynecology, their absorption in this event is not surprising. But perhaps no one understood the true nature of this public theater better than the *Eagle's* editors, who elaborated often on the prurient and compelling content of the drama and even used the term "audience" when referring to the trial attendants. "The medical language of the trial," the newspaper observed, "is as blunt as Shakespeare or even the Bible, and the printed reports can give but an imperfect idea of what the witnesses and the lawyers really say, but the hearing is not more suggestive than the sight of a dissecting room, and it has a good deal of the same feverish combination of attraction and repulsiveness. . . ."[4]

The lawyers spent the opening day of the trial selecting the jury. While the *Eagle's* defense team seemed content with a range of men who had not formed opinions of the case in advance, Dixon Jones's lawyers chose with greater care. Dixon Jones's side excused several men who were young and single and, not surprisingly, anyone who expressed discomfort with women surgeons. The doctors' counsel asked a number of jurors whether they were church-affiliated and which one they attended. He seemed to prefer married men with a few children, though he dismissed one man with seven, because three of them were girls. He probed for general medical knowlege, concerned that none would be opposed to laparotomy. All were asked about their experience with doctors and who attended their families. In the end, the jury represented a comfortable cross-section of Brooklyn's middle class. Nine out of the twelve jurors indicated occupation: There were two manufacturers, two clothiers, an insurance broker, a printer, a hatter, a coal dealer, and a gentleman in the oil business.[5]

Both sides in the contest milked the dramatic, the sensational, and the sentimental for all it was worth. The tone was set on the very first day, when lawyers for the plaintiff and the defense opened their cases with lengthy and vivid grandiloquence. The statement for the defense began with Mr. Dykman, one of the *Eagle's* lawyers, admitting that the newspaper wrote the articles about the Woman's Hospital in 1889, reiterating the story of the editors' decision to investigate the institution, recapitulating its dramatic accusations of fraud, misrepresentation, and fiscal dishonesty, and restating its insinuations regarding Mary Dixon Jones's bad character. Representing the *Eagle* as a courageous champion of the public's interest and alleging the exposé "on information and belief" to be true, Dykman gave notice that he would, in the course of the ensuing weeks, give justification thereof.[6] Charles A. Jackson, attorney for the plaintiff, countered by depicting Dixon Jones as a mature, socially responsible, and motherly woman, with strong ethical principles and a powerful desire to aid her suffering sisters, who had fallen afoul of a venal, vindictive, and powerful business corporation, one willing to destroy careers and slander innocents in order to sell newspapers.

Jackson opened with a polemic against the inordinate power of the press. He reminded the court that the present contest was a "vastly unequal" one, a struggle between a maliciously self-promoting corporation with abundant financial resources behind it, and a lone individual who was a blameless victim. Her practice and her character had been ruined by the *Eagle*'s charges, leading, indeed, to the ignominious obligation to defend herself in a criminal trial. "When a great newspaper has done what we shall show this paper has done, there is no other recourse left" but to seek reparation before a jury of one's "countrymen." Dixon Jones justifiably sought $150,000 in damages.[7]

Jackson went on to reconstruct Dixon Jones's biography in a carefully moderated language of women's rights, one that linked female emancipation to the more traditional values of duty and good works. He no doubt hoped that to the modern and broad-minded in 1892, Dixon Jones's concern for suffering women would overshadow the possible discomfort generated by her independence and professional success.

Born in Maryland and educated in female seminaries, where her abilities advanced her rapidly to the rank of principal, the Dixon Jones Jackson portrayed was a woman of impeccable character and outstanding intelligence who early in her education deplored her own ignorance of "health and its laws." Self-accomplishment and the grander aim of "the advancement of her sex" compelled her to continue her education. As she "went on studying the question of woman's health there developed before her vision a vast field of usefulness of American woman." This realization brought her to the study of medicine and surgery at the "only college whereat woman could then study medicine." Here she learned how "to treat her sister, found sick and fainting by the wayside." Graduating with "high distinction," more than entitled to the "high degree of doctor of medicine" that she earned, she lectured to women on health topics, opened a successful practice, and actively performed charitable work. Using Christlike imagery, Jackson described Mary Dixon Jones's "binding up the wounds of helpless and suffering [*sic*], restoring the deformed to straight-limbedness," and exercising "that skill which makes it possible for suffering humanity to bear the burden of advancing years."[8]

It was the same penchant for self-sacrifice, Jackson argued, that prompted Dixon Jones to leave a lucrative practice in Brooklyn for another grueling three-year course in medicine at the Woman's Medical College of Pennsylvania. Becoming "a humble student again," she "deliberately" threw away "gain" for "the advancement of her profession."[9] She studied with "the most eminent surgeon of the day," practicing technique in the hospitals, and emerging, for a second time, with the degree of "doctor of medicine." Her return to Brooklyn was in fact a triumph, taking up once more "the labor of her life" as people "flocked to her," allowing her to increase her earnings so steadily that by the time the *Eagle* took action against her, she was making $9000 a year. But lucre was beside the point. "Always a charitable woman," she "mingled . . . her charities with her work in her profession . . . contributing always, not a mite, but . . . a princely gift." And this is how she came to be associated with the original Woman's Hospital located on Debevoise Place. But when, in 1883, "by reason of some disagreement among the directors . . . the entire medical staff of the hospital was dismissed," Dixon Jones, gathering about her "reputable citizens [who] contributed to help it and to aid it by sums of money," courageously reestablished a hospital for women where once again "the sick were healed and . . . the helpless and young were made to be able to go out in life." Throughout this time she continued to be a student of medicine, publishing "articles printed in medical journals of recognized standing" and becoming known to the wider profession at home and abroad for her surgical skill.[10]

Yet none of these accomplishments was achieved, according to her lawyer, at the sacrifice of a passionate commitment to motherhood. A desire for self-improvement and social betterment did not prompt Dixon Jones to shirk her maternal duties. She raised three children. Now grown, one son was a Harvard graduate and a "minister of God," a second learned "under his mother's example" and "embraced her profession," and the third, a daughter, was an educated and accomplished young lady. Turning dramatically to the jury, Jackson concluded, here sat a woman whose life could "bear the scrutiny of a microscope," one known to all men in 1889 as "a good wife, a good mother, a patient nurse, a resigned, Christian, charitable woman, embracing what was best in femininity, comely in heart and in person."[11] This was the woman the *Eagle* had maligned.

During Jackson's presentation, Mary Dixon Jones sat silently, dressed in "deep mourning," one black-gloved hand partially shielding her face, looking "weary." "The long day in court brought deep lines into her face," the *Eagle* observed, "and she did not look as prepossessing nor as able at the afternoon session as she did in the morning."[12]

Jackson ended his opening statement with a resounding crescendo. The "malignity and malice" of the *Eagle*'s headlines, "unparalleled in the history of journalism," spoke for themselves. As to their effects, the hospital, he confessed, has been paralyzed: "the place, once busy, is silent, the hands, once active in charity, are stilled." With the passage of time, people have begun to suspect "some fire with all this smoke," and, little by little, the patronage previously extended to Dixon Jones has dwindled. "Charged with every crime, hypocrisy, murder, with insanity superadded," she has had no recourse other than the courts. She was here, Jackson concluded, drawing as much as possible on biblical images, to "seek an eye for an eye and a tooth for a tooth" against a behemoth who had emptied its "vials of wrath on the head of a defenseless woman." Give us a verdict, gentlemen, he implored the jury, "that will teach the corporation to obey the commandment which was handed down by the Almighty, 'Thou shalt not bear false witness against thy neighbor.' "[13]

Following a lengthy public reading of the articles involved in the suit, all 69,000 words, and the distribution of a "package of yellowed Eagles" to the jury, the case began in earnest on the third day.[14] Judge Bartlett granted permission to Dixon Jones's attorney, Stephen Baldwin, to present testimony justifying the plaintiff's claim that she was entitled to special damages from malicious *Eagle* actions extrinsic to the publication of the articles themselves. In this day's testimony Baldwin interrogated several witnesses, including Dixon Jones herself, whose statements not only challenged the *Eagle*'s narrative, but suggested that the newspaper had really launched a witch hunt, in which Dixon Jones was tried before all the evidence was in. For example, Robert Payne, a lawyer engaged by Jones to negotiate with the *Eagle* for the suppression of the articles just after they had begun to appear in 1889, explained that he had visited the newspaper's editorial office and spoken with the city editor, George Dobson. Explaining to Dobson that he had looked into the allegations and felt the paper to be misled, he warned that continued insinuations would ruin Dixon Jones's career. Dobson challenged his conclusion as to Dixon Jones's innocence and referred Payne to Sidney Reid, the reporter assigned to the case. According to Payne, Reid had already made up his mind. "He said that the Woman's Hospital was simply an outrage; that Mrs. Jones was carrying on a most nefarious business, and that he intended to send her to State prison."[15]

Oliver P. Miller, the cashier at Williamsburg Savings Bank who had paid Dixon Jones $1100 to remove a cancerous tumor from his dying wife, was also questioned regarding the newspaper's aggressive stance. He reiterated and embellished on his 1889 interview with the Brooklyn *Citizen*, in which he had claimed Reid advised him not to pay the money he owed Dixon Jones because "they were going to drive her out the city" and that the paper had "a million dollars back of them" to make it happen.[16] Next came Alfred Strome, a housepainter who took a letter commending Dixon Jones's treatment of his wife to the *Eagle* office in May of 1889 and was allegedly harrassed by Reid, who threatened him with police action "for bringing such a letter as that." Eventually the letter was published, though the *Eagle* discredited it for being "translated" from his wife's Swedish by a family friend.[17]

Following soon after Strome was Inspector Williams of the New York City police, who came all the way to Brooklyn to answer questions about Hungry Joe, the "bunco steerer." After several objections from the *Eagle*'s lawyers, Inspector Williams was allowed to explain for the benefit of the jury that a "bunco steerer" could be loosely translated as a confidence man with a bad reputation in the community. The *Eagle* had accused Dixon Jones of acts that would "make Hungry Joe stare," and Baldwin wanted to be sure the jury did not miss the sensationalist and vilifying nature of such a comparison in 1889.[18]

But Baldwin's star witness was the plaintiff herself, who was led fulsomely through her biography on the stand. During this narrative she recapitulated her youthful general and medical education, highlighting the latter, including her trips to Europe, her involvement with the first Woman's Hospital on Debevoise Place, and completing the narrative with an overview of her income from 1884 through 1891. She claimed that between 1884 and the time of the *Eagle*'s articles she had performed between 200 and 300 capital operations with only twelve deaths. The interview ended with the identification of a letter to her from Lawson Tait, England's famous ovariotomist, with whom she claimed an active correspondence. Clearly Baldwin's purpose here was to emphasize the contradiction between her stellar professional reputation and the *Eagle*'s portrait of a common criminal.[19]

Dixon Jones began the testimony "confident and smiling," but the cross-examination by the defendant's senior attorney, Colonel Albert E. Lamb, set the tone for future interrogations of Dixon Jones by the *Eagle*'s lawyers throughout the trial. Unfortunately, Dixon Jones was prone to losing her temper, making her a poor witness on her own behalf. The *Citizen* reported that "Judge Bartlett had to repeatedly call Mrs. Jones to order and severely reprimand her for her outbursts of imperiousness."[20] Indeed, the *Eagle* claimed that, when questioned, she often wandered from the point, so dangerously that once her own counsel even cut her off "in a way that would have seemed remarkably brusque had she not been his own witness and client." In addition, she began to make comments under her breath, trying the patience of the judge, who, after two unsuccessful attempts to call her to order, finally lost his temper. "Madam," he began, addressing her sharply, "you should not make such remarks. They are not proper, and the fact that you are a lady should not lead you to indulge in them. You did not do so in the previous trial, and I do not think you should do so now."[21]

Aggressive and deliberate in his attempts at character defamation, Lamb repeatedly searched for information that would reveal instability, unconventionality, or attempts to conceal the facts. From the very beginning of the encounter there was enmity in the air. For example, Lamb began by addressing her as Mrs. Jones, to which she immediately responded, "I am here as a physician, 'Dr.' Jones, if you please." "I beg pardon. I will not sin again," Lamb countered snidely. It was Lamb who uncovered the information that Dixon Jones spent long periods away from her husband, who lived with the family only "part of the time" after they settled in Brooklyn in 1865.[22]

On the fourth day of the trial, the *Eagle*'s lawyers launched their defense against the libel charges. Dykman's opening statement repeated the narrative of the Knapp concert, the complaints that had "poured into the *Eagle* office" against the hospital, including the discovery that its incorporation was faulty and its Board of Trustees and List of Consulting Physicians bogus. He reiterated the charge that the hospital was using public funds for private gain, and claimed for the *Eagle* the obligation to defend the people's interest. What the newspaper found in place of a public charity, he told the jury, was a hospital that "was

Jones, Jones—all Jones.'' Only then did it become "evident that there would have to be an investigation of the Joneses.''

Initially, the editors believed they were looking into financial misconduct only, but the deeper the newspaper probed into the matter, the darker and more suspicious were its findings. An interview with the Joneses revealed prevarication, concealment, and more misrepresentation. Likewise a visit to the hospital itself uncovered an institution full of discontented patients and poor facilities. In the meantime, after the publication of the first article, individuals from the community came forward, upstanding citizens like the Reverend Charles Cuthbert Hall, who volunteered information regarding Dixon Jones's medical practice and mishandling of patients. First, reporters investigated the Bates case, a story repugnant enough to incite them to continue the inquiry. In terms of the revelations found in the newspaper's article on the Bates incident, Dykman assured the jury, "Every word . . . will be proven to you to be absolutely true!'' But Bates's fate as a patient was not singular; the newspaper soon learned of others, concluding that many women did not know what kind of an operation was performed on them.

As reporters progressed from interviewing patients to examining death certificates, the paper "found everything pointing toward a desire and an intent to cover up the operation. And it seems to us, gentlemen, that the facts in relation to the surgical work of this hospital ought to be laid before the community.''[23]

For a second time in as many days, the *Eagle*'s lawyers, reminding their audience of the stakes in this case, played heavily on Brooklyn's sense of *amour propre*, its belief in itself as a worthy metropolis. "Gentleman,'' Dykman concluded, "there is more on trial here than the plaintiff and the defendant'':

> The public sentiment of the city of Brooklyn is here on trial. The kind
> of hospitals that we have in this city is on trial. . . . The charity of this
> city is on trial. . . . Our defense is, gentlemen, that we were performing
> our bounded duty, and that not only had we good and probable cause
> to believe these publications to be true, but they were and are true. [24]

It took thirteen days to present the newspaper's case to the jury, and a large number of witnesses—118 in all—were called to the stand. Their task was a simple one, and was stated baldly by Dykman at the end of his opening remarks: The jury must be convinced that the articles in question were statements of fact. "Justification'' became an important techno-legal term in the trial, because, according the the laws of libel, the *Eagle* could pursue only two lines of defense. Either it could argue that everything it printed was exactly true to the last detail, producing the creditable witnesses to prove it, or it could plead "mitigation'' in combination with justification. Mitigation allowed the *Eagle*'s lawyers to suggest that the plaintiff's character was generally bad "or was bad in respect to the general nature and subject-matter of the offense charged.'' A defense of mitigation might well entail the payment of damages, but if juries were convinced the plaintiff was unworthy, these could be minimal.[25]

Eagle lawyers would pursue both tactics in the newspaper's defense. They approached the task systematically, dividing the general accusations into a number of significant threads, including statements from trustees, narratives from several lady managers who attempted to disconnect Dixon Jones from the first hospital, witnesses who recounted their memories of the Annie Phillips incident, when Dixon Jones was accused of beating a servant girl, dozens of doctors who raised questions about her therapeutics, and a significant crowd of dissatisfied patients and their families, who poured out their tragic stories with great pathos and drama. The issue of Dixon Jones's alleged attempts to operate on the youthful members of her Sunday School class was also touched on, and saloon-owner and neighbor John Delany got the opportunity to describe for a third time the mysterious boxes that were secreted away from the hospital in the middle of the night.

As we look more closely at the proceedings, we will see that the evidence presented was overwhelmingly convincing, even if the *Eagle* had trouble proving truth down to the last detail. The trial testimony is rich, and the sight and sound of witnesses confirming and embellishing statements printed in the *Eagle* four years before added excitement and drama to the event. Ironically, the Brooklyn *Citizen* displayed remarkable restraint in its coverage of the case. Though it, too, reported on the events of the trial almost daily, it presented no verbatim statments and editorialized infrequently. Clearly the newspaper had ceased to be Dixon Jones's strong advocate as it was four years before, and one must surmise that the case no longer served as a convenient scourge with which the *Citizen* could attack its rival. Though the paper continued to sympathize with Dixon Jones's plight in small ways, the *Citizen* remained, for the most part, editorially silent on the matter.

Much of the ground covered in 1892 was, for those many who had followed the affair from the beginning, a replay of the controversy over the original 1889 articles and the issues raised in the manslaughter case of 1890. But there were also moments during the *Eagle*'s defense when witnesses embellished or added material that demands our attention if we are going to make any sense out of the multiple meanings of this trial. In this chapter we will re-examine and interpret this event in the light of the larger issues it raises, both for the actors in the drama as well as for historians: professionalism, class and gender tensions, relationships between the public and the medical profession, the self-appointed role of newspapers, and more.

NOBLESSE OBLIGE: CHARITY, MIDDLE-CLASS ASPIRATIONS, AND THE CULTURE OF PROFESSIONALISM

As *Eagle* lawyers called member after member of Brooklyn's resident elite to explain how their names came to appear on the Woman's Hospital's roster of trustees without their participation or consent, we learn that charitable giving, in the form of both money and time, legitimated an identification with the respectable classes that was as significant in Brooklyn as it was in other cities during this period. What type of cause one chose to lend one's name to, donate money to, or offer one's time promoting was socially significant and guided one's peers in the inevitable judgments made of a person's character.[26] This theme is illustrated over and over again in the testimonies of the respectable men the *Eagle*'s lawyers put on the stand to explain how they came to be members of a Board of Trustees that, in the operational sense, did not really exist.

Indeed, even *before* members of Brooklyn's finest classes were asked to testify, the appearance of Colonel William Hester, president of the *Eagle* corporation and manager of the newspaper, and St. Clair McKelway, the *Eagle*'s editor, made clear the role of social connections in both Dixon Jones's extraordinary success and her ultimate downfall. Taking the stand early in the *Eagle*'s defense, Hester admitted to two visits from Dixon Jones, in 1884 and 1885, for donations to the hospital, which he gladly gave. He also attended the fundraiser at the Knapps', where he met Dixon Jones again. The next day, in conversation with McKelway, who was also present at the concert and had also spoken to Dixon Jones, the latter remarked that he had heard suspicious rumors about the hospital. And there the matter lay for a month, until Dixon Jones's request for coverage from the *Eagle* and the anonymous note signed M.D. crossed the editor's desk on April 15. In his testimony, McKelway confirmed that the two of them discussed the matter again, admitting that he was discomfited by Dixon Jones's "expressed desire" at the party "to have [the hospital] favorably regarded by the press and the people." Moreover, McKelway also remembered that Dixon Jones was the individual that his friends, U.S. District Attorney A. W. Tenney and his wife, had accused of "cruelty toward an orphan child" roughly a decade before. This was a reference to the Annie Phillips incident, which took place in 1877, when a young ward in the Jones's household ran away to a neighbor, complaining that she had been mistreated. It was this consultation over recent events, which the city editor, George Dobson, was invited to join, that prompted the three to conclude that an investigation was worth pursuing.[27]

What is striking here is Dixon Jones's ability to tap into a certain set of social connections to bolster her initial success. However, those same social connections, specifically McKelway's relationship with A. W. Tenney and his knowledge of the Annie Phillips incident, would serve to undermine confidence in her honesty. And yet, as the testimony from a dozen prominent Brooklyn men whose names had been linked to the hospital's Board of Trustees reveals, her ability to manipulate the needs of the respectable classes to perform acts of charity *because others of their set were doing the same* was manifest. District Attorney Ridgway, for example, Brooklyn's leading prosecutor for the past eight years, admitted that Dixon Jones and her son were neighbors for a time, living on Ryerson Street in the Hill District, and that relations with the family were "pleasant" enough to prompt Ridgway to agree to draw up the articles of incorporation for the second Woman's Hospital free of charge. Again and again, leading men of the community affirmed a connection with the hospital that derived from the logics of their class responsibility, coupled with Dixon Jones's persistent method of recruitment.[28]

Although D. W. McWilliams, secretary and treasurer of the Manhattan Railway Company, remembered signing the articles of incorporation and gave money to Jones when she visited him at home several times, he never acted as a trustee or in any other capacity. Yet he was "friendly" toward the institution because of his "knowledge of the work which was being done in other cities." But most revealing and typical were the remarks of Joseph C. Hendricks, president of the King's County Trust Company and former president of the Brooklyn Board of Education. His positive response to a visit from Dixon Jones soliciting his aid was easy enough for him to explain. She told him "that a number of gentlemen, whose names she mentioned at the time, whom I knew very well, were associated with her in that enterprise." He agreed to be a member of the advisory board, but, because he was so busy at the time, only "on condition that [he] should not be called upon to perform any service." The other witnesses Dykman called regarding this matter, including not only prominent businessmen but Brooklyn's present as well as a former mayor, affirmed various versions of this story.[29]

Many physicians testified to a similar form of trust generated by the gentlemanly values of emerging professionalism. While most of the doctors the *Eagle*'s lawyers called to the stand were there to affirm the questionability of Dixon Jones's status prior to the publication of the articles, enabling the newspaper to claim mitigating circumstances in its defense, we can glean other insights from their remarks about how one built a reputation and generated collegial credibility, not only in Brooklyn, but in the profession at large. Especially telling was the testimony of Dr. Arthur M. Jacobus, a physician and surgeon practicing in New York City. He had been asked by Charles Jones to become a consultant at the Woman's Hospital and visited the institution perhaps four or five times in 1887, assisting at several of Dixon Jones's laparotomies. He knew Charles as a member of the King's County Medical Society and simply assumed that the mother belonged as well. Because of Dixon Jones's professional connections in New York, Jacobus implicitly trusted her knowledge and skill. "I knew that Dr. Jones, Sr. was a member or understood that she was a member, of the New York Pathological Society and took that as certifying to a certain extent to her qualities as a physician; and I knew that Dr. Jones, Jr., was an assistant to a New York institution in New York and I believe the academy of medicine." Baldwin, who elicited this information from Jacobus in the cross-examination, then asked, "They are both eminently respectable societies in your profession?" "Yes, sir," Jacobus confirmed.[30]

Several physicians who testified for the plaintiff had developed relationships with Dixon Jones in a similar manner. Indeed, the evidence this trial provides about the workings of professional networks is quite rich. Henry Garrigues, a leading New York gynecologist, explained that he had known Dixon Jones for roughly twelve years, had "read her articles in various medical papers," and knew her reputation to be "excellent." When Dykman asked in the cross-examination whether his opinion was derived solely from reading her publications, Garrigues replied that "to a large extent it was," but that he had also met her "on some three different occasions." "That was in New York," he added, and "he did not know so much of her reputation in Kings County."[31] H. Marion Sims, the son of the revered gynecologist J. Marion Sims, founder of the New York Woman's Hospital, was quite forthright about his membership on the consulting staff of Dixon Jones's hospital. He had known her for six years and her professional reputation was excellent. He had been asked often to come to Brooklyn to visit the hospital but considered it simply too far to travel. Dixon Jones had several times brought patients to consult with him, however, and he had heard his New York colleagues, "Dr. Wylie, Dr. Wyatt and Dr. Colt," speak favorably of her. Like Jacobus, he simply assumed that she was a member of the medical society. Similarly, William Polk of Bellevue met Dixon Jones several times through visits, consultations, and professional gatherings.[32]

Finally, Mary Putnam Jacobi, probably the most well-respected woman physician in the profession, testified to Dixon Jones's good reputation with New York doctors. She herself had been Dixon Jones's preceptor for three months, and in the last several years she had participated in conversations on the subject of Dixon Jones with a number of physicians who admired Jones's work, doctors in New York, Philadelphia, and "eight in London at a dinner, upon whom Dr. Mary Jones had made a marked impression when she was abroad." In what could only be interpreted as a slight to the Brooklyn medical profession, confirming the existence of a certain rivalry between New York and Brooklyn physicians that perhaps echoed the competition between the two cities mentioned in Chapter 2, Putnam Jacobi, who was known for her blunt manner, added that "we don't talk much about Brooklyn physicians in New York."[33]

Indeed, it appears that to be asked to sit on the consulting staff of a hospital was an honor that many physicians felt flattered to accept.[34] Testimony from a number of New York physicians, including Charles C. Lee and George Henry Fox, spells out the meaning of such a position, and the *Eagle*'s editorial staff commented particularly on the remarks of Dr. Lee, a mature and well-known New York surgeon connected with the Woman's Hospital of New York. Lee, although listed as a consultant to the Brooklyn hospital, seemed quite unfazed by the fact that he did not know its location. These staffs in most hospitals were "ornamental," he explained, and members were "very seldom called in." In principle, of course, they were expected to be active, but in practice, consultations "are frequently held in all hospitals when important operations are to be performed, but they are consultations between the operator and his immediate colleagues," who could be conveniently reached. Formal consultants were "not very often called." Fox corroborated Lee's characterization.[35] The *Eagle*'s deprecatory comments on these connections reflected tensions between professional procedure and public assumptions, with the *Eagle* championing public needs and expectations. "It is hardly likely," the newspaper observed, "that Dr. Lee's will be the last word upon this subject and taxpayers will watch the case with interest to learn if the consulting staffs of other Brooklyn hospitals are made up 'for ornamental purposes only.' "[36]

It is interesting to note here that most of the doctors who testified to Dixon Jones's good reputation resided outside Brooklyn. These were colleagues who did not encounter her on a daily basis, and who interacted with her only within the framework of the distant and formalized contacts of professional networks. In these venues, which could to a large degree be controlled by her, she might be careful to be on her best behavior, a fact that helps explain why such individuals might offer the most favorable impressions. In contrast, Brooklyn physicians were not only in direct competition with her, but often saw patients who had consulted with her or, perhaps more difficult to swallow, had lost patients to her surgical solutions when these women became discouraged with their more conservative treatments. The *Eagle* understood some of this dynamic when its editor, commenting on Putnam Jacobi's testimony regarding the favorable impression Dixon Jones made on her New York colleagues, observed, "It was not the same kind of an impression she made upon her professional brethren of this city where her patients were."[37]

In spite of the testimony of New York physicians like Putnam Jacobi, the *Eagle*'s lawyers presented damning evidence from Dixon Jones's colleagues in Brooklyn. Doctor after doctor confirmed that he had heard negative things about her before the exposé was published, while the respectable matrons who were involved in the organization of the first hospital on Debevoise Place recounted in dramatic detail why they attempted to sever her connection with the institution.[38]

First came the Brooklyn physicians Jerome Walker, John Shaw, John E. Richardson, Andrew Otterson, and others, who had discovered from the original *Eagle* articles that their names appeared on the hospital consulting staff. Each of them recounted a brief and ambiguous meeting with Dixon Jones that apparently encouraged her in the conviction that she could appoint them without giving offense.[39] Next came a number of physicians with stories of rumors about or explicit encounters with unprofessional conduct. Z. Taylor Emery, for example, recounted the incident he described to the *Eagle* reporter in 1889, when Dixon Jones abruptly walked out of the operating room because it appeared a patient was not taking the ether well. The common talk before the *Eagle*'s exposé, he insisted, was "that she was unscrupulous."[40] Landon Carter Gray had initially supported acceptance of Dixon Jones into the King's County Medical Society, and promoted her candidacy to several members in 1883. He was involved as a physician with the first women's hospital on Debevoise Place, and it was only after the trouble she had with the lady managers there that his opinion of her began to change. He could not cite any specific instance of unprofessional conduct, but he knew several of the lady managers considered her disreputable. Moreover, he had talked with "quite a number" of physicians about her. The medical community was certainly divided in its opinion, but he believed a "considerable majority" were "opposed" to her before the *Eagle* articles were published.[41]

But perhaps the most incriminating of all was the statement of Dr. Caroline Pease, a graduate of the Woman's Medical College of Pennsylvania and, in 1892, resident physician at the State Hospital for the Insane in Poughkeepsie, New York, who had worked with Dixon Jones briefly in 1886. There is interesting evidence of Pease's state of mind regarding this case, because, just before the trial began, she wrote to Dr. Clara Marshall, dean of her alma mater. She told Marshall of being approached to testify by an attorney for the *Eagle*, and of her hesitation to accept. Neither the newspaper nor Drs. Skene or Raymond— two principal witnesses—were hostile to women physicians, she explained, of that Pease was absolutely certain. She then shared with Marshall her own experience as Dixon Jones's assistant, an experience from which she came away utterly disgusted with the woman's "lack of principles."[42]

In the end, Pease did testify, and many considered her deposition crucial to the case. In response to Dykman's question about methods of procedure, not only did she detect "a very marked discrimination in favor of surgical cases," she lost confidence in her employer's judgment for other reasons as well. For example, the hospital had a very small supply of drugs, often inadequate to cover patients' needs, and, while working for Dixon Jones, she was instructed, when the pharmacy came up short, to sell patients bottles of glycerine and colored water in place of medicine at ten cents a bottle, labeling the bottles with the prescribed compound, and recording the transaction in a record book "as . . . if we had the medicine there." In addition, if dispensary patients were discovered to have the financial resources to pay, they were often told they were too sick to visit the hospital and would be attended to by one of the doctors at home for $1 a visit. As to Pease's experience as a surgical assistant, she stated that during a leg operation, perhaps for a cancerous growth, there was insufficient ether. On another occasion, when she was assisting at a laparotomy, Dixon Jones told her that "she didn't find what she expected to find." Although in his cross-examination Baldwin attempted to paint Pease as primarily a medical specialist whose inexperience in surgery might have colored her judgment, Pease remained unflustered and stuck to her story.[43]

Dr. William Wallace's testimony was also significant. A well-respected physician who had practiced in Brooklyn for twenty-eight years, he chaired the King's County Medical Society Board of Censors during the time that Dixon Jones's application was rejected. This committee examined the professional credentials of prospective candidates and inquired as to their general reputation. Wallace remembered that Dixon Jones was rejected unanimously. "The general impression," he explained, "was that she would be no credit to the society," though this was "not in reference to her skill." It is interesting to note that Wallace could give nothing more specific on this score, and for this reason remained vulnerable to Baldwin's cross-examination.[44]

For example, when Baldwin pressed Wallace, it became clear that the committee depended entirely on the informal comments of colleagues. He could cite only three physicians by name who spoke to him regarding Dixon Jones, though he remembered the negative feeling among members as being quite widespread. But he could recall only one specific instance of what he interpreted as unprofessional conduct on Dixon Jones's part. This involved a story from "Dr. Freeman," who told of consulting with a patient on whom Dixon Jones had urged a major operation for fibroid tumors. When he examined her, Freeman noticed only one tiny fibroid that he snipped off then and there, without the patient's consent or knowledge. It was an odd and troublesome example to be used as evidence of Dixon Jones's unprofessional conduct, though the implication was that she was trumping up excuses to operate. But the incident gave rise to more than one reading, and, knowing this, Baldwin pressed Wallace mercilessly as to whether he considered Freeman's act, which involved executing a minor procedure without informed consent, to be permissable within the bounds of professional behavior.[45] Though in Wallace's opinion Freeman acted perfectly within accepted expectations, the example stands as confirmation of the disparity in understanding regarding physician-patient communication, to say nothing of a hint of different standards for male and female practitioners. We will encounter this subject again in the course of exploring this trial.

This exchange also stands as a good example of the complexity and subtlety of the gender discrimination perpetrated by the male professional community in Dixon Jones's case. Though Wallace vigorously denied overt prejudicial intentions, stating to Dixon Jones's attorney that "[they] have a large number of ladies" in the medical society, we cannot reconcile certain facts without interpreting her rejection as an example of how a woman's perceived public misconduct more easily incurred censure than a man's. Wallace admitted in response to Baldwin's probing that, throughout the entire period of Dixon Jones's application and rejection from the King's County Medical Society, her son Charles had been a member in good standing. Indeed, the council minutes of the society list him as nominated and accepted in October 1882. From 1887 to 1889, he had been not only a member of the council, the society's governing body, but also served as assistant secretary of that group. Certainly we have learned enough to see that Charles was implicated in many of the complaints mustered against the hospital and against Dixon Jones's therapeutics. Why, then, was there never any attempt to reconsider his membership? Indeed, why was he admitted at all?

The fact that Charles Dixon Jones was accepted as a colleague and a gentleman can be ascertained by other bits of evidence embedded in the council minutes. For example, his mother's name came up in council meetings only twice, first in April, and again in May 1884. At the April meeting, probably as a way of avoiding giving offense, the group decided to table her request for membership, noting that "inasmuch as her name had not been proposed during the past year, it was not properly before them." But by May it became clear that action needed to be taken, and her admittance was postponed indefinitely. More interesting was secretary Z. Taylor Emery's record of the discussion, in which there was open recognition of and palpable distaste expressed for the possibility of slighting her son. "In regard to the nom [sic] of Dr. Mary D. Jones," he wrote in the minutes, "it was thought best to have Dr. Wallace give her son the explanation that there is so much opposition to her name that it would be well to postpone action for the present."[46] Gentlemen and colleagues owed each other certain courtesies. The gentlemanly code produced the generosity with which Charles, who was, after all, a graduate of Long Island Hospital Medical College, Brooklyn's proud and cherished medical school, was treated, standing as a powerful demonstration of the workings of old-boy networks.

The timing of the medical society's decision suggests that rumors of Dixon Jones's bad character must have emerged at least in part out of the dramatic breakup of the first Woman's Hospital in February 1884. Indeed, in their attempts to raise questions about her professional and personal integrity, the *Eagle*'s lawyers milked that incident for all it was worth. There were a variety of themes teased out of this imbroglio, including Dixon Jones's questionable skill as a physician, her financial irresponsibility, her secretiveness, her imperious manner, and even the possibility that she performed abortions. The first witness asked to describe events leading up to that occurrence was Cornelia W. Plummer, who had joined the Board of Lady Managers in the spring of 1882. Plummer recalled that complaints from various sources about Dixon Jones's "illegal practices," some from staff doctors, others from patients, came to the attention of the board in the fall of 1883. Most of these were verbal, given to various board members at different times, but there were also three incriminating letters the board had received that Plummer had given to the *Eagle*'s reporter, Sidney Reid, when he interviewed her in 1889. The first letter, written by Mrs. Seth Low, accused Dixon Jones of using contributions given to her and earmarked for the Woman's Hospital to support the private dispensary on Prince Street that Jones ran with another woman physician and member of the hospital staff, and of deliberately misrepresenting the status of that institution by conveying the impression that it was intimately connected with the hospital. The other two letters, one from a Mrs. Bartol, the other from Mrs. A. L. Lawrence, herself a member of the Board of Lady Managers and, like Bartol, an articulate and active constituent of the elite charity circuit, complained bitterly of poor treatment at the hospital. Mrs. Lawrence had reluctantly undergone two operations at the hands of Dixon Jones, and felt the doctor to have been overbearing in her insistence that they were necessary. She complained of acute pain and a slow recovery, adding that her health had not improved. "I consider Dr. Jones wholly unfit for the place she holds in your institution, for I have found her untruthful, unscrupulous and by no means the skilled practitioner she claims to be. . . ." The letter added that Lawrence was prepared to substantiate all charges in a personal interview with members of the board if necessary.[47]

As if the Lawrence letter was not damning enough, Plummer also told the court that Mrs. Lindsay, also a respectable member of the female elite who had been a patient in the hospital, confided that Dixon Jones had performed an abortion on her, and that Plummer had conveyed this information to Reid in 1889. Apparently Reid had already heard the story from another source, and asked Plummer to confirm it. She told Reid at that time that the hospital board had knowledge of the case, and that "our matron had stated that when the woman had entered the hospital she left a trail of blood all the way from the entrance to her room," adding that Mrs. Lindsay had arrived in Dr. Jones's carriage. In light of these complaints, the lady managers had organized a Visiting Committee to investigate conditions at the hospital.[48]

Was Dixon Jones likely to have performed an abortion? It is impossible to know for certain. Clearly she was not an abortionist, though one can imagine a variety of reasons why she might have been willing to go through with the procedure for selected patients whose health was threatened by pregnancy. Her public stance was staunchly against the practice, and in 1894, she published an articulate article condemning criminal abortion, perhaps as a defense against the accusations of Plummer at the trial, but also because it was a required position for a physician at this time.[49]

In the wake of such grumbling and discontent among the lady managers, several meetings were called to discuss matters, but the fateful one came in February 1884, when there was a complicated attempt by the opposition to sever Dixon Jones's relationship with the hospital. Various versions of this event were recounted during the trial, but Mrs. Plummer's description focused on the attempt of the board to institute a new rule dismissing any doctor from the staff who was not a member of the King's County Medical Society. When this was proposed, the meeting erupted in chaos, with supporters and detractors of Dixon Jones attempting to assert control. Mrs. Plummer and others were especially emphatic about Dixon Jones's unpleasant behavior. She allegedly became very angry and "stamped her foot and held the floor" for hours, until she finally stormed out, taunting the board to find someone else to treat the hospital's patients. The image Plummer presented, perhaps aided somewhat by the *Eagle*'s reportage, was of a collection of timid and proper ladies being streamrolled by an aggressive, angry, and outspoken woman, given to tongue-lashings and skilled at the art of harangue.[50] The struggle resulted in the disbanding of the hospital and its reincorporation a year later under the tight control of Dixon Jones.

UNBRIDLED AMBITION AND PATIENT CREDULITY

The *Eagle*'s lawyers culminated their efforts to detail Dixon Jones's unscrupulousness by drawing evidence from a staggering number of dissatisfied patients. This phase of the trial proved exceptionally theatrical, and in its depiction of events, the *Eagle* went out of its way to provide its readers with seductive commentary. After a few days of such testimony, the newspaper editorialized, under the headline "Continuing the Melancholy Tale of Lives That Have Been Wrecked Under the Gleaming Blade of Mrs. Jones." "To a sense as delicate as Thoreau's the circuit court room, part I, might well smell of ether and blood and reflect the gleam of the surgeon's knife from its dark corners," the newspaper announced, "so many of the surgical operations of Mrs. Dr. Mary A. Dixon Jones have been described there this week."[51] Calling the stories of ex-patients and their relatives "dismal," the *Eagle* commented at length on the "thin, sallow" appearance of the women, who allegedly still "showed the traces of ill health in their drawn faces."[52]

"Tragedy is never very far removed from this remarkable trial," the *Eagle* opined a week later, in a presentation of itself as the defender of the poor, ignorant, and defenseless:

> Pathos abounds in the long story of operations . . . and subsequent deaths . . . and yesterday contrasting social conditions were added. . . .
> Graham Avenue and Henry Street are a good way apart, literally, and

in their social significance, but yesterday both of them contributed to the grim record of the Jones knife, which is being spread out before a patient and attentive jury. . . . One of the pathetic revelations of the trial has been the number of poor and ignorant women who have fallen under the influence of Mrs. Dr. Mary A. Dixon Jones and who have come forward to tell how and why they regretted their acquaintance with her. Some of these women could not speak the language of the country and most of them were thin faced and accustomed to toil. The impression produced by the trial so far would be that Mrs. Dr. Jones' patients were from this class almost wholly had it not been for the cases of Mrs. Oliver P. Miller and Mrs. Bates. . . . The tone of voice and the language in which Mrs. Gale [Mrs. Bates's sister] told her story marked her as from a cultivated family, and although the suffering of a woman of that sort is no more moving than that of a simple and ignorant sister, the wonder that she should suffer in the same way cannot hardly fail to impress the listener.[53]

The array of patient testimony was dizzying. Over fifty witnesses were called in connection with Dixon Jones's surgical treatments, and they recounted tales of poor communication, dramatic and fearful diagnoses, repeated operations, unrealistic promises of restored health, and unhappy outcomes. Many verified stories printed in the 1889 articles, while others, whose stories did not make their way into print, were called upon to justify the newpaper's accusations of unprofessional behavior, poor surgical judgment, and overeager operating. Again and again women told of diagnoses that terrified them, tales of tumors that would result in insanity or sudden death if they were not removed. The Ida Hunt and Sarah Bates cases formed the centerpiece of this testimony, but there were other poignant stories from bereaved family members of the deaths of loved ones in the wake of operations. These narratives appealed "to the sympathy of women with peculiar force," drawing more and more female spectators into the courtroom crowds during the third week in February.[54]

In summing up the patient testimony, the *Eagle* editorialized on Dixon Jones's powers of persuasion. It was obvious, the newspaper noted, "that Dr. Mary A. Dixon Jones was a woman of strongly magnetic personality." Witnesses had attested to "the caressing terms and tones with which she induced them to undergo operations of whose seriousness they had little idea, and it has been shown that patients who had met Dr. Jones trusted her implicitly in the face of vigorous protests from friends and relatives."[55]

Two other accusations were carefully linked by the *Eagle*'s lawyers to the theme of patient maltreatment, both of them attempts to represent Dixon Jones as hardhearted and without normal female feelings. The first was an allegation regarding Dixon Jones's exploitation of a servant girl in 1877, and the second explored rumors that she had urged members of her Sunday school class to undergo operations. As to the latter, the *Eagle*'s lawyers failed to prove their case. They produced only one witness, William A. Bedford, Superintendent of the Sunday school at Hanson Place Methodist Church, who could do no more than confirm the existence of gossip about the matter and allege that Dixon Jones gave up teaching there to avoid further talk. We know she gave physiological lectures to young women; it is plausible to speculate that one or two of them were offended and complained, giving rise to exaggerated stories. Whatever the real truth, Dixon Jones's lawyers produced five women witnesses who had been students in the class, all of whom swore to her "excellent" reputation, praised her selflessness for volunteering to teach, and claimed never to have heard even a "whisper of complaint."[56]

More undermining of the generosity and gentle maternalism her lawyers attempted to associate with Dixon Jones were the details of the Annie Phillips incident, which were brought to the attention of the jury and the public when Judge A. W. Tenney and several former neighbors of the Joneses testified on the *Eagle*'s behalf. Tenney, a former U.S. District Attorney and a man with an impeccable reputation in Brooklyn, explained that he had lived next door to the doctors in 1877. He recalled that Phillips was at the time perhaps eleven or twelve years old, a small, frail, "thinly clad" and poorly fed girl who performed all manner of work at the Jones household, including washing, cleaning, shoveling snow off the stoop, the walkway, and in the backyard, driving Mrs. Jones to see patients in the carriage, and placing the ash barrels in the back of the house. She was, Tenney believed, the only servant. He verified what he had told reporter Reid regarding her running away to his house, her story of mistreatment, his decision, based on Annie's complaints in the form of a written statement made to him, coupled with things he had himself witnessed, to write Dixon Jones a letter stating that he would not return her to the doctor's care. Included in Annie's written statement were vivid accounts of physical abuse, such as beatings with a broomstick over the head and being thrown "about the room by the hair of her head." When Dixon Jones heard from Tenney she and her husband came to see him at his office. Claiming that Annie was lying, she explained that the girl had been indentured to her by the Brooklyn Orphan Asylum. But Tenney answered that parts of the girl's story could be verified by both himself and neighbors, who had witnessed some of the abuse. He then suggested that Dixon Jones seek redress in the courts, letting her know that he was prepared for such an eventuality. She never did so. Annie lived with the Tenneys for a year and a half, proving to be "an excellent girl in every way— excellent in disposition, and in manners, and in truthfulness." Three other neighbors, Mary E. Pendleton, Mrs. Annie Peabody, and Harriet Van Benshoten, validated Tenney's story.[57]

In Dixon Jones's defense, Baldwin put William O'Brien, the Jones's "colored" coachman, on the stand, who testified that Annie was treated like Dixon Jones's own daughter. The three Jones children—Charles, the Reverend Henry O. Jones, and Miss Mary Jones—all claimed that Annie was smothered with kindness. Dixon Jones stated that the girl was "kindhearted" but "careless," and that the neighbors meddled.[58] Apparently neither side attempted to call the adult Annie, now married and living in New Jersey, to the stand. The *Eagle*'s lawyers perhaps felt that Tenney's statements and corroboration of neighbors were sufficient. On Dixon Jones's side, Annie's exoneration of her would have been enormously helpful. That she did not appear suggests that at least some of the testimony may have been true. Clearly Tenney's status and narrative power dominated the retelling of this incident, and it could hardly have failed to impress the jury with its implications. Indeed, in a protracted discussion over the fine points of the law that occurred in the middle of this portion of the defense's case, Dixon Jones's lawyer admitted that the plaintiff did not consider the Phillips story libelous, only a deliberate attempt to defame Dixon Jones's character.[59]

MALIGNING NEWSPAPERS, JEALOUS RIVALS, AND GRATEFUL PATIENTS

On February 20, the defense rested, and lawyers for the plaintiff took up their work. Their main strategy was to question the truth of as many of the allegations against Dixon Jones as possible, contradict the image of her the newspaper had fashioned, and demonstrate malice whenever possible. Stephen Baldwin began by returning to the dissolution of the old hospital, and called six witnesses to the stand who claimed that this event was the result of a conspiracy against Dixon Jones by a collection of ungrateful women, who steadfastly refused to acknowledge her Herculean efforts on the institution's behalf. Three of these, Esther E. Baldwin, Horatio B. Elkins, and Sarah J. Millette, were members of the "Committee of Five," the body rapidly organized in May 1889 to issue a statement vindicating Dixon Jones of all wrongdoing in the face of the *Eagle*'s accusations. Esther Baldwin affirmed her longstanding friendship with Dixon Jones, as did Sarah Elizabeth Elkins, who called the doctor a "sweet sister of charity." So, too, did Sarah J. Millette, who had also been a patient and at one time a member of the Board of Lady Managers of the first Woman's Hospital. All three disputed Mrs. Plummer's version of the events of Feburary 1884. The three male witnesses were William R. Taylor, a manufacturer who had been an incorporator and served as treasurer of both the first and the second hospital; Horatio Elkins, who became president of the hospital association in 1889, after the *Eagle* articles were published; and the Reverend Dr. Joseph Pullman, now of Connecticut, who also remained a loyal supporter after the exposé. All three praised her work on behalf of the Woman's Hospital and supported her in the reestablishment of the institution when the first one disbanded.

Unfortunately, some of this testimony was marred by the behavior of Mrs. Elkins, whose eagerness to defend Dixon Jones led her to violate courtroom decorum by making disparaging and unsolicited remarks about those who opposed Dixon Jones. After admonishing her several times to follow the rules of testimony, Bartlett lost his patience, and warned her that if it were not "for your sex I should not allow such answers to be made. You are plainly endeavoring to disregard the cautions of the court in regard to the acts of others."[60] The *Eagle* made much of this incident in its summary of courtroom events, noting that neither of these witnesses "had the faintest idea of the legal rules limiting the scope of evidence." The image of another unruly woman, just like Dixon Jones, could not have failed to cross the minds of a few members of the jury and the audience.[61]

Following testimony regarding the disbanding of the first hospital came former patients of Dixon Jones's who told of successful operations, kindly and competent treatment, adequate communication between doctor and patient, and miraculous cures. Dixon Jones's lawyers called to the stand even more satisfied patients than the defense had disappointed ones, close to sixty of them. The *Eagle* noted that the women were "plumper and more healthful looking than most of the patients of Dr. Mary A. Dixon Jones whom the defendant put upon the stand." A couple of days later the newspaper again commented on the appearance of Dixon Jones's supporters, noting that they were a "less wretched looking lot than those who have told so touchingly of the wreck of their womanhood."[62]

Many of these women were pleased to report that Dixon Jones had sought consultation regarding their cases with prominent New York physicians, such as T. Gaillard Thomas, Lewis Pilcher, W. Gill Wylie, Mary Putnam Jacobi, Henry J. Boldt, and Augustus P. Dudley.[63] Scores of men and women testified to Dixon Jones's excellent reputation, many admitting that they referred friends to her without a second thought.[64] Mrs. Gedney noted that Dixon Jones had advised *against* an operation, while Mrs. Hannah Carlton, who had undergone surgery, took the stand with an infant in her arms, an eloquent counter to the stories of patients who accused the doctors of leaving them sterile. Several patients also spoke of Dixon Jones's kindness and generosity, especially in her concern for family finances. Mrs. Maggy Kalbrenner recalled that she was asked if she could afford the $60 she paid for her operation, and Mrs. Eliza Schlagel affirmed that the doctor did not charge her anything because her husband was out of work. According to the *Eagle*, Dixon Jones paid close attention to these witnesses, "nodding and smiling when testimony goes to suit her and shaking her head when she doesn't agree."[65]

MAKING THERAPEUTIC UNCERTAINTY PUBLIC

Throughout the first several weeks of the trial, the attorneys for both sides became involved in a protracted discussion with Judge Bartlett regarding whether the original articles impugned Dixon Jones's surgical skill. The *Eagle*'s lawyers, having lost this battle at the manslaughter trial, claimed that her proficiency was never at issue, but Baldwin, arguing a point of law, showed Judge Bartlett several of the newspaper's statements that could easily be interpreted as undermining confidence in Dixon Jones as a surgeon. Early in the trial Bartlett sided with the *Eagle*, for example, when he refused to let Dr. Arthur Jacobus answer questions relating specifically to her surgery, and left the question of deciding the admissibility of such testimony to a later date.[66]

By the time the plaintiff's case commenced, however, the judge was ready to allow testimony regarding medical decision-making and technique. In response, Dixon Jones's lawyers pulled out all the stops and introduced a distinguished array of reputable and knowledgeable physicians and surgeons. These men had much to say of interest, and this portion of the trial contextualizes for us some of the debates in the field of gynecological surgery. Witnesses put in the foreground two burning issues in particular: first was the question of when to operate, with Dixon Jones being painted by most of her Brooklyn colleagues as too aggressive a surgeon, dangerously neglectful of the more conservative course of palliative treatment.[67] Second, taking their cues from the many patients testifying to that effect on behalf of the *Eagle*, doctors debated whether Dixon Jones had habitually abstained from obtaining adequate informed consent from either her patients or their families.

The *Eagle* partially understood the professional impact of the trial. Calling this moment of testimony "the expert stage," it attempted to titillate its readers with vivid descriptions of events.[68] Samuel King verified that he had told the *Eagle* that Dixon Jones had a "mania" for the knife, and stood by this opinion. George Drury repeated his conviction that Dixon Jones's operation on a shared patient, Mrs. McCormick, was unnecessary. Dr. A. W. Shepard, whose offices were located in close proximity to Dixon Jones's dispensary, claimed that "tumors and similar troubles in his neighborhood became unduly frequent" after the Joneses located there, and he often advised patients against submitting to surgery.[69]

On March 3, the newspaper called attention to the "introduction of a peach basket . . . brought by the mysterious old man with the flowing beard . . . from the Jones mansion." The basket, laden with bottles of surgical specimens preserved in alchohol, made the courtroom look "like a section of a pathological museum, so many bottles of preserved specimens were scattered about." A couple of days later the newspaper cited "two big brass mounted compound microscopes" as "prominent features of the stage setting of the court room." One had been left by Charles Heitzman, Jones's mentor in pathology, and was readied to allow him to describe the slides he and his son had made from her surgical specimens. "The other was on the table of the counsel for the defense and was the property of Dr. J. M. Van Cott, an expert who is following the case for the defense and sits with the defendant's counsel."[70]

Eight distinguished gynecologists and three pathologists contributed relevant testimony regarding these questions. Robert T. Morris was the first to give evidence, stating that he knew Dixon Jones, had seen her operate several times, and had consulted with her on many occasions. He admitted to identifying with Dr. Lawson Tait and a more aggressive school of surgery, but he also revealed that the schools "had come together in the last year." Asked to examine the contents of the peach basket, he confirmed quite forcefully that "in almost every case immediate removal would be required," though in the cross-examination he was pushed to admit that he had not done extensive pathology work in more than a decade.[71]

More intriguing were the statements of Henry Clarke Coe, because his remarks prompt speculation on the role of the Dixon Jones trial in shaping medical therapeutics. We remember Coe from Chapter 4 as an extremely thoughtful practitioner, who charted a moderate course between radical and conservative surgical approaches and whose knowledge of surgical pathology and belief in its usefulness was extensive. His attempts to answer questions honestly and in careful detail hint at the possibility that standards of diagnosis and treatment for operations of the type Dixon Jones was doing in the late 1880s were in a noticeable state of flux.

Coe had known Dixon Jones for some years, and had himself performed 150 laparotomies. He testified that opening the abdomen had become more common in the past decade because of dramatic reductions in the death rate due to antisepsis. Commenting on Dixon Jones's working-class patients, he pointed out that "among the laboring classes" from 10 to 15 percent of women were afflicted by the diseases she diagnosed at the Woman's Hospital. Moreover, before 1889, "the surgeon would not have hesitated to operate" in many, if not all the cases whose specimens he was asked to examine. Letting Dixon Jones off the hook in significant ways, Coe even admitted that "before 1889 there was, in popular acceptation, a craze for the sort of operation involved in this case, among a certain class of physicians, and that operations were performed then in cases in which no gynecologist would think of operating now without long palliative treatment." However, since that time, there had been a marked change. "Palliative treatment was now usual." Though, as the *Eagle* pointed out, "the general effect of his testimony was to support that of Dr. Morris in most cases," he also "emphasized more strongly than other witnesses have done the strongly conservative turn of the practice since 1889, *when the attention of the profession was so pointedly turned upon the Jones methods.*" Here we have evidence not only of shifting guidelines, but of the possibility that the Dixon Jones affair actually helped catalyze some of these changes.[72]

To complete testimony regarding the pathology of the organs removed, the plaintiff's lawyers called Dr. Charles Heitzman and his son Louis, who merely confirmed that he had made the slides on exhibit. Both were pathologists, and Heitzman had been Dixon Jones's research mentor for almost twenty years. A Hungarian-born immigrant trained in surgery and microscopy who had settled in Brooklyn in 1874, he had a respectable local reputation and was one of the founders of the American Dermatological Association.[73] Heitzman praised Dixon Jones's expertise and confirmed her diagnosis of "gyroma" in several of the specimens he was shown. He then enthused over her "discovery" of the diseases "gyroma and endothelioma" in 1888 and 1889. In the cross-examination, Dykman attempted to bring out that both of these conditions were merely normal states recognized by most pathologists and physicians, but Heitzman did not agree and would not allow himself to be contradicted.[74]

This line of questioning was obviously the result of advice given to the defense by Dr. Joshua M. Van Cott, a thirty-year-old pathology professor and junior colleague of A. J. C. Skene at Long Island Hospital Medical College who had studied with "Virchow and Coht [Koch] in Berlin and . . . belonged to various societies and hospitals. He had studied microscopy for seven years and had made 600 autopsies." Van Cott was called to the stand by the defense the following day, and his testimony discredited Heitzman's in two ways. First, Heitzman had been somewhat flustered when he realized that he had initially failed to notice three organs instead of two in one of the bottles. He finally admitted that there was one too many. Van Cott commented immediately that this was not the case, "one had simply been pulled apart into two pieces," making Heitzman look a little silly.

But more dramatic was his decided contempt for the doctors' pathology. Commenting that the specimens were improperly cut and "unfavorable for examination," and that it was "important to see the tissue fresh," he nevertheless expressed grave doubts regarding the seriousness of their diseased state. "As to Dr. Jones's disease with the six syllable name, endothelioma, he had read Dr. Mary Jones's articles in the medical journals, and he believed the condition so nearly as he could make out what she meant, to be very rare, and not one of disease." In fact, "the only pathologists he knew who believed in the existence of the two Jones's diseases were the Drs. Heitzman, in whose laboratory they were said to have been found." Indeed, since the *Medical Journal* published her articles on gyroma and endothelioma, he had been so disappointed in its editorial standards that "he stopped taking the paper from that time."[75]

A. J. C. Skene, probably the most well respected of all Brooklyn physicians, also cast doubt for the defense on Dixon Jones's pathological diagnoses. But in many ways Skene's testimony merely revealed his conservatism. While Van Cott was an up-to-date pathologist, trained in Europe, Skene was a reluctant participant who dragged his feet in terms of accepting the relevance of microscopical work to surgery. Indeed, he admitted that he did not use the instrument and found the microscope "useless in this class of disease because it could not be used on the living patient." Again we are reminded that routine biopsies were still a thing of the future. Moreover, unlike Lawson Tait and his followers, he opposed exploratory surgery as too dangerous.[76]

These highly technical debates, in which both Charles and Mary Dixon Jones participated when they were recalled to testify, provided the *Eagle* with another opportunity to impugn Dixon Jones's authenticity as an icon of femininity. As the various indications for operations were being discussed during a rather lengthy rebuttal of a large number of both specific and general accusations in regard to the nature of her patient care, she took the opportunity, while discussing the case of one patient in particular, to offer what the paper called a "physiological lecture . . . to the jury." "Mrs. Dr. Jones stood down by the rail in front of the stenographers table,"

and, holding the manikin up before her with her right hand, she pointed with her left hand at the organs under discussion. . . . Soon after this a jar containing the specimens removed from one of the Memmen girls was handed to Mrs. Dr. Jones. She hastily unlaced her glove—the other one had been removed—drew from her hand sachel [*sic*] a pair of shining nippers, with handles like scissors, and removed the specimen from the bottle. Then she dropped the specimen into her hand, laid down the nippers and, after asking the court's permission to go nearer to the jury, walked outside the railing to the box and explained to the jurors what the alleged defections in the organs were on which she had based the opinion that an operation was necessary.

The implication, of course, is that her cold scientific gaze stood in noticeable contrast to her feminine self-presentation. As if to drive home the point, the *Eagle* went out of its way at that same descriptive moment to point out what she was wearing: "a handsome black silk dress, with puffed sleeves, a small black bonnet and gold bowed eye glasses, which she held with a handkerchief in her black gloves." In this instance, the paper insinuated, clothes did not make the woman, but merely masked her true nature.[77]

In terms of struggling with the issue of informed consent, there was a wide range of opinion on how much information doctors should share with patients before surgery. Two key witnesses for the plaintiff, Gill Wylie and Abel Mix Phelps, offered strikingly candid opinions, which contrasted markedly with some of the defense testimony given early in the trial. Dr. Augustus Buckmaster, Dr. Samuel King, Dr. John Rushmore, A. J. C. Skene, and others confessed themselves to be uneasy about Dixon Jones's poor communication with patients.[78] Indeed, Skene had insisted that "the effect of such operations" be explained to "all patients except children and insane people." He always sought the consent of the husband and relatives as well, and "he didn't think you could find a surgeon who would operate on a woman if her husband objected." He was "especially careful to make himself understood by an ignorant woman."[79] In contrast, Phelps rarely discussed procedures with "extremely nervous women incapable of understanding a scientific explanation." Nor was it usual for him "to explain beforehand to ignorant patients" what would occur during "such operations as were performed at the Jones' hospital." For patients like these he merely told them "they must put themselves in his hands." On cross-examination he added that charity patients especially "might be frightened off the operating table" if told what would happen to them. Gill Wylie agreed with Phelps. He had had extensive experience with Dixon Jones and had visited the Woman's Hospital in Brooklyn. "The danger from laparotomies had now become so slight," he declared, "that much less ceremony was observed than there used to be, about obtaining consents, securing assistants, and the like."[80]

RESOLUTION

Skene's comments marked the end of the medical testimony, and here the plaintiff rested its case, concluding the substance of the trial. The following day, Colonel Lamb spoke for three hours, summing up the *Eagle*'s defense with a canny eloquence that touched on all the themes the newspaper's legal team tried to bring out at the trial, but playing especially to his audience's gender anxieties. He sincerely regretted, he began, that the plaintiff was a woman, because to speak the truth about her would not be pleasant. Recalling for the jury his caustic exchange with Dixon Jones at the beginning of the proceedings over how she should be addressed, Lamb feigned satisfaction that she had demanded to be called "Doctor Jones." Happy to be relieved now of the "consciousness of her sex," Lamb cautioned that "in so doing she has placed herself in the ranks of men in a learned and honored profession." She now had the same obligation as her brothers to do right. "She has consented to be judged as a man," warned Lamb, "and as a man I shall treat her."

Lamb went on to recount once more the history of the case. He reminded the jury that Dixon Jones herself had originally requested that the *Eagle* write something about the institution. But when letters incriminating the hospital arrived, and these charges were investigated, the Joneses sent Mr. Payne to reconcile the parties. But the newspaper refused to be silenced, not out of malice but out of a sense of public responsibility. Lamb then revisited Dixon Jones's various misrepresentations, regarding the history of the hospital, the existence of the board of trustees, its shadow advisory board, and its pretentious consulting staff. Why did the hospital issue only one report? Why were its articles of incorporation irregular? Why were prominent names connected with it under false pretenses? Why, if Dixon Jones were trustworthy, would Dr. Caroline Pease, such a "prominent physician, connected with one of the largest institutions in this state," give incriminating evidence against her? "If I cannot make clear to you that this was a private institution supported by public money," Lamb concluded in this section of his peroration, "then I do not understand the value and bearing of evidence."

Next, Lamb turned to the accusation that Dixon Jones had "a craze" for the knife. Indeed, her unnatural passion for surgery at an age when a man of comparable experience might be thinking of retirement should be taken as proof of her mental instability. A craze, he explained "is a strong passion for a certain line of conduct." Did Dixon Jones have it? "Let us see":

> At a time when most men are looking around to retire, this lady takes up a difficult and dangerous branch of surgery. She was 56 years old, a time when the arm which interprets the brain begins to stiffen, when she began this course of laparotomies. No man at that age would have thought of it. Compare her statement of 100 laparotomies at this little hospital with the statistics from St. Peter's, St. Mary's, and the women's hospitals in New York and Philadelphia. I think we shall show you that she took in, as we charged, every woman who complained of a pain in the back or abdomen and operated on them. . . . One by one they went in and one by one . . . they were borne back outside the door either dead or half alive. . . . Hadn't she a craze to operate . . . and so get the practice? . . . We have shown you patient after patient who went here well and strong, doing their own housework, and came out crippled.

It is true, Lamb continued, that the Joneses offered specimens in defense of their diagnoses. But many were missing, and several that were offered were "brought in a mutilated condition." Though the Jones's experts and their "New York doctors" swear that they "found gyroma" in three of these cases, physicians for the *Eagle* do not consider gyroma a disease at all. "I insist," he asserted, "that this woman was operating on every woman she could get on her table to get more specimens in which Heitzman could find gyroma. Had she a craze for such operations or had she not?"

In closing, Lamb took up the question of Dixon Jones's reputation. The first evidence of her bad character ("and reputation is character") was "her treatment of little Annie Phillips." And what was her reputation among neighbors after 1877, and again, in 1884, "when "fifteen women got out of a hospital because Mrs. Jones was connected with it"? Or when the Saturday and Sunday Association refused her application for funds after a thorough investigation? "What was her reputation when twelve doctors of the highest standing have told you that it was bad?" "Reputation," Lamb reminded the jury, "does not rise above character."

"I ask a verdict for this defendant," Lamb concluded, "because it has rendered a great service to the community." It closed the doors of a "bastard" hospital and "staid the uplifted knife of this old woman," who, in obedience to an "unholy craze," was "sacrificing every marital right and all hope of posterity of all the trusting women whom she could coax within its reach." If you examine the *Eagle*'s articles, Lamb pleaded with the jury, "you may find a few weak lines here and there on which to base another verdict," but if you punish the defendant for doing right, "you will bolster up institutions like this and you will throttle a bold press, the only agency through which such abuses can be investigated."[81]

Compared with Colonel Lamb's vivid imagery and forceful language, Stephen Baldwin's concluding statement appeared lifeless; the *Eagle* seemed almost sympathetic as it described him as the individual who had borne the greatest burden of the trial, who had "almost lived in the Jones case for two years" and had endured the last "weary six weeks in the courtroom." Baldwin reminded the jury at the outset that Dixon Jones had already been acquitted of criminal wrongdoing, and that she had already been vindicated by the law. He reiterated his description of her as a simple woman who had to "work for a living," and hence became a doctor in order to do good. In opposition to this innocent individual, he once again drew a picture of a huge, rich, and malicious corporation, a newspaper that had the reputation of being a "mendacious, lying sheet" even before its attack on Dixon Jones. Now the *Eagle* had viciously accused her of every "every crime in the calendar"—murder, manslaughter, and abortion, this last dismissed as by far the "commonest rumor about every doctor." Unfortunately, because the plaintiff was a woman, "nothing could be more natural" than such a rumor "springing up about her." But have the newspaper's lawyers given justification of these charges? Not in the least.

Instead, knowing that their case was weak, they represented the *Eagle* as a defender of conservative surgery, a ploy that would not work any better than its accusations of abortion would. For if opposing radical surgery was their object, why did the newspaper "not attack Dr. Gill Wylie of New York or Dr. Lawson Tait of Birmingham, England, who performed ten such operations to Dr. Mary Jones['s] one?" This was a case of "sensational and malicious journalism" pure and simple, and the jury must put a stop to it. The *Eagle* had destroyed the only reputation that was dear to the plaintiff, that for good works among the poor and needy. Indeed, he concluded, the paper had left the Dixon Jones family doubly bereft, taking from them everything—present as well as future, when they would have "nothing left but a mother's memory." Conspicuously absent from his summary of the facts was an attempt to address the accusations of financial mismanagement, misrepresentation, and deceit.[82]

Following Baldwin's summation, Judge Bartlett gave his charge to the jury. It was a lengthy and clear explication of the law in which he also attempted to recapitulate the highlights of this complicated and protracted case. His statement clarifies a number of issues for the historian as well, and it is particularly intriguing in light of the jury's verdict in the case. As is typical, he began by elucidating the definitions of libel and the points of law that should guide the jury in its decisions.

The alleged libelous material consisted of over twenty-eight articles, the judge began, and not all of them were indictable in part or in full. Libel is the publication in writing of something untrue that brings an individual into "public hatred, ridicule, or contempt." It was the jury's role to deal with questions of fact, while the judge monitored what evidence the law permitted to be laid before them as an aid to passing on questions of fact. The plaintiff has alleged that her professional conduct had been libeled and wants damages.

Charges of libel must involve serious behavior, such as criminal wrongdoing, dishonesty, or unprofessional conduct. The claim that a woman stamped her foot, or engaged in a heated discusssion, Bartlett cautioned, may raise some eyebrows, but it did not fall into the category of libel. Libel involved behavior that was more serious. And there were only a few ways of defending an individual accused of this charge. The first was justification—proving that the allegations were true. In justification, the proof had to be absolute. It would not do, Bartlett explained, for a newspaper to charge a person with murder and prove in court that it was only manslaughter, nor could it allege to the forging of a $20 check, only later to learn that the amount was only $15. This was not adequate justification. However, Bartlett explained, if the jury believed the person being libeled was guilty of *something*, it could, "notwithstanding the strict rule of law," award only *nominal* damages, indicating its lack of sympathy with the plaintiff and its suspicion that he or she was not entitled to compensation.

The newspaper also had the right to argue a defense of mitigation, which, in the Dixon Jones case, consisted of "many elements." Bartlett emphasized four in particular that were utilized by the *Eagle*'s lawyers. First, they argued that the information the newspaper published came from many sources believed to be trustworthy, and from people who were known to tell the truth. Second, the newspaper attempted to prove the existence of rumors in the community affirming Dixon Jones's guilt in performing certain acts in advance of the publication of the *Eagle*'s allegations. Third, the newspaper could claim that its agents were aware of the plaintiff's bad reputation previous to the printing of the articles. And finally, the defendant could plead "absence of malice," claiming that personal spite was not a motive for the *Eagle*'s exposé, a component of the paper's defense that goes a long way toward explaining why Stephen Baldwin chose to underscore the paper's maliciousness in his opening and closing statements.

The judge went on to review what he felt to be the salient issues, high-lighting for the jury aspects of the case on which they should focus their attention. First came the question of whether the hospital truly was a private institution improperly receiving public funds, or a charity of considerable benefit to the community. In connection with this question was Caroline Pease's testimony, vigorously denied by Dixon Jones, that she was instructed to dispense colored water in place of medicine. "That allegation, if true," Bartlett noted, "bears directly and distinctly on the charge that this institution was not conducted for the public benefit." But who is telling the truth? "It is difficult to escape the conclusion that there is perjury on one side or the other," the judge warned. "It is for you to say which of these women told the truth." As for the accusation in the Bates case that the plaintiff made out the death certificate while Bates was still living, there was no dispute that the undertaker found himself in Bates's room before she died. The issue was, how did he get there? Did Mrs. Jones send for him, or was he instructed to come by the family? Again the jury was obligated to determine which story was more believable.

In the case of Ida Hunt, Bartlett felt it would be wrong to assume that she did not know she was to have an operation. The question at issue was why Dixon Jones summoned the woman's husband and parents to the hospital. Was it out of friendship and kindness, as Mrs. Jones contends, or because, according to Hunt's family, the doctor wanted the dying patient removed? Moreover, in the case of Elizabeth Bruggeman, it seemed clear that the body was removed without a permit. But was Dr. Jones aware of this fact?

Did Dixon Jones have a "mania" for the knife? Here Bartlett felt there was evidence to sustain both views. The testimony of a number of doctors supported allegations of unnecessary operations. Yet others gave evidence to support Dixon Jones's claim to the contrary. Expert testimony often involved such "contradictions," he cautioned. Once again the task was the jury's to decide.

Finally, there were four charges for which Bartlett was "inclined to think . . . there is no evidence tending to show that they are true." These included the allegations, based on the statement of Dolly Brown, that Dixon Jones performed an abortion, the charges concerning her treatment of Mrs. Tweeddale and Mrs. Steinfeldt, and the suggestion that the doctor was asked to leave her Bible class because she had urged students to undergo operations. In these instances at least, the newspaper did not muster adequate "evidence to prove the truth." "If I am right in this view," the judge continued, "then . . . so far as these matters are concerned, the plaintiff is entitled to recover nominal damages, and if you think the publication of the articles has injured her, more than nominal damages."

In closing, Bartlett was careful and clear. Mary Dixon Jones was entitled to damages in connection with those four instances where the newspaper failed to give justification. The question for the jury was to determine what sort of damages the doctor was entitled to, nominal or substantial? The rule of thumb in such decisions was "the better the character, the more the damages; the worse the character the less the damages." The jury's opinion of Dixon Jones's character, then, was to be a key element in their decision, and a determining factor in ascertaining the extent of the damages to be awarded. Bartlett made a final comment on the right of the press in a free society to expose all manner of abuse, but cautioned for the last time that such action could be taken only within the limits of the truth. "Take this case, gentlemen," he exhorted, in an inadvertent reminder to us that the jury was all-male, "consider it carefully":

> Try to decide it justly. Do not be influenced by any consideration as to the wealth or poverty of these litigants or by the relative position of the plaintiff and defendant, but pass upon these questions just as though you had never heard of them before you entered court, and as though you never expected to hear of them after leaving court.[83]

The following day the *Eagle* pointed out in an insightful editorial that the only verdict that could vindicate Dixon Jones was the awarding of exemplary damages. Rendering only nominal damages or finding "no cause of action" would indicate that the newspaper had in substance proved its case, failing only in a handful of technical details to justify its charges completely. As the public waited for the decision, the atmosphere in the courtroom remained one of "suspense," according to the *Citizen*, as "leading lawyers and prominent newspapermen" and "public men and distinguished citizens" came and went, mingling with an anxious crowd of "spectators . . . waiting with unflagging interest for the final scene in the trial that has so long been the centre of attraction in various circles in this city."[84]

The jury's task was not an easy one, and there was dissension in the ranks, though none, it appeared, favored awarding Dixon Jones the damages that would have completely vindicated her. A preliminary vote revealed six for the *Eagle* and five for giving Dixon Jones nominal compensation.[85] Unable to move the discussion along, the foreman sent a message to Judge Bartlett, asking that the jury be excused. Bartlett emphatically "declined to comply with the request," and they doggedly returned to their work. Polling each other hourly, they assumed deliberations would be carried into Sunday morning. "We were, therefore, surprised when the clerk told us we would be called into court at midnight," reported one member of the group. "At about ten minutes of 12 this notice was brought to us, and we were told to prepare. Before going in we decided to cast a final ballot. This was done and the result was a verdict for the defendant."[86] The decision had taken thirty-seven grueling hours of debate.

When it was announced, whispers of surprise "culminated in a low whistle of astonishment from the back of the courtroom." Stephen Baldwin, "already pale from six weeks['] exhausting work, turned a shade paler," and rose slowly, asking that the jury be individually polled. The courtroom was quiet as one by one each member affirmed his vote. The judge thanked the jury, rewarding them with extra pay for their "arduous labors," and "Clerk Carr hurried around and dropped a silver dollar into the hand of each." Bartlett then adjourned the court. Mary Dixon Jones had left the room when the jury retired, but Charles waited through the night with Baldwin, showing no emotion when the verdict was read.

The two departed together, and, outside the building, Baldwin, "much taken aback" and hidden from view by a turned-up overcoat collar, "acknowledged his disappointment frankly," speaking of his intention to appeal.[87]

The trial was over, and reactions to it came from all sides. The *Eagle*, of course, was ecstatic, and saw the decision as a victory for the popular press, noting that because juries are notoriously hostile to newspapers, the event represented full vindication of its position and a "moral defeat" for "the woman Jones."[88] On March 14, Judge Bartlett denied Stephen Baldwin's request for a new trial. A week later the Brooklyn Health Commissioner revoked the permit of the Woman's Hospital and Dispensary. On Sunday, March 20, the Brooklyn Woman's Homeopathic Hospital changed its name "to avoid confusion with the Jones hospital." Mrs. J. H. Bartis, president of the board of managers, in a telling interview, announced that the staff included twenty-three women physicians, and that membership in the King's County Medical Society was required. "Under no circumstance," Mrs. Bartis told the *Eagle*, "do we permit an operation until it has become perfectly clear that no other course will give the patient a chance." So far none of the women physicians had ventured to take charge of a capital operation, not because they are not competent, but "because we desire to take every possible precaution." Asked by the reporter whether the Dixon Jones case had proved to be an embarrassment, Bartis replied: "Not in the least." Indeed, women physicians had received a great deal of attention because of it, and have had the opportunity to demonstrate their good character. "We are no more to be judged by the actions of any single individual than any other member of any other profession would be under similar circumstances. One by one the obstacles to woman's advancement as physicians have been removed and she is now very much the arbiter of her own success."[89]

What began with a bang, as a spectacle of uncommon proportion that drew Brooklynites out their homes and into the courtroom to witness a very public discussion of a number of pressing topics of the day—medical treatment, female health, the canons of medical professionalism, scientific and technological innovations, the relationship of personal ethics and middle-class responsibility to public order, and women's roles in a changing society—ended in a whimper. The verdict, a resounding defeat for Dixon Jones, virtually terminated her surgical career. Eventually, she and Charles moved to New York City, and Dixon Jones continued to publish extensively in pathology and surgery, revisiting former operations and case studies and utilizing the specimens and slides she had gleaned from them. But, like Imlach before her, her counterpart in England, her active role as a clinician was over. Even if the affair had not damaged her reputation as a practitioner, she would have been unable to compete with the many renowned male surgeons in New York whose reputations eclipsed hers. She is to be commended for retaining a place in the profession in spite of these setbacks. Throughout the 1890s, male practitioners continued occasionally to refer to her work. Active until her death, Dixon Jones penned one of her last publications after a trip to Chicago in 1905. In it she complained about the difficulty of doing good microscopical work in "smoky cities."[90] She died three years later. No obituaries have been found.

9

Meanings

Sensational public trials tell at least two stories at once. The first belongs primarily to the characters involved. The second, perhaps even more compelling and instructive than the first, mirrors the wider field of politics and culture in which the trial takes place. I have argued from the outset that the Mary Dixon Jones affair was never simply the story of a remarkable and eccentric nineteenth-century woman physician, but should be understood as a public event that opens a window onto Victorian society. Indeed, the trial not only aired significant issues being addressed in the public sphere, but informed and molded the opinions of its audience. It exposed to public debate contentious matters of medical professionalization in various guises, including the emergence of modern scientific values, new technology, specialization, novel medico-legal develop-ments, and innovative approaches to disease, diagnosis, and patient care. The widely attended court proceedings highlighted topics like the nature of class respectability and the problem of middle-class social responsibility, as the ac-countability of private elites in monitoring quasi-public cultural and charitable institutions was considered. Questions about the role of government and the press in guarding the public interest threaded throughout the *Eagle*'s spirited self-defense. Finally, because its central character was a woman, gender and its various connotations at the end of the nineteenth century proved a salient theme throughout, transforming points of community concern in provocative ways.

How might the various meanings of Dixon Jones's career and trials be assessed? I will first address medical issues, asking what these events revealed about professional tensions in Brooklyn and elsewhere. I will then return briefly to the question of middle-class urban culture, highlighting the dilemmas the affair raised for Brooklyn's professional and entrepreneurial elites. Finally, I will take up the issue of gender for the last time, exploring how anxieties and assumptions about changing sex roles shaped the affair in particular ways.

AFTEREFFECTS: SURGICAL DECISION-MAKING, PROFESSIONAL
SELF-REGULATION, AND THE LAW

Both trials highlighted topics that divided the medical profession: indications for surgery, what constituted malpractice, questions of informed consent, radical versus conservative approaches to therapy, grounds for judging operative and diagnostic competence, and the role of pathology in diagnosis. In defense of Dixon Jones came an array of prominent surgeons from New York City and Philadelphia. A. M. Phelps, W. Gill Wylie, H. Marion Sims, Robert T. Morris, and others each confirmed that they had completed hundreds of laparotomies of the type performed by the plaintiff, and that they had consulted with her on numerous occasions. But what is particularly striking about their testimony is its subtext. Though trial transcripts and newspaper accounts do not convey tone of voice or facial expression, my reading of these statements is that the speakers were not particularly close to Dixon Jones or necessarily invested in promoting her career. Yet quite a few distinguished practitioners, some of them at the pinnacle of their careers, traveled across the Brooklyn Bridge at considerable personal inconvenience to give evidence on behalf of a woman who was at best an acquaintance. There is no evidence that these men were more accepting of women physicians than other of their male colleagues.[1] What motivated them? The answer lies in their astute perception that it was not simply Dixon Jones's surgical practice that the *Eagle*'s campaign brought to trial, but theirs as well. In this instance, gender antagonism played second fiddle to rivalries between newer and older conceptions of medical professionalism, catalyzing the urgent obligation of radical surgeons to defend their achievements.[2]

To illustrate how some of these tensions played themselves out, let us explore the issue of malpractice. Contemporaries were acutely conscious of the increase in malpractice suits throughout the nineteenth century, especially those for surgery. Indeed, by the 1880s, many worried that these cases were becoming so frequent that some of the most qualified "medical men are considering the propriety of refusing to attend surgical cases, and confining their practice to that of medicine alone." Difficulties arose partly because definitions of malpractice were in flux and partly because innovative and sometimes experimental techniques raised expectations of a cure and were improperly understood by the lay public. Ironically, it was not the unqualified who were most vulnerable, but doctors like Dixon Jones and her colleagues, who attempted new methods of cure. "As a general rule," complained one practitioner, "malpractice suits are not brought against disreputable and incompetent men, but against our most capable and accomplished practitioners."[3]

Although malpractice law was not uniform and judges and lawyers drew on English precedents in forming American standards, by the mid-nineteenth century experts were in general agreement that, in treating patients, physicians were not required to guarantee a cure, but merely to exercise *"ordinary* care and skill." This standard did not require a doctor to be the best in the field, nor did it preclude making an honest mistake in diagnosis. But it did demand from a physician an accepted level of knowledge and good judgment. Typically in such cases, juries played an important role. While judges were careful to explain clearly to them the legal standards by which they were required to render opinions, much like Bartlett had done at the trial, it was the jury that determined questions of fact, including assessing the standards of the profession at large and deciding what constituted carelessness in specific instances.[4]

Physicians increasingly resented lawyers and juries. Exhortations to the profession to defend its honor appeared frequently in the medical press. Indeed, reading some of these helps us to understand why Dixon Jones, emboldened by her victory in the manslaughter trial of 1890, might decide to bring suit against the *Eagle.*[5] Dixon Jones was a person who clearly failed to perceive how her aggressive and self-congratulatory manner grated on individuals expecting more feminine reserve from a woman practitioner. Nor was she able to predict that public sympathy with her plight was muted by her own demeanor during the trial. Given these blind spots, one can easily see how she might have come to view her own case as a battle fought for important professional principles, particularly when several of her colleagues interpreted the proceedings exactly the same way.

For example, many practitioners struggling with the issue of malpractice gave the Dixon Jones manslaughter trial of 1890 significant attention. The *New York Medical Record*'s undisguised relief at the acquittal was noted in the previous chapter. Others commented on the case as well. For example, at the section on Medical Jurisprudence at the annual meeting of the AMA in 1890, Albert Vanderveer discussed "The Medical-Legal Aspect of Abdominal Section," referring specifically to Dixon Jones's case, as well as to another in which the surgeon performed a laparotomy without realizing that his patient was pregnant. Vanderveer was especially concerned about the ways in which the press might interfere with the legal process. "We all may at any moment be placed upon our defense by clamor of the public press," he observed, "which seldom, very seldom, gets down on the right side of any medical question. Dr. Mary A. Dixon Jones is a conspicuous example of newspaper persecution, which happily she overwhelmed." Yet Vanderveer also expected the public to have "proper protection." He sought a system whereby justice could be rendered "to all concerned in these cases."[6]

Others used the Dixon Jones affair to think through these difficulties. W. W. Potter pointed out how the manslaughter suit highlighted both the attraction and dangers of hospital treatment in abdominal cases. On the one hand, the surgeon is attracted to the advanced equipment and other conveniences that "facilitate the work." But although management of patients in the hospital setting is "conceded to be the best," these methods are "little understood, speaking generally, by the physician in whose charge they have been previously, or for that matter by the general practitioner commonly." Often the result can be criticism arising out of ignorance "excited both against the hospital and the surgeons connected with it." This difficulty, Potter observed, "was lately illustrated in a trial of a prominent operator . . . for manslaughter." He went on to discuss the details of the Ida Hunt case. A woman who had been operated on "desired to go home on the fourth or fifth day." Her friends "cooperated with her," and "she died of septic peritonitis soon afterwards, hence the indictment and trial."[7]

Potter also had something to say about the use of specimens in the courtroom. He felt that they often provided misleading evidence. Experts knew that after a growth was preserved for some time in alchohol, "it becomes distorted, decreases in size, and . . . the original lesion for which it was removed is often unrecognizable." If specimens of this sort happened to fall into the hands of an ignorant and gullible patient, "one capable of being wrought upon by a malevolent medical or surgical 'brother'—Heaven save the name—untold mischief may result."

Potter, like Vanderveer, also worried about interfering newspapers. "It may be proper to add," he wrote, completing his narrative of the Dixon Jones indictment, "that a prominent journal, of a hitherto reputable standing, lent its influence to accomplish the ruin of this surgeon, thus compromising the good name of legitimate journalism. The surgeon happily was vindicated by the court and jury."[8]

The Dixon Jones affair thus also animated the uneasiness of physicians who had already recognized the power of the press to do harm. Two years previously, after Dixon Jones's manslaughter trial, the *Brooklyn Medical Journal* worried about the negative effects of sensationalized reporting of medical stories in the lay press. Only a few months earlier Edwin A. Lewis had complained bitterly of the ramifications of the recent interest of "the secular press" and "some of the better magazines" in "medical matters." The information offered was "so unscientific, if not positively untrue" that it was "harmful rather than of use," with the result being a general public either "over-educated" or "badly educated'' on "matters medical and surgical.'' Unfortunately, ignorance did not prevent people from having an "opinion to offer in every case,'' thwarting the freedom of doctors to make decisions without "interference and disregard of directions."[9]

Detectable in the undercurrent of anxiety about malpractice was not simply a fear of the depradations of unscrupulous lawyers, ungrateful patients, antagonistic juries, and lying newspapers. Perhaps most disturbing of all was the way in which such cases raised fears of a disunited and disorganized profession. One disgruntled practitioner, B. H. Detwiler, complained in a paper delivered before his colleagues at a meeting of the Pennsylvania Medical Society that "no designing lawyer or ignorant jury can convict an honest practitioner, if a dishonest doctor is not behind it all.'' Doctors in the audience agreed. "We ought to abstain from all criticism upon operations performed by regular physicians,'' responded W. T. Bishop of Harrisburg. From Philadelphia, W. E. Hughes added that "in the schools of medicine the students should be taught to support one another, to treat each other as brethren; and an endeavor should be made to inculcate a more kindly, friendly feeling. . . .''[10] Over and over again physicians worried about how to "bury our little petty jealousies and present a united front.'' "Until physicians have that sense of honor which will make them refrain from giving invidious opinions on the work of other physicians,'' Dr. J. H. Etheridge observed, "malpractice suits will thrive.''[11]

Some of this dissension emerged as a by-product of the antiquated expert witness system inherited from the English.[12] According to those procedures, court officials had the power, but were not required, to consult medical experts in any case they deemed fit. When they chose to exercise that right, physicians were subpoenaed to give advice or complete postmortems without the expectation of compensation. Most attempted to avoid such responsibility. But even when compelled to participate, few American physicians had the forensic expertise to perform their duties skillfully. In addition, physicians could be hired to testify by the adversaries in a particular case, which meant their opinions were solicited "not as neutral seekers of the whole truth, but as advocates for one side or the other.''[13]

As suits involving medical testimony rapidly multiplied in the latter half of the nineteenth century—one contemporary estimated that by 1876 the number had soared to approximately 20,000 trials a year—the system reached a crisis. Although, as a Brooklyn physician observed in 1879, "most physicians in active practice are frequently called to testify,'' the increasing dysfunctionality of the procedure proved to have especially negative effects on the medical profession's status and public image.[14] Little wonder that the plight of the expert witness emerged as the most popular topic of medical jurisprudential discussion in medical societies "from coast to coast.''[15]

Complained the *Boston Medical and Surgical Journal* in 1872, "scarcely a trial in the civil or the criminal courts occurs, requiring the assistance of a medical expert, that does not bring into unenviable notoriety, not the medical witness alone, but the medical profession which he represents.'' During these debates, doctors expressed a number of significant concerns. First, many understood the professional risks of medical testimony. A poorly answered question or, worse, a mistake in judgment expressed on the witness stand, could ruin an individual's career. More unsettling was the fact that the hefty compensation paid some individuals threatened to corrupt testimony by making expert opinions purchasable in the marketplace. The pressure on witnesses to tailor their statements flagrantly to meet the needs of patrons had understandably harmful effects on doctors' reputation for integrity. Such a situation not only undermined a sincere desire by leaders of the profession to make a helpful contribution to the field of medical jurisprudence, but generated vociferous mistrust in the public sphere. By the end of the 1870s, newspapers questioned the value of outside medical experts, lawyers opened examinations of physician witnesses with questions about how much they were being paid to testify, and the entire unsavory process made "physicians look scientifically weak, internally divided, and dangerously unprofessional."[16]

One much-discussed solution for dealing with the problem was a revision of the procedures for presenting evidence from experts in court. Doctors were enormously sensitive to the difficulties inherent in being medical witnesses, not only because of the implications of disloyalty to colleagues, but also because they understood quite clearly that their opinions were "used by lawyers on both sides to prove their case" and were "not impartial." As one physician put it, "of all the cant that is canted in this canting world expert medical cant is the most pernicious."[17] In the course of debates over the issue, medical societies began to organize funds to help their members bear the financial burden of malpractice suits and the negative effects of expert testimony that such suits often invoked.[18] But critics also understood that expert testimony had its place. The "fact of the matter is," admitted Judge W. S. Kerr, in an article published in the *Journal of the American Medical Association*, when medical witnesses "appear as members of a great and entlightened profession, to aid in the administration of the law . . . their expertise is needed."[19]

In Brooklyn, among members of the King's County Medical Society, the problem of expert witnesses was being discussed at the very moment that the *Eagle*'s exposé regarding Dixon Jones's hospital first appeared. Indeed, in May of 1889, the *Brooklyn Medical Journal* published a paper on expert testimony given by Justice Willard Bartlett before the Society of Medical Jurisprudence. Throughout the rest of that year and for several years following, the medical society participated in an ongoing discussion of expert witnessing. A number of suggestions were made, including having medical experts appointed by the court, rather than by the lawyers representing each side. Ironically, one of the key actors in stimulating discussion on this topic was Dr. Landon Carter Gray, a practitioner who testified against Mary Dixon Jones at the libel trial and who, in 1893, published a paper carefully reviewing the problem of expert testimony and the various solutions being considered.[20]

Practitioners understood, of course, that differences in medical testimony also indicated changing standards of care and newly emerging styles of practice. Indeed, the successful ascendancy of surgical treatment led to a decided power shift in the medical hierarchy. The aggressive and entrepreneurial approach to professional disputes displayed by younger gynecological surgeons prompted more traditional physicians to lament the passing of an older, gentlemanly image. Suspicion of the new professional style can be detected in the outcry against specialization as elitist and dehumanizing; indeed, similar accusations were hurled against laboratory science. But how did one explain these disagreements to patients when such tensions were aired in public?

Echoes of these controversies and the anxiety they produced reverberate frequently in the 1892 trial testimony. Dixon Jones's critics, almost all of whom practiced in Brooklyn, focused often on the uncertain validity of her therapeutics, but even more powerfully on her questionable professional "character," perhaps in an effort to play down authentic disagreements and present a united front. The testimony of A. J. C. Skene was typical. Known to be a staunch conservative on the subject of ovariotomy, Skene was a recognized authority on women's diseases. He acknowledged that he had known Dixon Jones for fifteen or sixteen years, that she had operated on two of his patients against his wishes, and that he no longer consulted with her. When Dixon Jones's lawyer tried to characterize Skene as a member of the "conservative" as opposed to "radical" school of gynecology, Skene demurred, essentially papering over heated therapeutic disputes with the comment that with good surgeons, "surgery was never resorted to except in cases where life would be in danger if no operation should be performed." Though he and Dixon Jones were close in age, his comment underscores the fact that they were a generation apart therapeutically, because Dixon Jones and her surgical colleagues had been doing exploratory surgery for almost a decade. We remember that others among her detractors questioned Dixon Jones's pathological diagnoses, implying that she had invented them after the fact merely to justify her resort to the knife.[21]

Folded into these questions regarding professional style and therapeutic decision-making was the issue of informed consent, which was both implicit and explicit in discussions of malpractice. The very term "informed consent" is a modern construction, and the wide disagreement among practitioners, even on what it meant, is certainly clear from the trial. Some of the physicians who testified felt that Dixon Jones explained to patients as much as was practical; others said that she was not explicit enough. Increasingly, the medical literature appeared to be suggesting that there was only one way to avoid devastating lawsuits, and that was to be more open and honest with patients. "Do not claim," warned F. J. Groner, "more than you can perform." David W. Cheever agreed. "Do not operate without the full consent of the patient and friends, if possible," he cautioned. "See that some responsible party understands what operation you intend to do, and what may be reasonably expected from it."[22] Perhaps most intriguing, however, was the statement of Joseph Price, a leading radical surgeon in Philadelphia, most probably inspired by his recent experience testifying on Dixon Jones's behalf at the 1890 manslaughter trial.

Reporting on his latest surgical exploits in an article published in the *Annals of Gynecology*, he ventured a comment on the subject of physician-patient communication. Too many single and married women are told by their physicians that "nothing short of an operation will cure them, but without being told the nature, object, and results of the operation," he cautioned. The only excuse for such neglect is the doctor's "supposition that an explanation will scare away the patient and an operation will be lost. Operators so eager for work as this . . . involve themselves in the extremest of contradictions. . . ." As far as his own patients were concerned, "none were operated upon without fully explaining, so far as it was possible, the general nature of the operation to which they were about to be subjected, its reasons, its advantages, its dangers, with honorable carefulness to friends and patient."[23]

Certainly the Dixon Jones affair stimulated these discussions, if for no other reason than because of the way it exposed professional discord to public scrutiny. The response of the editor of the *Journal of the American Medical Association* suggests that most of Dixon Jones's surgical colleagues were embarrassed by her suit for libel and would have preferred a more private venue to air their disagreements. *JAMA*'s comments represented a carefully crafted effort not to take sides, and reflected discomfort with the sensationalizing of what were at the time serious rifts within the professional community. Headlining its remarks "A Triumph for Conservative Gynecology," the journal expressed doubts "whether it is wise or expedient for members of the profession to seem to assent to be publicaly [*sic*] designated as conservatives, and radicals or liberals, in surgery, no matter what may be its branch or specialty. . . . These pseudonyms are misleading to the public."[24]

JAMA's hesitation to publicize dissension was dramatically evident in the city of Brooklyn among leading members of the medical profession during the entire Dixon Jones affair. But there is irony here as well. One thing the affair made clear was the inability of local professional networks then in place to police, discipline, or even adequately monitor individuals within their ranks. Members could be expelled from the medical society, or not admitted at all, as was the case with Dixon Jones. Doctors could refuse to consult with a particular practitioner, and cease to refer patients. But the evidence suggests that Dixon Jones was impervious to such tactics, in part because they were not punitive enough, but also because female patients had their own powerful networks of referral, and they did not always listen to their male physicians. Often women came to Dixon Jones because they preferred being treated by a woman, and she was the leading female surgeon not only in Brooklyn, but in the greater New York area.

The difficulty the Brooklyn medical community experienced in putting a stop to what they believed was irresponsible practice prompts speculation that a number of individuals resorted to cooperating clandestinely with the *Eagle*, willingly feeding the newspaper's reporters information "on background." This would explain the many anonymous letters calling for an investigation that the *Eagle*'s editors claimed to have received in 1889. Indeed, after the trial was over, the *Eagle* flamboyantly ran a headline reading "Doctors Gain by the Verdict in the Jones Case," alleging that "the cooperation [from the medical profession] which the *Eagle* received was of the strongest kind."[25]

In the trial's aftermath, the comments of A. J. C. Skene are again worth noting. Interviewed in his office at Clinton and State streets, he voiced satisfaction with the verdict, making two important points. First, with regard to the best venue for airing medical controversy, he graciously accepted the role of the *Eagle* in creating precedent, despite the suspicions of colleagues nationally that the press could also prove an adversary. But in light of the outcome, how could Skene behave otherwise? "I believe the medical press and the medical societies are the proper media through which to settle all questions under discussion which require settlement," Skene began.

> At the same time, when doctors of medicine get into court in order to try certain causes involving questions of medicine that are largely decided by medical experts, then the decisions carry as much weight as those arrived at in medical societies or in the medical press. So far as the Jones case is concerned, the verdict is as it should be—on the side having the preponderance of superior medical authority. More than that it gave the medical profession of Brooklyn an opportunity of placing themselves on record as being among the most conservative and progressive of scientists who value national reputation more than self-advancement.[26]

The second part of Skene's statement suggests that he had special reasons to be grateful to the newspaper, because in crushing Dixon Jones, it also fought *his* battle against radical surgeons. Its aftermath would surely give Dixon Jones's imitators pause. "The trial has . . . been one of the most notable in the history of medicine in this country," Skene admitted. This was so because it involved "a branch of science not frequently in litigation. The majority of all cases upon which expert testimony is called are fractures and other injuries from accident. So a great deal of light was thrown upon a new field of jurisprudence in the trial of the Jones case. . . . It has shown how the law looks upon our work."[27]

THE PROBLEM OF SOCIAL RESPONSIBILITY: POLICING THE PUBLIC SPHERE

The collaboration between the *Eagle* and Brooklyn's medical profession in monitoring public and professional behavior highlights larger issues raised by the Dixon Jones affair. The *Eagle*'s exposé presumed and proclaimed the function of newspapers to be providing common intelligence to concerned citizens. In that guise, the *Eagle* had wielded a great deal of power, but it also took its cues from what it perceived to be pressing public issues, and throughout the decade of the 1880s the paper cultivated its image as watchdog on behalf of the people of Brooklyn.

We remember that the *Eagle* supported the reform mayor, Seth Low, and began to fancy itself an independent publication with a commitment to civic responsibility. In that role the newspaper took up various political topics, including the ongoing struggle with the inadequacies of the prevailing system of private charity, a subject that engaged many members of the professional middle class. The issue had special resonance in Brooklyn, because the city built its self-image on its residential attractiveness to morally upright families fleeing the depravity of New York. Thus, in the minds of its best people, stories of corruption hurt, and a reputation for scrupulousness appeared even more crucial to Brooklyn's boosters than it did to leaders in a city of New York's size and diversity.

Given what we know about the rapid growth of Brooklyn in these years, its smallness and intimacy was, by 1892, increasingly a useful fiction. The close relations among members of its elite and entrepreneurial classes worked in some ways to Dixon Jones's advantage. There were fewer people to get to know; indeed, some of the gentlemen who initially supported her hospital, like District Attorney Ridgway, were neighbors. It also meant that she lived in a city where women doctors could open viable practices and not be as vulnerable to competition from the powerful leading male practitioners in New York. Yet, just as the genteel could easily cross the bridge to shop, Dixon Jones lived close enough to that premier urban medical center to take advantage of its modern professional facilities and burgeoning opportunities for continuing education.

Moreover, the special reputation of Brooklyn as a "woman's city" suggests that middle-class women there were more visible or influential in the public sphere in a variety of venues. The networks of female patients described in Chapter 6 provide one significant example. Another was the group of female spectators who daily attended the trial. A third is the wives and daughters of the entrepreneurial elite, many of whom supported Dixon Jones in the establishment of her first hospital. Her easy accessibility to key members of the reformist middle class depended, in part, on women taking seriously the idea that a hospital for their sex similar to the one founded by J. Marion Sims in New York was needed, and it is clear from the *Eagle*'s reports that Dixon Jones gathered around her a committed group of prominent women "overflowing with loyalty and devotion" who supported her until the end.[28] We do not know enough about female communities in other cities to do more than speculate about Brooklyn's typicality in this regard. But women's presence in public contributed significantly, not only to the attention focused on Dixon Jones at the earliest stages of the crisis, but to shaping the outcome of the event in the longer term.

In addition, revelations of Dixon Jones's haphazard and casual financial record-keeping, coupled with a larger public discussion of the antiquated role of hospital boards of trustees, spoke eloquently to the increasing complexities of hospital administration. The Dixon Jones affair became a forum for the consideration of such inadequacies in an age increasingly enamored of professionalism and efficiency. The last decade of the nineteenth century was a time when institutions of this kind began moving toward fresh managerial ideals, which included financial reorganization, cost management, business enterprise, and attention to the dictates of the market. Increasingly, hospital administrators were hired who were not necessarily trained in medicine or nursing, but had experience in business and displayed the professionalism and corporate orientation deemed necessary to transform small, idiosyncratic private charities into major urban health care facilities. Although community hospitals like Dixon Jones's performed important transitional work toward a fully modernized system capable of handling more efficiently the needs of a growing multi-class city, they were "flawed institutions," sometimes egregiously so.[29]

Measured against the casual oversight of other small charitable institutions in the city, Dixon Jones's own failures appear much less conspicuous. "They were generally underfinanced and understaffed places where cruel treatment and suffering seemed omnipresent," David Rosner has observed.

> Depending upon the sponsorship and purpose of the hospital, patients were treated with varying combinations of compassion, condescension, and scorn. Often the community's most paternalistic members would organize a hospital with a view toward reforming patients. Treatment sometimes bordered on punishment for working-class patients, considered by some trustees to have "underdeveloped or ill-developed character." Because scientifically based medical services were minimal or nonexistent, physicians and surgeons in training quite literally "experimented" or "practiced upon" these patients.[30]

Given the almost universal inadequacies of these institutions, one can imagine that the *Eagle*'s condemnation of Dixon Jones's facility accomplished several things at once. For the elite, and for physicians involved in similar community hospitals, the exposé separated "good" institutions from "bad," thereby obscuring the failings of all such charitable enterprises and allowing Dixon Jones to take the blame for problems that should have been monitored by the entire community of political and professional leaders. Once Dixon Jones was isolated, and the extent of her deception brought into the open, the slight embarrassment that key figures among Brooklyn's professionals and entrepreneurs might have felt for allowing themselves to be deceived by the use of their names could easily be dismissed as they closed ranks.

In the end, the libel trial is a story very much about Brooklyn's emerging middle class, a community that was extremely conscious of its reputation and the importance of living up to its image vis-à-vis New York. In the *Eagle* articles, the working class and the poor appear primarily as abstractions, and when poor women are described, they are mentioned with a paternalistic concern that emphasizes their difference, gullibility, and subordination. The success of reform politics in Brooklyn, coupled with the recurring edginess of the *Eagle* around the financing of medical charities, suggests that the animosity to Dixon Jones that gathered momentum throughout the life of the affair had much to do with a perceived need to police unruly members of the respectable elite, staking out guidelines of behavior for everyone, but particularly for middle-class women. After all, accusations that Dixon Jones did not behave like a lady represented class anxieties as much as they did any collective disapprobation of poorly behaved and overbearing women.

For Dixon Jones's patients, the opportunity to speak out was especially welcome. Scholars have explored a variety of interesting literary evidence to support the contention that Victorians gendered notions of spectatorship and unbridled emotionalism as female, just as they gendered conceptions of scientific

rationality male. Athena Vrettos's work on late nineteenth-century attitudes toward sickness and health argues that Victorians often viewed disease as a metaphor for larger social conditions and characterized women as particularly vulnerable to "neuromimesis," a tendency to imitate disease symptoms after
reading or hearing about them. Practitioners who discussed its effects saw it as
"a threat to the detached clinical gaze deemed essential for doctors." But there
is evidence that female spectatorship, especially of the sort produced by the libel
trial, offered additional satisfactions to women having little to do with neuromimesis. The trial affirmed their perceptions of their own bodies. These satisfactions could be only dimly understood by contemporary medical theorists and
are easier for the historian to identify in retrospect.[31]

In addition, the trial provided an unusual and opportune public forum to
air disappointments and complaints about the female condition in a manner that
gave those who testified—whatever their class status or convictions about Dixon
Jones as a practitioner—a sympathetic and captive audience. Middle-class
women and poor immigrant women came together to speak in public about the
burdensome experience of their own bodies. This suggests that gynecological
surgery took on a special urgency at the end of the nineteenth century, as advances in medical technique turned ill women's "wants," namely, the desire
for good health, into "needs," the right to demand it from their doctors.[32] The
trial afforded a rare forum for such conversation outside medical journals, to
which lay women had little access. For those who were not just sick, but poor,
and might conceivably have harbored deep and cumulative resentments over the
cavalier treatment they received from the often inadequate and punitive private
charity system and its paternalistic dispensers, the trial offered an opportunity
to complain in public, or at least to identify with and feel validated by the
testimony of those who did. Of course we will never know how accurate the
newspaper's allegations really were, nor what motivated certain patients to testify against her. But scapegoating a woman physician, especially one as "out-
of-bounds" as Mary Dixon Jones was portrayed as being by the *Eagle*, was a
relatively safe way of speaking truth to power.

In addition, as we reflect on the significance of the female body and its
ailments as a potent organizing theme throughout the court proceedings, it is
possible to speculate that, for her detractors, the vulnerable female body and the
obligation of civilized gentlemen to protect it became a cogent and convincing
metaphor for Brooklyn itself, that "city of homes and churches," where carefree
schoolchildren paraded down tree-lined streets, and respectable families lived in
stability and comfort. This is decidedly *not* the adorned and eroticized female
body characteristic of Manhattan's "Ladies' Mile." In making this distinction
I wish to emphasize yet again Brooklyn's representation of itself as a city where
the "Lady Bountiful" image of female gentility overshadowed newer incarna-
tions, especially those that combined "sensuality, publicity, and refinement"
and were projected by frequenters of Manhattan's commercialized zones of pleasure and profit.[33]

In Judge Bartlett's courtroom, the female body (and its parts) could be held
up to full view without incident. It could be discussed scientifically by medical

experts as a decorous public looked on. This fact alone suggests that, by the close of the Gilded Age, the sequestering of Victorian women in the chaste and modest privacy of the domestic sphere was rapidly coming to an end. But for respectable observers of these changes, the body in question was always the one earmarked for motherhood, and decidedly not the one slated for erotic display. The personal tragedy for the women who told of their physical trials was not simply their chronic pain. Even more pathetic, indeed, was the melancholy fact that disease and its cure rendered them incapable of having children. If the female body stood in for the city in the minds of Dixon Jones's enemies, then her alleged violation of patients' bodies represented an even more egregious attack on the social body—indeed, on motherhood itself—and spoke pointedly to the true nature of her shameful breach of Brooklyn's trust.

GENDER AND ITS MEANINGS AT THE TRIAL

Imbricated in the social and professional questions featured in this trial is the role of gender anxieties in shaping both problems and resolutions. The court proceedings offered up the spectacle of a woman physician accused of misusing professional power and expertise to manipulate and harm her female patients. While Dixon Jones's lawyers employed her sex in her defense, urging that her work embraced the "best in femininity," many detractors found her behavior particularly heinous because she was a woman. These critics described her as difficult, imperious, and determined to go her own way. Colonel Lamb's closing statement is revealing in this regard. In choosing to repeat his encounter with her at the beginning of the trial, when she refused to be called Mrs. Jones and claimed for herself the professional appellation of "Doctor," Lamb implied that she had unsexed herself. Elsewhere in his argument he drew on images of witchery, pronouncing her "an old woman" with an "uplifted knife" who rendered women childless inside the doors of a "bastard" hospital, while giving in to an "unholy" craze.[34] These images were powerful and familiar ones in American culture, and by successfully articulating for jurors familiar stereotypes, Lamb may well have helped create a context for their verdict.[35]

In an editorial after the decision was handed down, the *Eagle* repeated and even embellished some of these themes. In addition, the paper painted a portrait of science gone mad. Against the "nullifying industry to which the knife has been perverted" the *Eagle* represented itself as the protagonist of "enlightened science," the guardian of the "lured, the credulous, the illiterate and the self defenseless" and "the champion of children yet to be."[36]

The refrain of science perverted is worth exploring further. Though Americans tended to exhibit more faith in science and technology than their English counterparts, an awareness of the dark side of science was not wholly absent from popular consciousness on this side of the Atlantic.[37] One has only to reflect on the approval in this country of literary works such as *Frankenstein, Dr. Jekyll and Mr. Hyde*, and the Sherlock Holmes stories of Conan Doyle, where the evil Dr. Moriarty was forever being thwarted by calm rationality, to be reminded that scientific progress, when unbounded by social reponsibility, could easily be imagined as destructive. American authors produced no full-length novels exploring such themes, but a respectable collection of short stories about evil or misguided doctors—including Nathaniel Hawthorne's "Rapuccini's Daughter," Stephen Crane's "The Monster," and Charlotte Perkins Gilman's "The Yellow Wallpaper"—suggests that cultural anxieties regarding the misapplication of the healer's art dwelt just below the surface calm.[38]

Anxiety over the meaning of masculinity and femininity structured these larger cultural concerns about medicine and science. Rationality and objectivity, the thought processes of modern scientific endeavor, increasingly represented the province of men, while emotion, passion, and intuitive thinking, now a contaminant to proper scientific endeavor, became identified with the feminine. One interesting theater for the public expression of such ideas was the courtroom, where prescriptive notions of gender were played out in especially dramatic fashion. I refer here to a handful of sensational Victorian murder trials where women were accused of crimes of passion. Again and again lawyers for these women crafted a defense strategy that required the acceptance of a naturalized feminine irrationality. Using new biological theories about sex differences, they painted the perpetrators as victims of passions and emotions more powerful than human volition or will, and the majority were acquitted.[39] These increasingly familiar portrayals of women in the courtroom served as subversive counterimages to the figure of Mary Dixon Jones, who made valiant efforts to identify herself with rational science during her own trial, as when she lectured the jury on the condition of the various organs displayed before the court, or calmly discussed the nature and technique of the gynecological operations she performed. The *Eagle* described her at these moments as cold and unfeeling, allowing the newspaper to typecast her in a painfully ironic way. It both refused her the opportunity to identify with rational science and represented her as disrupter of social order for her valiant attempts to do so.[40]

There is yet another way that the Dixon Jones trial can be linked to general cultural anxieties about changing gender roles. The Mary Dixon Jones affair should be considered in light of an expanding list of late nineteenth-century public scandals that historians of Gilded Age culture have recently explored.[41] David Scobey has suggested that the era's taste for such sensationalism represents a telling example of its "renegotiation of respectability."[42] Angus McLaren adds that the crime of blackmail multiplied in this period specifically because Victorians were especially concerned with reputation in a commercializing world where wealth and gentility were increasingly bifurcated. Indeed, Gilded Age Americans witnessed more than their share of infamous public events. These included political and financial crises of corruption and graft as well as sensational sex scandals, among which Brooklyn's Beecher-Tilton adultery trial, with which the Dixon Jones's imbroglio was compared by an enthusiastic newspaper reporter anxious to make a point, remained prominently at the head of the list.

Although the libel trial was decidedly *not* a sex scandal, it manifested a number of the qualities Scobey notes were crucial to the meaning of the other trials. It provided a public forum for the discussion of sex roles and women's lives, just as exposing the erotic transgressions of male and female members of the elite forced respectable society to reexamine shifts in social sensibilities surrounding the "lady in public." Moreover, the trial had socially "*regulative* effects." The sex scandals "made a spectacle of *both* the pleasures and the dangers of desire, containing the fantasy transgression within a drama of surveillance and shame."[43] The libel trial played a similar role in chastising a woman doctor whose dreams of success were fraught with a different kind of danger. Though it can be argued that Dixon Jones brought opprobrium upon herself specifically because her ambitions compromised her professional integrity, her achievements demonstrated what a determined woman could accomplish, even as she was disciplined for the means she used to attain them.

An additional instance of Dixon Jones's defiance of accepted boundaries, this time professional as well as gendered, was her penchant for self-advertisement. Dr. Reuben C. Moffat, president of the Saturday and Sunday Association, the charitable organization that had denied Dixon Jones's hospital's solicitations for funds, testified that he had been struck by the "pretentiousness of the institution" in offering a consultants' list including Lawson Tait, "who," he explained, "is the first gynecological authority in the world" and would surely have no interest in "this relatively petty hospital in Brooklyn."[44]

Moffat's remarks indicate that, by the end of the century, self-promotion was considered a serious violation of accepted medical professionalism. But while a man could and often did get away with such behavior, Dixon Jones clearly could not. The point is best illustrated by looking at the career of John Benjamin Murphy, a slightly younger contemporary of Dixon Jones's who, as a general surgeon, helped perfect the operation for acute appendicitis and was Professor of Clinical Surgery at the College of Physicians and Surgeons in Chicago. Tall, spare, and "commanding," Murphy nevertheless had a difficult personality, and is recalled as someone with "a singular ability to arouse envy, distrust and dislike."[45] In the 1890s, he continually offended colleagues with repetitive efforts to steal the public and professional limelight, each infraction appearing worse than the last. He aroused such ire in colleagues that his admission to the American Surgical Association was denied for almost four years. One physician, who opposed his membership, insisted that "the self-laudatory egotist who seeks, after the manner of the charlatan, to impress upon an unenlightened and gullible public his superiority to all others, who covets the notoriety which the frequent appearance of his name in the public press may bring, must be persona non grata. . . ."[46] Such a description might have been used verbatim by the prosecution at Mary Dixon Jones's trial.

Yet despite the continual controversy and resentment that Murphy's self-promotion aroused, he is remembered primarily as a "superb clinician, an engaging teacher, and a very skillful surgeon."[47] He remained Chief of Surgery at Chicago's Mercy Hospital from 1900 to 1916, held a professorship at Northwestern University Medical School, and served a term as president of the Chicago Medical Society (1905), the Illinois State Medical Society (1910), and the American Medical Association (1911). He is described extensively in several medical reminiscences and has been the subject of two biographies. In contrast, until now Dixon Jones's achievements have been lost to the historical record.[48]

Not only men questioned Dixon Jones's professional character. Although Mary Putnam Jacobi testified in her defense, other women physicians took the stand and publicly voiced their reservations regarding her medical reputation. We have already reflected on the testimony of Caroline S. Pease, but Pease was not the only woman physician who refused to be associated with Dixon Jones. Annie Brown, practicing in Brooklyn since 1880, also left her employ in 1881, after a period of only nine months, while Eliza Mosher and her partner, Lucy Hall Brown, feared that Dixon Jones would give all women physicians a bad name. Annie Brown claimed that she and another "lady physician" connected with Jones "concluded it was better for us professionally to leave her."[49] Mosher and Lucy Hall Brown explained that they heard about Dixon Jones's bad reputation in 1884, soon after they set up practice in the city. In a letter to Elizabeth Blackwell written the week Dixon Jones's first case report appeared in the *American Journal of Obstetrics*, Mosher stated that

> there are several regularly graduated women who are already members of the Kings Co. Med. Socy. There is one who, judging from her paper read before the Pathological Socy not long since, is rather an able woman, but her manners are beyond description—we could not identify our selves with her safely and she is an element of evil because of her coarseness.[50]

Criticism of Dixon Jones by these women physicians represented much more than discomfort with her personal style. Like some of their more traditional male colleagues, they were suspicious of her willingness to embrace the new ideology of medical professionalism. It has already been emphasized how this ideology was increasingly characterized as masculine at the end of the nineteenth century. The gendering of professional behavior animated by an activist, empiricist, and experimental stance evoked a materialist conception of the body that encouraged the practitioner to think in terms of not the whole patient but specific organs of local infection. In contrast, women like Eliza Mosher and her mentor, Elizabeth Blackwell, one of the leaders of the women's medical movement in the United States and England, held fast to a more familiar approach to patient care—one shared by both sexes earlier in the century—that was now being identified as feminine. In sketching out their concept of the good practitioner, they drew on past holistic relationships to disease and crafted a version of female professionalism that utilized the language of fellow-feeling and sympathy.[51]

Ironically, Dixon Jones troubled the cultural boundaries that they helped erect. One might indeed argue that, in the final analysis, it was not for attending medical school that she was condemned, or for treating women with surgery, or even for running her own hospital. What made Dixon Jones a "persona non grata" was her failure to live up to the feminine images even she and her lawyer endeavored to project. This understood, we must not reduce her complexity to a crude stereotype. Dixon Jones embodied *competing* images of the woman doctor, one a nurturing caregiver, who taught Sunday school in a respected Methodist church on the side, the other a hard scientist. In that sense, she remains a troubling figure, and one not easily contained. Her story demonstrates how far women physicians had progressed by the end of the century as well as how, why, and in what ways they could also be penalized for their achievements.

On the face of it, Caroline Pease displayed absolute sincerity when in a letter written in 1892 she reassured the dean of her old medical school, the Woman's Medical College of Pennsylvania, that the Brooklyn *Eagle* focused idealistically on Dixon Jones's individual infractions, and was not out to embarrass women physicians as a group. Unfortunately, Pease did not have our hindsight. Like Dixon Jones, Pease had boldly chosen to step out of her sphere by becoming a physician and taking up the cause of women's advancement. Her success and the respect she garnered for it from male colleagues likely obscured her recognition of the gendered nature of the professional values she had embraced with such enthusiasm when she became a doctor. Nor, from the vantage point of the late nineteenth century, could she possibly comprehend the ways in which she and women physicians like her participated in the castigation of one particularly unruly member of their sisterhood, whose ungovernable behavior reflected badly on them all.

Dixon Jones appears curiously unaware or impervious to these fast-developing but unspoken prescriptions for female professionalism. Her apparent willingness to forsake the relatively safe but always professionally marginal women's medical community to pursue her self-interest in the world of men not only made the female physicians of Brooklyn uncomfortable, but also allowed the Brooklyn *Eagle* to paint her as a monster rather than a simple anomaly, as a woman who resorted to "the surgeon's knife on any and all occasions, not stopping to consider the small matter of necessity." The *Eagle* implied that her "mania" for surgery reflected monetary greed, an unnatural desire to acquire more laboratory samples for her research, or a twisted urge to deprive women of their childbearing capacities. There was no room in these gendered notions of the woman physician to accept that her interest in radical surgery might have grown out of sincere intellectual and therapeutic judgment. In relation to public assumptions about proper female behavior and the emergent models of comportment for women physicians that we have discussed, Dixon Jones had truly stepped out of bounds.[52]

Verbally aggressive and unwilling to defer to male colleagues, perhaps even dishonest in the financial management of her hospital, Dixon Jones was the nineteenth-century version of the "difficult woman." Hers was an uneasily negotiated identity, one which even some of her female colleagues found unpalatable. Yet while most of them hovered on the margins of medicine, Dixon Jones forced male colleagues to take notice of her accomplishments. For this reason the notion that she probably was unaware of her shortcomings is especially poignant. In several brief digressions in articles published after the trial, she referred vaguely to the persecution of women physicians. In one she wrote, obviously referring to herself, "Women physicians sometimes have very little quarter, and many suffer most seriously, when doing their best, and the best that can be done."[53]

Indeed for much of Dixon Jones's career subsequent to the libel trial she endeavored mightily to erase its effects. In 1894, she reconnected with the female medical world by becoming an associate editor for the *Woman's Medical Journal*, where she began reprinting some of her articles in surgery and pathology. When she was introduced to readers by the editor, she was described as "Mary Dixon Jones of Brooklyn, N.Y., . . . surgeon to the Woman's Hospital," despite the fact that the institution had been disbanded and she was already living in New York. A biographical sketch, probably written by one of the editors from information she provided, appeared a year later, reading very much like a brief in her defense. Dr. Jones, it began, was "descended from one of the first and most artistocratic families in the southern part of Maryland." It proceeded to highlight her early genius, while still a child of "six or seven," when she demonstrated the ability to "carry on long and elaborate mental calculations." It moved on to record a brilliant educational career begun in her early teens at "what was then considered the best college for women in this country." Two letters, one from a fellow teacher at Wesleyan Female College, the other from the wife of the headmaster of the Baltimore Female College, where she taught briefly, sang her praises, as a student, a teacher, a physician, and, perhaps most interestingly, as a mother. "Her highest reach," commented one, "is motherhood—her children are her greatest triumph." The other correspondent called her hospital "the noblest work that God could inspire in a woman's heart."[54]

Yet no amount of Monday morning quarterbacking could alter the painful verdict. In the end, Dixon Jones's inconsistent behavior became a significant factor in determining the outcome of the libel suit. In one way or another, all trials become a forum for the telling of competing stories, and they proceed by "constructing, presenting, and interpreting narrative versions of past events." Laura Korobkin reminds us about the nature of these proceedings, that, from the moment Dixon Jones filed the original complaint in 1889, to the trial testimony, the arguments of counsel, and even the verdict itself,

> litigants, lawyers, and judges are engaged in a constant process of . . . shaping and presentation. To win a case, a litigant must transform the complex and ambiguous data of subjective experience into a persuasive narrative. Not only must that narrative be coherent, consistent, and believable, but it must be unambiguously moral, must demonstrate the litigant's entitlement to win (or to defeat) the case.[55]

In this very important sense, the Dixon Jones affair was no exception. It is clear throughout the case that Dixon Jones's lawyers were hard at work to convince the "jury-audience" of the legitimacy of their story, using, as do all litigants, "what they know or infer about jurors' and judges' values, education, and literary familiarity.'' How and what they chose to emphasize represented ''the teller's best guess about what will persuade the specific audience for whom it is constructed.''[56]

The clarity and believability of the narrative is especially crucial in lengthy and complicated proceedings producing a lot of contradictory evidence, and the Dixon Jones trial was particularly remarkable in that regard, as Judge Bartlett's final comments to the jury made clear. Korobkin's observations are especially acute when she notes that the party who supplies the most believable and persuasive formulation of the facts ''has gone a long way towards winning the case.'' She adds that ''many of the bitterest courtroom conflicts are, at bottom, about which party will control the story framework through which the jury 'reads' the case.''[57]

In accomplishing this task, Dixon Jones and her lawyers floundered, partly because her behavior in court too often contradicted the sentimental narrative they constructed to win the case. While they attempted to represent her as a motherly, selfless, self-sacrificing Lady Bountiful whose only desire was to end the suffering of poor women, a genteel lady whose need to support herself and her three children ended in a malicious and randomly motivated attack by a wealthy newspaper corporation hungry for good copy, Dixon Jones's demeanor eroded the power of those images to persuade. She spoke out of turn on the stand, made comments under her breath, demanded that the prosecuting attorney address her as ''Doctor,'' and began the trial as such an uncooperative and sarcastic witness that, in its opening days, Judge Bartlett felt it necessary to admonish her. Her self-presentation as a rational and objective scientist whose colleagues were all male, her *apparent* calm in the midst of the pathos engendered by the tragic stories of female patients, could hardly have helped to win an ordinary middle-class male jury to her cause.[58]

Ironically, the *Eagle*'s lawyers prevailed by the skillful use of a competing sentimental narrative. Dixon Jones was even an unwitting aid to their side, playing the part they scripted for her better than she played her own.[59] In their hands, she became a mad and unruly old woman—a witch, in fact—determined to rob unfortunate patients of their child-bearing capacities and use their bodies for science, performing experiments geared not to the advancement of truth, but to the selfish promotion of her ill-begotten career. This projection of her power to do evil undermined all her efforts to gain sympathy. She failed egregiously in the attempt to represent herself as the real victim.

Despite the contemporary verdict, however, our own judgment need not be as harsh. History can be kind, and a hundred years have passed since Dixon Jones struggled to achieve great things. Today we enumerate her accomplishments with greater ease and certainty than even she did, despite her fulsome efforts late in life. History is also indebted to transgressors. But for her early missteps, that anonymous M.D.'s note, and the excessive zeal of a newspaper eager to claim its own place in the historical record, Dixon Jones might have received an entry in the *Dictionary of American Medical Biography* as glowing and as unblemished as that of her arch-rival, A. J. C. Skene. Instead, her life opens a window onto Brooklyn, surgery, gender tensions, and American history that might never have appeared had she been as well behaved as Eliza Mosher or Caroline Pease. In the final analysis, such an outcome may be small recompense to Dr. Mary Dixon Jones herself. But with hindsight, we can mark this, too, as one of her many achievements.

Appendix
Bibliography of Dr. Mary Dixon Jones's
Medical Writings

1. "A Case of Tait's Operation," *American Journal of Obstetrics and Diseases of Women and Children* 17 (November 1884): 1155–1161. This is her first operation. The article was presented originally by B. F. Dawson at the May 15, 1883, meeting of the Obstetrical Society of New York. (See *Proceedings* 16 (November 1883): 1191–1193.)

2. "Removal of the Uterine Appendages—Recovery," *Medical Record* 27 (April 1885): 399–402.

3. "Removal of the Uterine Appendages: Nine Consecutive Cases," *Medical Record* 30 (August 21, 1886): 198–208.

4. "Ovariotomy and Disease of the Fallopian Tubes," Letter to the Editor, *Medical Record* 30 (August 28, 1886): 252.

5. "Seven Cases of Tait's Operation," *Transactions* of the Alumnae Association of the Woman's Medical College of Pennsylvania 11 (1886): 33–41.

6. "A Report of Five Laparotomies," *Transactions* of the Alumnae Association of the Woman's Medical College of Pennsylvania 12 (1887): 65–69.

7. "Removal of Uterine Appendages: Five Cases," *American Journal of Obstetrics and Diseases of Women and Children* 21 (February 21, 1888): 159–175.

8. "Two Cases of Removal of Uterine Myoma: One, Suprapubic Hysterectomy; the Other, Complete Hysterectomy. A New Method of Disposing of the Stump. Microscopical Examination of the Appendages. Remarks on the Treatment of Uterine Myoma by

Electricity," *New York Medical Journal* 49 (August 25, 1888): 198–205. Also published in the *Woman's Medical Journal* 4 (April, May 1895): 97–108, 123.

9. "Carcinomatous Degeneration of the Ovaries," *New York Medical Journal* 49 (January 19, 1888): 79. This is a presentation of several specimens at the December 12, 1888, meeting of the New York Pathological Society, and is also noted in its 1888 *Proceedings*, 141–143, and in the *Medical Record* 36 (February 16, 1889): 190–191.

10. "A Hitherto Undescribed Disease of the Ovary: Endothelioma Changing to Angeioma and Haematoma," *New York Medical Journal* 50 (September 28, 1889): 337–345.

11. "Misplacements of the Uterus; History of Cases Showing How in Many Instances They Are Produced; The Accompanying Condition; Microscopical Examinations," *The Pittsburgh Medical Review: A Monthly Journal of Medicine and Surgery* 3 (October 1889): 301–309. Also published in the *Woman's Medical Journal* 2 (January 1894): 1–6.

12. "Another Hitherto Undescribed Disease of the Ovaries. Anomalous Menstrual Bodies," *New York Medical Journal* 51 (May 10, 1890): 511–551.

13. "Suppurating Endothelioma—Myofibroma in a Condition of Necrobiosis—Remarks on the Treatment of the Pedicle, etc.," *Medical Record* 38 (September 6, 1890): 262–269. Also published in the *Woman's Medical Journal* 1 (July 1893): 137–143.

14. "Sterility in Woman—Causes, Treatment, and Illustrative Cases," *Medical Record* 40 (September 19, 1891): 317–336. Also published in the *Philadelphia Times & Register* 25 (August 1892): 170–184, as "Why Women Do Not Become Mothers—Causes of Sterility in Women."

15. "Changes in the Ovary as a Result of Menstruation and Gravity," *Philadelphia Times & Register* 25 (April 30, 1892): 446–451.

16. "Microscopical Studies in Pelvic Peritonitis," *Medical Record* 41 (May 18, 1892): 597–604.

17. "Letter to the Editor: Retroversion in Pregnancy," *Philadelphia Times & Register* 25 (August 6, 1892) 167–168.

18. "A Talk on Subjects Relating to Parturition," *Philadelphia Times & Register* 25 (August 6, 1892): 159–164. This article was subsequently reprinted in the *Woman's Medical Journal* 4 (November 1895): 281–288.

19. "Review of Recent Gynecological Literature," *Philadelphia Times & Register* 25 (August 20, 1892): 227–239.

20. "Shall Mothers Nurse Their Babies?" *Philadelphia Times & Register* 25 (August 1892): 220–221.

21. "Diagnosis and Some of the Clinical Aspects of Gyroma and Endothelioma of the Ovary," *Buffalo Medical and Surgical Journal* 32 (November 1892): 197–214.

22. "Carcinoma of the Floor of the Pelvis," *Medical Record* 43 (March 11, 1893): 292–297. Also published in *Woman's Medical Journal* 4 (April 1895): 179–188.

23. "Colpo-Hysterectomy for Malignant Disease—Some Considerations in Regard to the Operation, Technique, etc., with a Report of My First Five Cases," *American Journal*

of Obstetrics and Diseases of Women and Children 27 (April, May 1893): 525–540, 650–688.

24. Letter to the Editor in Response to Editorial, "Who Was She?," *Philadelphia Times & Register* 26 (December 16, 1893): 1167–1169.

25. "Oöphorectomy in Diseases of the Nervous System," *Medical and Surgical Reporter* 68 (May 1893): 796–806; subsequently published in *Woman's Medical Journal* 4 (January 1895): 1–11; (Feb. 1895): 30–36, 39, 50–52.

26. "A Consideration and Some Criticisms," *Woman's Medical Journal* 2 (April 1894): 80–82.

27. "Microscopical Investigation in the Minute Structure of the Human Organism," *Woman's Medical Journal* 2 (April 1894): 89–90.

28. "Early Operations," Editorial in the *Woman's Medical Journal* 2 (May 1894): 110–111.

29. "The Minute Anatomy of the Fallopian Tubes," *American Journal of Obstetrics and Diseases of Women and Children* 29 (June 1894): 785–802.

30. "Endothelioma of the Ovary," *Woman's Medical Journal* 3 (July 1894): 20–22.

31. "Criminal Abortion—Its Evils and Its Sad Consequences," *Medical Record* 46 (July 1894): 9–16; also published in *Woman's Medical Journal* 3 (August 1894): 28–31, 60–70.

32. "A Report of Some Operations by Dr. George M. Edebohls at the St. Francis Hospital, New York City," *Woman's Medical Journal* 3 (November 1894): 133–136.

33. "Surgical Problems," *Women's Medical Journal* 3 (December 1894): 164–165.

34. "An Open Letter—The Summing Up," *Woman's Medical Journal* 3 (December 1894): 145–149. On abortion.

35. " 'Round the Library Table," *Woman's Medical Journal* 4 (January/February 1895): 19–23, 30–36, 39.

36. "Dilatation of the Cervical Canal," *Woman's Medical Journal* 4 (September 1895): 234–235.

37. "A Series of Thoughts on Abdominal Work," *Woman's Medical Journal* 4 (November 1895): 290–292.

38. "Intra- or Extra-Peritoneal Treatment of the Pedicle, or Total Hysterectomy," *Medical Record* 48 (August 24, 1895): 260–63. Also published in *Woman's Medical Journal* 4 (October 1895): 255–260.

39. "The First Total Removal of the Fibroid Uterus," *American Journal of Obstetrics and Diseases of Women and Children* 23 (March 1896): 405–414.

40. "Laparotomy for Diseases of Women from 1879–1889," *American Journal of Obstetrics and Diseases of Women and Children* 26 (July 1897): 74–91.

41. "A Third Hitherto Undescribed Disease of the Ovaries, with a Review of the Two Former," *Transactions* of the Alumnae Association of the Woman's Medical College of Pennsylvania (1897): 64–70.

42. "Personal Experiences in Laparotomy," *Medical Record* 52 (August 7, 1897): 182–192.

43. "Diseased Ova," *American Journal of Obstetrics and Diseases of Women and Children* 26 (August 1897): 175–201.

44. "Hysterectomy for Fibro-Myomata—Some Early Records—Remarks," *British Gynaecological Journal* 13 (August 1897): 502–565.

45. "Editorial," *American Journal of Surgery and Gynecology* 12 (January 1899): 146–148. This is an odd collection of comments on women physicians.

46. "The So-Called 'Total Hysterectomy' of Dr. R. E. Haughton, of Richmond, Ind.," *American Journal of Surgery and Gynecology* 12 (January 1899): 133–135.

47. "The Third Hitherto Undescribed Disease of the Ovary: Myxomatous Degeneration," *Medical Record* 55 (May 6, 1899): 632–638.

48. "The Fourth Hitherto Undescribed Disease of the Ovary: Colloid Degeneration," *Medical Record* 56 (November 1899): 657–667. Also published in *British Gynaecological Journal* 15 (February 1900): 398–441, 555–578.

49. "Insanity, Its Causes: Is There in Woman a Correlation of the Sexual Function with Insanity and Crime?" *Medical Record* 58 (December 15, 1900): 925–937.

50. "The Origin of Ovarian Cysts," *American Journal of Obstetrics and Diseases of Women and Children* 42 (October 1900): 519–535.

51. "The Origin of Fibroid Growths of the Uterus," Letter to the Editor, *Medical Record* 59 (February 16, 1901): 267.

52. "Studies in the Normal and Pathological Structures of the Ovary. No. 1: The Graafian Follicle," *Annals of Gynecology and Pediatry* 14 (September 1901): 825–845.

53. "Fibroid Tumors of the Uterus, Their Relation to Diseased Adnexae. Origin of Fibroid Tumors. When Is the Proper Time for Their Removal?" *Annals of Gynecology and Pediatry* 14 (April 1901): 460–469.

54. "The Origin and Formation of Fibroid Tumors of the Uterus," *Medical Record* 60 (September 14, 1901): 401–406.

55. "The Opinions of Different Surgeons and Pathologists as to the Origin and Cause of Fibroid Tumors," *Medical Record* 62 (August 30, 1902): 323–331.

56. "Tumors of the Uterus: Their Etiology," *Medical Record* 64 (October 10, 1903): 561–572.

57. "Difficulties in Microscopical Work in Smoky Cities," *Medical Record* 67 (April 29, 1905): 667.

Notes

INTRODUCTION

1. The *Eagle's* 1889 articles on Dixon Jones ran almost daily from April 24 to May 31, 1889. The newspaper covered the manslaughter trial from February 18 to 25, 1890. Reports on the libel trial appeared from February 1 to March 17, 1892.

2. *Eagle*, February 2, 1892.

3. *Citizen*, March 14, 1892.

4. *Eagle*, March 11, 1892.

5. *Citizen*, March 12, 1892.

6. *Brooklyn Medical Journal* 6 (May 1892), 302, and the *Journal of the American Medical Association* 18 (April 1892), 431–442; *Brooklyn Eagle Almanac*, 15 March 1892, for coverage by several presses, including the *Tribune* quote; "Dr. Raymond Horsewhipped," New York *Times*, May 3, 1892; for other *Times* coverage see February 2, 4, 12, 13, 15, March 17, May 10, December 30, 1892. The Brooklyn *Citizen* covered the trial almost daily from February 1 through March 14; New York *Daily Tribune*, February 2, 4, 9, 10, 11, 16, 18, 24, March 12, 14. The Beecher-Tilton scandal involved accusations first published in October 1872 by the women's rights and free love advocate Victoria Woodhull in her newspaper, *Woodhull and Claflin's Weekly*. She accused the most renowned minister of the age, Henry Ward Beecher, of committing adultery with Elizabeth Tilton, the wife of his friend and congregant Theodore Tilton. Although Beecher and powerful members of his Brooklyn-based Plymouth Church succeeded in suppressing the story for almost three years, Tilton eventually filed criminal charges, and, in 1875, a six-month trial ensued that created a national sensation. In the end, Beecher was acquitted when the jury could not agree to convict.

7. See the New York *Times*, May 3, 10, 1892.

8. Howard Kelly and Walter Burrage, eds., *Dictionary of American Medical Biography* (New York: D. Appleton, 1928), 677.

9. One juror was excused halfway through the trial because he was experiencing financial hardship.

10. Robert Darnton, *The Great Cat Massacre and Other Episodes in French Cultural History* (New York: Basic Books, 1984), 3. There are many works that can be cited here, and my list is far from definitive and will be confined to works that influenced me. Natalie Zemon Davis's *The Return of Martin Guerre* (Cambridge, Mass.: Harvard Univ. Press, 1983), is a good place to begin, and inspired me to write about Mary Dixon Jones. Also influential are Carlo Ginsburg, *The Cheese and the Worms: The Cosmos of a Sixteenth-Century Miller* (New York: Penguin Books, 1982); Jonathan Spence, *The Question of Hu* (New York: Random House, 1988); Gene Brucker, *Giovanni and Lusanna: Love and Marriage in Renaissance Florence* (Berkeley: Univ. of California Press, 1990); Robin Wagner-Pacifici, *The Moro Morality Play: Terrorism as Social Drama* (Chicago: Univ. of Chicago Press, 1986); Angus McClaren, *A Prescription for Murder: The Victorian Serial Killings of Dr. Thomas Neill Cream* (Chicago: Univ. of Chicago Press, 1993); Altina Waller, *The Reverend Beecher and Mrs. Tilton: Sex and Class in Victorian America* (Amherst: Univ. of Massachusetts Press, 1982).

11. See Robert Hariman, ed., *Popular Trials: Rhetoric, Mass Media, and the Law* (Tuscaloosa: Univ. of Alabama Press, 1990), Introduction, 3.

12. For a very helpful review article which links the new work in science to the history of medicine, see John Harley Warner, "The History of Science and the Sciences of Medicine," in Arnold Thackray, ed., *Constructing Knowledge in the History of Science. Osiris* 10 (1995), 164–193. The other essays in this volume are also exemplary. For feminist-inspired histories of science and the body, see Londa Schiebinger, *The Mind Has No Sex? Women in the Origins of Modern Science* (Cambridge, Mass.: Harvard Univ. Press, 1989); Thomas Laqueur, *Making Sex* (Cambridge, Mass.: Harvard Univ. Press, 1990); Cynthia Russett, *Sexual Science* (Cambridge, Mass.: Harvard Univ. Press, 1989); Ludmilla Jordanova, *Sexual Visions: Images of Gender in Science and Medicine between the Eighteenth and Twentieth Centuries* (Madison: Univ. of Wisconsin Press, 1989); Joan Jacobs Brumberg, *Fasting Girls: The Emergence of Anorexia Nervosa as a Modern Disease* (Cambridge, Mass.: Harvard Univ. Press, 1988); Barbara Duden, *The Woman Beneath the Skin* (Cambridge, Mass.: Harvard Univ. Press, 1991). For the way such work helped me rethink some of my own approaches to the history of women physicians, see Regina Morantz-Sanchez, "Feminist Theory and Historical Practice: Rereading Elizabeth Blackwell," *History and Theory*, Beheft 31 (1992): 51–69.

13. Regina Morantz-Sanchez, *Sympathy and Science: Women Physicians in American Medicine* (New York: Oxford Univ. Press, 1985).

14. Cynthia Russett's *Sexual Science* (Cambridge, Mass.: Harvard Univ. Press, 1989) is the best single volume on these developments.

15. Much of this work has been stimulated by efforts to elaborate on Jurgen Habermas's notions of the public sphere. Scholarship has emerged in a variety of disciplines and directions. For a clear statement of Habermas's theories and how they are being developed, see Craig Calhoun's introduction and the other articles in Craig Calhoun, ed. *Habermas and the Public Sphere* (Boston: MIT Press, 1992).

16. Stuart Blumin, *The Emergence of the Middle Class: Social Experience in the American City, 1760–1900* (New York: Cambridge Univ. Press, 1989), 138–140. There is a vast literature on this subject, and I will cite only representative examples here:

Katherine C. Grier, *Culture and Comfort: People, Parlors and Upholstery, 1830–1930* (Northhampton: Univ. of Massachusetts Press, 1988); Susan Strasser, *Never Done: A History of American Housework* (New York: Pantheon Books, 1988); Margaret Marsh, *Suburban Lives* (New Brunswick, N.J.: Rutgers Univ. Press, 1990); Gwendolyn Wright, *Moralism and the Model Home* (Chicago: Univ. of Chicago Press, 1980) and *Building the Dream: A Social History of Housing in America* (New York: Pantheon Books, 1981); Steven Mintz, *A Prison of Expectations: The Family in Victorian Culture* (New York: New York Univ. Press, 1985); Mary Ryan, *Cradle of the Middle Class: The Family in Oneida County, New York, 1790–1865* (New York: Cambridge Univ. Press, 1982); Karen Haltunnen, *Confidence Men and Painted Women: A Study of Middle-Class Culture in America, 1830–1870* (New Haven: Yale University Press, 1982). For the English context, Leonore Davidoff and Catherine Hall, *Family Fortunes: Men and Women of the English Middle Class, 1780–1850* (Chicago: Univ. of Chicago Press, 1987).

17. Blumin, *Emergence of the Middle Class*, 138–140. For associational life, see Davidoff and Hall, *Family Fortunes*, 416–450. For the larger context, see Geoff Eley, "Nations, Publics, and Political Cultures: Placing Habermas in the Nineteenth Century," in Craig Calhoun, ed., *Habermas and the Public Sphere* (Cambridge, Mass.: Harvard Univ. Press, 1992), 289–339, 292. For the withdrawal of the elite from formal politics, see Mary Ryan, "Gender and Public Access: Women's Politics in Nineteenth-Century America," in Calhoun, ed., *Habermas*, 258–288, 276, 277.

18. Nancy Fraser critiques Habermas's basic categories of social analysis, in which economic and state apparatuses are distinguished from the "lifeworld," or private sphere of the family. See "What's Critical About Critical Theory? The Case of Habermas and Gender," in Seyla Benhabib and Drucilla Cornell, eds., *Feminism as Critique* (Minneapolis: Univ. of Minnesota Press, 1987), 31–55, 45.

19. The ground-breaking reconceptualization of white middle-class women's associational activity came with Paula Baker, "The Domestication of Politics," *American Historical Review* 89 (June 1984): 620–648, but the work on female quasi-political activity in the nineteenth century was already quite rich and continues to be vibrant.

20. Quote from James J. Walsh, "Women in the Medical World," *New York Medical Journal* 96 (1912): 1324–1328, 1324. For an extensive discussion of these arguments, see Morantz-Sanchez, *Sympathy and Science*, 47–63.

21. Morantz-Sanchez, *Sympathy and Science*, 90–265. On women doctors, see Mary Roth Walsh, *"Doctors Wanted: No Women Need Apply"* (New Haven: Yale Univ. Press, 1977), passim; Gloria Moldow, *Women Doctors in Gilded-Age Washington* (Urbana: Univ. of Illinois Press, 1987); Barbara Sicherman, *Alice Hamilton: A Life in Letters* (Cambridge, Mass.: Harvard Univ. Press, 1984); Virginia Drachman, *Hospital with a Heart* (Ithaca: Cornell Univ. Press, 1984); Thomas N. Bonner, *To the Ends of the Earth: Women's Search for Education in Medicine* (Cambridge, Mass.: Harvard Univ. Press, 1992).

22. For a helpful historical discussion of the transition to the linguistic turn and its effects on social history, see Geoff Eley, "Is All the World a Text? From Social History to the History of Society Two Decades Later," in Terence McDonald, ed., *The Historic Turn in the Human Sciences* (Ann Arbor: Univ. of Michigan Press, 1996).

23. Kelly and Burrage, eds., *Dictionary of American Medical Biography*, 677. Webster's Dictionary defines "obliquity" as "deviation from moral rectitude or sound thinking" (*Webster's Ninth New College Dictionary*, 1985). "The Nestor of surgery" is probably a reference to Dr. A. J. C. Skene, whom we will meet in the course of this narrative.

NOTES TO CHAPTER ONE

1. Reflex theory dominated medical thinking in the latter half of the nineteenth century, although there were numerous challenges to it by this period. "Reflex irritation" as Glover meant it was that nervous connections between the pelvic region and the brain may have been causing Hunt's headaches, triggered by minor inflammation of the uterine or ovarian region. Radical surgeons took pelvic inflammation seriously and advised the surgical removal of the source, perhaps a diseased ovary or fallopian tube. Conservative physicians sanctioned operations only in the most extreme and obvious cases of diseased organs, while psychiatrists tended to reject surgery altogether as an effective solution. See Edward Shorter, *From Paralysis to Fatigue: A History of Psychosomatic Illness in the Modern Era* (New York: Free Press, 1992), 40–68, for a summary of reflex theory, and Nancy Theriot, "Women's Voice in Nineteenth-Century Medical Discourse: A Step Toward Deconstructing Science," *Signs* 19 (Autumn 1993): 1–31, for disagreements between surgeons and psychiatrists.

2. *Eagle*, May 3, 1889.

3. Ibid.

4. Ibid.

5. Raymond Schroth, *The Eagle and Brooklyn* (Westport, Conn.: Greenwood Press, 1974), 92, 95.

6. On Knapp see the New York *World*, February 23, 1890, p. 18, and the *Eagle*, June 9, 1889, p. 10. Knapp was widely known for his presidential connections, and often held parties for former national leaders.

7. *Eagle*, April 24, 1889.

8. Ibid. The *Eagle* later retracted this claim and admitted instead that the two had donated money to the institution.

9. Both of these notes are printed verbatim in the *Eagle*'s first article on Mary Dixon Jones, April 24, 1889.

10. Ibid.

11. Ibid.

12. Actually, the hospital published only one report, for the year 1886 (Brooklyn: Eagle Book Printing, 1887). It was extremely impressive, claiming the special work of the institution to be the treatment "of poor women suffering from those many distressing diseases to which women are liable." It argued that a hospital was more suitable than their homes to restore the health of "these mothers, wives and daughters." According to the report, the hospital had five objects: an In-Department for the treatment of women's diseases, a special building for the performance of gynecological surgery, an In-Department for other types of surgery, an In-Department to treat surgical and noninfectious diseases of children, and an Out-Patient Department for the ambulatory care of women and children; see p. 4. The report does not say which of these goals had yet been attained. It was this report that listed a number of leading Brooklyn businessmen and politicians as "Trustees and Incorporators" and advertised a group of "consulting Surgeons and Physicians" that was a veritable *Who's Who* of leading practitioners in New York, with Lawson Tait, of Birmingham, England, in a category by himself as "Honorary Consulting Surgeon." The hospital claimed to have seen 4,525 patients in the outpatient department in 1886. Eleven abdominal sections were performed with a mortality rate of 5.2%, compared with the "reports of general hospitals" as between "25 or 50 per cent . . . for this class of operations," 13–14. The treasurer (William R. Taylor) attested to receipts from all sources at $7,030.17, expenditures at $5,550.22, with a balance of $1,479.95. A copy of the hospital report is in the New York Pathological Society Papers at the New York Academy of Medicine Archives.

13. Ibid. For reasons that will become apparent later in this chapter, a subcommittee investigating the affair authorized by the New York Pathological Society was given a copy of the trustees' minutes, and took extensive notes. Although few trustees showed up for meetings, the minutes appear quite official, and the hospital seems to have transacted its affairs in businesslike fashion. See New York Pathological Society Minutes, New York Academy of Medicine Archives.

14. For a detailed account of the closing of the first hospital and the conflict that occurred between Dixon Jones and the Board of Lady Managers, see *Eagle*, May 4, 1889, and February 5, 8, 1892. It is noteworthy that the hospital report published in 1887 in no way acknowledged this complicated history and led readers to believe that there was only one hospital, founded in 1881. See p. 3: "The Hospital was founded in 1881 for the reception and treatment of poor women suffering from those many distressing diseases to which women are liable." See report in New York Academy of Medicine Archives.

15. The information cited above can be found in the April 24, 1889, edition of the *Eagle*, entitled "YES OF COURSE! The Eagle Will Examine the Woman's Hospital."

16. Ibid. District Attorney James Ridgway actually drew up the second hospital's Articles of Incorporation in 1884, charging no fee. See notes on Trustees Minutes, New York Pathological Society MSS, New York Academy of Medicine, 3. For information on Ridgway's career, see Henry R. Stiles, ed., *The Civil, Political, Professional and Ecclesiastical History and Commercial and Industrial Record of the County of Kings and the City of Brooklyn, N.Y. from 1683 to 1884* (New York: W. W. Munsell, 1884), 2: 1254; Henry W. B. Howard, ed., *The Eagle and Brooklyn: The Record of the Progress of the Brooklyn Daily Eagle, Issued in Commemoration of its Semi-Centennial and Occupancy of its New Building: Together with the History of the City of Brooklyn From Its Settlement to the Present Time* (Brooklyn: Brooklyn Daily Eagle, 1893), 426–428.

17. See April, 25, 1889. "Hungry Joe" was the nickname of a notorious Brooklyn criminal and confidence man, and the headline became one of the many libelous phrases cited by Dixon Jones's lawyers in the 1892 court case.

18. Ibid.

19. Ibid.

20. See April 26 and 27, 1889. For other articles briefly touching on the *Eagle*'s accusations of misrepresentation and financial dishonesty see May 8, 10, 12, 1889.

21. *Eagle*, May 2, 1889.

22. Ibid.

23. Ibid. See Morris Vogel, *The Invention of the Modern Hospital, Boston, 1870–1930* (Chicago: Univ. of Chicago Press, 1985), 75–77.

24. Ibid.

25. May 6, 1889.

26. May 7, 1889.

27. May 9, 10, 1889.

28. May 10, 1889. The physician who saw Tweeddale after Dixon Jones's operation was Dr. Matthew Howard. Dixon Jones also told Tweeddale that her two daughters, both in their early twenties, were ill, and that they, too, should submit to ovariotomy. Howard believed that they were perfectly healthy.

29. May 11, 1889. See also the similar case of Mrs. Margaret Fisher, the wife of a carpet salesman who was told she needed a "slight operation" for retroversion and laceration. When it was over Dixon Jones told her she could still have children, but she later learned from Charles that she could not (*Eagle*, May 14, 1889). Mrs. A. E. Schultz also testified that she had not authorized the ovariotomy performed on her (*Eagle*, May

19, 1889), as did Dr. C. Lundbeck, on behalf of his patient Mrs. Hutton, the wife of a shoemaker, who had come to him for treatment after she had been operated on by Jones. See *Eagle*, May 11, 1889.

30. *Eagle*, May 9, 1889.

31. See also the comments of Mr. Henry Hall, Mr. Charles A. Dayton, Mr. Samuel Pelgrift, and Mrs. Albert Miller, *Eagle*, May 8, 1889. It is interesting that their middle-class aspirations did not extend to being uncomfortable with a saloon in the neighborhood.

32. See the very end of the article appearing in the *Eagle* on May 12, 1889. For an excellent discussion of the meanings of vivisection in this period, see James Turner, *Reckoning with the Beast: Animals, Pain and Humanity in the Victorian Mind* (Baltimore: Johns Hopkins Univ. Press, 1980); and, more recently, Susan Lederer, *Subjected to Science: Human Experimentation in America before the Second World War* (Baltimore: Johns Hopkins Univ. Press, 1995).

33. *Eagle*, May 8, 1889.

34. *Eagle*, May 9, 10, 1889. Actually, after investigating the matter, the *Eagle* reported that two separate death certificates had been made out for Bruggeman. The first indicated heart disease as the cause of death; the second, heart disease complicated by a fibroid tumor. When he received the death certificate, Bruggeman's husband was distressed to learn that the Order of Chosen Friends, to which his wife belonged and with which she held an insurance policy, would not pay out with heart disease as the sole cause of death. Believing that his wife died because of the surgery, Bruggeman understandably went to see Dixon Jones about the matter. Dixon Jones allegedly agreed to alter the death certificate *for a fee*, which Bruggeman paid. The first document remained on the file with the Health Department, while the second was sent to the Order of Chosen Friends, which eventually paid out on the policy.

35. *Eagle*, May 10, 1889. See also May 6, 1889, for a lengthy discussion of her charges to O. P. Miller, which the *Eagle* clearly implied were excessive. Mrs. John McCormick told the *Eagle* that the Joneses had misrepresented their fees to her. See May 11, 1889. The *Eagle* was appalled that Dixon Jones tried to bill Sarah Bates's husband $750 for her fatal operation. See May 2, 1889. See May 12, 1889 for a clear summary of these charges.

36. May 4, 1889. Water cure offered an alternative therapeutics to regular, allopathic medicine. It involved the use of water in a variety of ways, both internally and externally, and was highly critical of the harsh measures of what it termed "heroic medicine." Water cure spas existed in various resorts in the East and Midwest, and water cure was very popular with women because of its emphasis on self-help, diet, and exercise as an alternative to drugs. But by the 1880s public interest in sectarian medicine was waning.

37. This history is inaccurate. Dixon Jones was from Maryland and settled in Brooklyn after the Civil War. She had earned a diploma from the New York Hygeio-Therapeutic College in New York and it was perfectly legal. She had also read medicine with two prominent physicians in Maryland. Her practice did cater to women and children, as did the practices of most women physicians at the time. See Chapter 3.

38. *Eagle*, May 4, 1889.

39. Emphasis mine.

40. The *Eagle* reported that Annie Phillips "is now a happy young wife and mother, living in Hoboken," May 4, 1889. More details of this incident came out in the 1892 libel trial. See Tenney's testimony, February 9, 1892, and the testimony of Charles

Dixon Jones and his sister, Mary, March 1, 2, 1892. They claimed Annie was always treated kindly, like a member of the family. On Tenney, see *The Eagle and Brooklyn*, 483; *The National Cyclopaiedia of American Biography* (n.d., n.p.), vol. 2: 334–335; and *Appleton's Cyclopaiedia of American Biography* (New York: T. Appleton & Co., 1900), vol. 7: 261.

41. This individual was George C. Moffat, who was affiliated with the Women's Homeopathic Hospital of Brooklyn. Mentioning his homeopathy was Dixon Jones's attempt to taint him with sectarianism, in spite of the fact that the AMA had voted to allow regular physicians to consult with homeopaths by this time, just as the *Eagle* had hoped to delegitimate her by dredging up her water cure connections.

42. May 4, 1889. For more on Moffat see William Harvey King, ed., *History of Homeopathy and Its Institutions in America* (New York: Lewis Publishing, 1905), v. 1: 102, v. 4: 59, 278, and Thomas L. Bradford, ed., *Homeopathic Bibliography of the United States* (Philadelphia: Boericke & Tafel, 1892), 209.

43. May 10, 1889.

44. May 14, 1889.

45. May 10, 1889. Among the group were Drs. Carolan, Barber, Grover, Howard, and Shepard, all of whom made statements to the newspaper. See also Skene's testimony at the libel trial, February 19, 1892. On Skene see later chapters and Harvard Kelly and Walter Burrage, eds., *American Medical Biographies* (Baltimore: Norman, Remington, 1920), 1058–1059.

46. Ibid. The paper erroneously calls the woman Dr. DeForest, but in the 1892 libel trial it is made clear that she was Dr. Caroline Pease. See Pease's testimony, *Eagle*, February 9, 1892. On Emery, see Irving A. Watson, *Physicians and Surgeons of America* (Concord, N.H.: Republican Press Association, 1896), 433.

47. *Eagle*, May 18, 1889. Performing an abortion was an accusation that carried with it significant public and professional disapprobation. By the end of the nineteenth century physicians had come out emphatically opposed to abortion, as it had been criminalized, and women doctors especially were careful to avoid the sullying association because earlier in the century the term "doctress" was usually a synonym for "abortionist."

48. "Dr. King Thinks That Insanity Is at the Bottom of It," *Eagle*, May 10, 1889. Sims was J. Marion Sims's son. See Floyd Elwood Keene, ed., *Album of Fellows of the American Gynecological Society, 1876–1930* (Philadelphia: Wm. J. Duncan, 1930), 538. For Mundé, see Kelly and Burrage, eds., *American Medical Biographies*, 833, and "Paul F. Mundé: In Memoriam," *American Journal of Obstetrics* 45 (April 1902): 556–561. On King, see Thomas Herringshaw, ed., *American Physician and Surgeon Blue Book* (Chicago: American Blue Book Publishers, 1919), 266.

49. May 12, 1889.

50. May 14, 1889.

51. Ibid. On May 19 the *Eagle* published a letter from Dr. Lundbeck asserting that Mrs. Strome was not competent even to dictate the communication credited to her.

52. May 17, 1889.

53. June 14, 1889.

54. Ibid.

55. Ibid.

56. Note, in contrast, the *Eagle*'s attorney arguing in 1892: "And, gentlemen, the hospital was Jones, Jones—all Jones!" *Eagle*, February 4, 1892.

57. Ibid. This is a separate article from the one on the Committee of Five and appears at the end of the newspaper, rather than on the front page, under the headline

"A Board of Five Made Up to Whitewash Mrs. Mary Ann [*sic*] Dixon Jones. Mr. Moss Makes a Candid Admission—He Lent His Name for Three Weeks. . . ."

58. The *Eagle* had a daily circulation of 45,000, the *Citizen* a circulation of 25,000. For purposes of comparison, the New York *Tribune* had 75,000 readers and the New York *Times* 30,000. Statistics are for 1892. *Remington Brothers' Newspaper Manual* (New York: 1892), 139, and N. W. Ayer & Son's *American Newspaper Annual* (Philadelphia: N. W. Ayer & Son), 1892.

59. This editorial was not written in connection with the Woman's Hospital controversy, but was printed in defense of one of its original incorporators, S. V. White, a banker who apparently was suing the *Eagle* for libel. There was a story on Dixon Jones that day as well, covering her public denial in a suit for $50,000 in damages brought against her by Mrs. Steinfeldt, one of the unhappy patients referred to in the *Eagle*'s series. The tone of the article was to take Dixon Jones at her word. See *Citizen*, May 26, 1889.

60. *Citizen*, May 31, 1889. The *Eagle* does not mention the libel suit in its articles.

61. *Citizen*, June 4, 1889.

62. *Citizen*, June 7, 1889.

63. June 2, 7, 1889.

64. See Harold Syrett, *The City of Brooklyn, 1865–1898: A Political History* (New York: Columbia Univ. Press, 1944), 159–161, who notes that when the paper "was not defending the ring, it was attacking the *Eagle*." For information on McLean, see obituary in New York *Times*, December 6, 1922, 19; *The National Cyclopaedia of American Biography* (New York: James T. White and Co. 1906), 552–553; Henry W. B. Howard, ed., *The Eagle and Brooklyn*, 209; Schroth, *The Eagle and Brooklyn*, 97.

65. *Citizen*, June 8, 1889.

66. See editorial, ibid. The Packer Institute was a local institution well respected by the Brooklyn elite. Many compared it to Vassar in quality of education and training. See a report of the Packer Commencement in the *Citizen*, June 12, 1889.

67. Ibid.

68. See editorial, June 8, 1889.

69. *Citizen*, June 9, 1889. It is hard to tell what the *Citizen*'s motive was here, but it might have been a case of the pot calling the kettle black. Whereas the *Eagle* was founded in 1840 and had a well-established reputation, the *Citizen* was the "new kid on the block" and had been in existence only four years. While the *Eagle*'s circulation was clearly the greater, the *Citizen* had done extremely well, building to a figure of 25,000 by 1892. See *Remington Brothers' Newspaper Manual*, 139. See also *Citizen*'s editorial of June 10, 1889, where it describes the writer of the articles in the singular, hinting that perhaps it was the reporter, presumably Sidney Reid, who was "concocting stories out of his own foul and mischievous imagination," that "even the editor of the paper must have been startled by." These comments are perhaps meant to imply that the *Citizen* knew more than it was willing to say in print.

70. *Citizen*, June 10, 1889. See editorial as well as the article.

71. Emphasis mine. Editorial, *Citizen*, June 11, 1889.

72. This letter was printed in full in the *Citizen* on June 8, 1889, and was allegedly sent to the *Eagle* and initially suppressed.

73. *Citizen*, June 10, 1889. For additional patient testimonies, see *Citizen*, June 17, 1889.

74. Note this statement from the *Citizen*: "The dispensary in Fleet place has an average of thirty patients a day, or about 5,000 a year. Yesterday 70 cents was collected from fifteen patients" (June 11, 1889). On June 12, the *Citizen*'s reporter wrote of a

visit to the hospital, where it interviewed convalescing patients, all of whom testified to kind treatment and excellent medical and nursing care.

75. *Citizen*, June 11, 1890.

76. Ibid.

77. See news article and editorial in *Citizen*, June 14, 1889.

78. See news article and editorial in *Citizen*, June 15, 1889. See also editorial, June 16, 1889, and a recapitulation of events around the report in an editorial, June 18, 1889.

79. *Citizen*, June 20, 1889.

80. A typical example of these letters was that from Dr. Paul F. Mundé, connected with the Woman's Hospital in New York (see Chapter 2), who wrote: "Dear Doctor: I beg to acknowledge the receipt of your letter of 20th inst. informing me of my election as consulting surgeon to the hospital. Permit me to express to the Board of Trustees through you my appreciation of the compliment and my acceptance of the position. Will you kindly send me a prospectus of the hospital with list of officers, etc." John A. Wyeth wrote: "My dear Doctor: Your letter informing me of my election as consulting surgeon to the Woman's Hospital of Brooklyn was duly received. I accept the position and feel honored in being appointed." The *Citizen* printed fourteen letters of acceptance, all from New York physicians (*Citizen*, June 22, 1889). On Phelps, a prominent orthopedic surgeon, see obituary, *Medical Record* 62 (1902): 583–584. On Dawson, see Chapter 3.

81. *Citizen*, June 24, 1889.

82. Ibid., news story and editorial.

83. *Citizen*, September 11, 23, 1889.

84. *Citizen*, June 24, 1889, also "The Jones Case Summed Up," June 23, 1889.

85. June 1, 1889. On the career of Eli Robbins, see Stiles, v. 2, 1102–3.

86. May 31, 1889.

NOTES TO CHAPTER TWO

1. Julian Ralph, "The City of Brooklyn," reprinted from *Harper's New Monthly Magazine* (April 1893), in Mary Ellen and Mark Murphy and Ralph Foster Weld, eds., *A Treasury of Brooklyn* (New York: William Sloane, 1949), 61.

2. George William Curtis in *Harper's* 67 (August 1883): 466. Quoted in Syrett, *The City of Brooklyn, 1865–1895: A Political History* (New York: Columbia Univ. Press, 1944), 154. See also Henry W. B. Howard, ed., *The Eagle and Brooklyn: The Record of the Progress of the Brooklyn Daily Eagle, Issued in Commemoration of its Semi-Centennial and Occupancy of its New Building: Together with the History of the City of Brooklyn From Its Settlement to the Present Time* (Brooklyn: Brooklyn Daily Eagle, 1893), 162–167.

3. *Eagle*, May 24, 1883, and Raymond A. Schroth, *The Eagle and Brooklyn: A Community Newspaper, 1841–1955* (Westport, Conn.: Greenwood Press, 1974), 89, 79, 83–89.

4. Ralph, "City of Brooklyn," 54.

5. "We have now in New York only the rich and the poor," Scribner's magazine declared. "The middle class, who cannot live among the rich, and will not live among the poor . . . go out of the city to find their houses" (*Scribner's* 6 (1873): 748), quoted in Stuart Blumin, *The Emergence of the Middle Class: Social Experience in the American City, 1760–1900* (New York: Cambridge Univ. Press, 1989), 275).

6. Harold C. Syrett, *City of Brooklyn*, 11.

7. One common story that particularly rankled was the humorous one about General Howe, the English military leader during the Revolutionary War who allegedly captured Brooklyn first "so that he might have a place to sleep in while taking New

York" (Syrett, *City of Brooklyn*, 12). A contemporary willing to speak candidly in 1893 wrote, "Every other city earns its own way, while Brooklyn works for New York, and is paid off like a shop-girl on Saturday nights." Ralph, "City of Brooklyn," 53.

8. For increasing middle-class membership of fire companies see Blumin, *Emergence of the Middle Class*, 216. On the growth of these city services in Brooklyn, see Howard, ed., *The Eagle and Brooklyn*, 162.

9. Howard, ed., *The Eagle and Brooklyn*, 162, 164.

10. Howard, ed., *The Eagle and Brooklyn*, 161–175, 181, 184, 186, 193. See also Henry R. Stiles, ed., *The Civil, Political, Professional and Ecclesiastical History and Commercial and Industrial Record of the County of Kings and the City of Brooklyn, N.Y. from 1683 to 1884* (New York: W. W. Munsell, 1884), 2: 633–667; Syrett, *City of Brooklyn*, 13–16, 139–140. Syrett's comment about Brooklyn being the storehouse of New York is found on 139.

11. Quoted in Syrett, *City of Brooklyn*, 236. Howard, ed., *The Eagle and Brooklyn*, 188.

12. Syrett, *City of Brooklyn*, 237, 236, 12–13, 141.

13. See David Rosner, *A Once Charitable Enterprise: Hospitals & Health Care in Brooklyn & New York, 1885–1915* (New York: Cambridge Univ. Press, 1982), 23–24. I thank Rosner for turning up these statistics.

14. Howard, ed., *The Eagle and Brooklyn*, 181.

15. Ibid., 181.

16. Ibid., 169–170. See also Julian Ralph's comment that Brooklyn was the home of "the married middle people of New York, Manhattan Island being the seat of the very rich, the very poor, and the unmarried" ("City of Brooklyn," 54).

17. For a wonderful exploration of the various contemporary debates over the meaning of the city, see Carl Smith, *Urban Disorder and the Shape of Belief* (Chicago: Univ. of Chicago Press, 1995). See Syrett, *City of Brooklyn*, 19, for Beecher's comments. John Kasson describes two prevailing views of the nineteenth-century city, the "bird's eye" view and the "mole's eye" view. The first "presented the city as a clearly legible text of unity and progress, flourishing markets and civic spirit," while the latter "showed cities ravaged by the single-minded devotion to gain. Material greed and the pressures of the marketplace, these writers insisted, had created new cities polarized between the greedy, snobbish upper class, and the degraded, often vicious poor." Brooklyn boosters obviously used the language of the "bird's eye view" to describe their own hometown, while New York was always characterized through the "mole's eye." John Kasson, *Rudeness and Civility* (New York: Hill and Wang, 1990), 72–77, 77.

18. See Howard, ed., *The Eagle and Brooklyn*, 942, 188.

19. According to Stuart Blumin, this lack of interest in politics was quite typical of the middle class in this period. See Blumin, *Emergence of the Middle Class* 138–140.

20. It is perhaps worth taking note of the use of the word "masculine" here; clearly this commentator accepted the notion that the comfortable domesticity that became the hallmark of Brooklyn's attraction for the middle class was powerfully associated with the feminine. This interpretation is borne out at the end of the quote. Ralph, "City of Brooklyn," 59. For the emergence of spaces, especially in New York and other cities, where genteel women could participate in publicly displaying their fashionable garments and liberalized manners, helping to create an erotic spectacle of desire associated with the new consumer society, see Elaine Abelson, *When Ladies Go A Thieving: Middle-Class Shoplifters in the Victorian Department Store* (New York: Oxford Univ. Press, 1989); William Leach, *Land of Desire: Merchants, Power, and the Rise of a New American Culture* (New York: Random House, 1993); T. J. Jackson Lears, *Fables of*

Abundance (New York: Basic Books, 1994); David Scobey, "Anatomy of the Promenade: The Politics of Bourgeois Sociability in Nineteenth-Century New York," *Social History* 17 (May 1992): 203–227.

21. Howard, ed., *The Eagle and Brooklyn*, 942–943.

22. Ibid., 943. On the significance of church membership to middle-class status in general, see Blumin, *Emergence of the Middle Class*, 218–219.

23. Eric Monkkonen, *America Becomes Urban: The Development of U.S. Cities and Towns 1780–1980* (Berkeley: Univ. of California Press, 1988), 109. There are numerous examples of early women's reform institutions eventually being taken over by city and state governments. The literature on the maternalist state makes this argument.

24. "Hospitals, dispensaries, 'homes,' training-schools, day nurseries, employment bureaus, work exchanges and other philanthropic enterprises" flourished, while "many fine new buildings have been reared and are being reared to give accommodations to the institutions already in existence." Howard, ed., *The Eagle and Brooklyn*, 191–192. The literature on women's participation in social welfare activity is extensive.

25. Kathleen D. McCarthy, *Noblesse Oblige: Charity & Cultural Philanthropy in Chicago, 1849–1929* (Chicago: Univ. of Chicago Press, 1982), 23, 27–32, 37–38, 49. The literature on hospitals in relevant here. See Morris Vogel, *The Invention of the Modern Hospital: Boston, 1870–1930* (Chicago: Univ. of Chicago Press, 1980); David Rosner, *A Once Charitable Enterprise: Hospitals & Health Care in Brooklyn & New York, 1885–1915* (New York: Cambridge Univ. Press, 1982); Charles Rosenberg, *The Care of Strangers: The Rise of America's Hospital System* (New York: Basic Books, 1987); Diana Long and Janet Golden, eds., *The American General Hospital* (Ithaca: Cornell Univ. Press, 1989).

26. Rosner, *A Once Charitable Enterprise*, 26–31, 22–23.

27. Ralph, "City of Brooklyn," 55, 54. Howard, ed., *The Eagle and Brooklyn*, 941. Indeed, the latter credits Brooklyn's women with beginning "the coalescence" of class relations even before club life and charity functions reached their peak.

28. Ralph, "City of Brooklyn," 55, 54. For middle-class women helping to shape discourse about the city, see Judith Walkowitz, *City of Dreadful Delight: Narratives of Sexual Danger in Late Victorian London* (Chicago: Univ. of Chicago Press, 1992). Margaret Marsh argues that the city also held out important opportunities for freedom, mobility, and self-improvement, and that until the 1920s middle-class women were reluctant to leave the city for the suburbs. Her argument suggests indirectly the attraction to women of Brooklyn's domestic image, because they believed it enabled a woman to enjoy the benefits of a city without its dangers. See Margaret Marsh, *Suburban Lives* (New Brunswick: Rutgers Univ. Press, 1990).

29. Ralph, "City of Brooklyn," 55–56.

30. Ibid.

31. Ibid., 56. Ralph is partially mistaken about selling pews. In the 1870s Henry Ward Beecher instituted the custom of renting pews to the highest bidder at the annual "pew auction" at Plymouth Church. This is one of many examples of the way Brooklyn's self-representation fell somewhat short of reality. See Altina Waller, *Reverend Beecher and Mrs. Tilton* (Amherst: Univ. of Massachusetts Press, 1982), 101.

32. Scobey "Anatomy of the Promenade": 203–227, 203, 204.

33. David Scobey, "Nymphs and Satyrs: Sex and the Bourgeois Public Sphere in Victorian New York," paper delivered at the Newberry Library, Chicago, November 1995, pp. 7, 18.

34. One might argue that the behavior of Brooklyn's middle-class women and men underscores the role of voluntary associations in bourgeois self-affirmation. The contrast

between Brooklyn and New York also dramatically illustrates how gender structured genteel activity and behavior. Geoff Eley, "Nations, Publics, and Political Cultures: Placing Habermas in the Nineteenth Century," in Craig Calhoun, ed., *Habermas and the Public Sphere* (Cambridge, Mass.: Harvard Univ. Press, 1992), 307–319; Mary Ryan, "Gender and Public Access: Women's Politics in Nineteenth-Century America," in Calhoun, ed. *Habermas and the Public Sphere*, 259–288.

35. Paul Starr, *The Social Transformation of American Medicine* (New York: Basic Books, 1982), 64, 68–69.

36. Willard P. Beach, "Specialists and the General Practitioner," *Brooklyn Medical Journal* 3 (1889): 222–224.

37. In 1870 there were 678 patients per physician; in 1880, 617; and in 1890, 663. See U.S. Government Printing Office, *Ninth Census of the United States*, 1: 75, 779; *Compendium of the Tenth Census of the United States*, Part 1, 229, *Statistics of the Population of the U.S. at the 10th Census* (1883), 865; *Report on the Population of the U.S. at the 11th Census* (1890), 1: 370, 640. See Louis F. Criado, "The Necessity of Medical Reform," *Brooklyn Medical Journal* 7 (June 1893): 366–373, 369.

38. "The Financial Results of Medical Practice," *Brooklyn Medical Journal* 2 (1888): 132–135, 134.

39. See Emmett D. Page, "The Dispensaries of Brooklyn," *Brooklyn Medical Journal* 2 (1888): 373–377; "The Abuse of Charity" and "Is the Medical Profession Overcrowded," editorial page, *Brooklyn Medical Journal* 3 (1889): 194–195. On the history of the dispensary, in which some of these anxieties are put in professional context, see Charles Rosenberg, "Social Class and Medical Care in 19th-Century America: The Rise and Fall of the Dispensary," *Journal of the History of Medicine and the Allied Sciences* 29 (Winter 1974): 32–54.

40. Criado, "Necessity of Medical Reform," 371.

41. "Medical Charities," *Brooklyn Medical Journal* 4 (1890): 431–432.

42. "The Changing Conditions of Professional Work in the City of Brooklyn, with Special Reference to Surgical Practice," *Brooklyn Medical Journal* 1 (January 1888): 1–11, 4.

43. Ibid., 9, 6.

44. Ibid., 8, 10.

45. According to Stiles's *History of the County of Kings*, the members of the consulting staff included J. H. Hobart Burge, Frank W. Rockwell, John Byrne, Arthur Mathewson, Landon Carter Gray, Francke H. Bosworth, and James Watt, all Brooklyn practitioners. The only New Yorker of the bunch was B. F. Dawson. Lady Officers were Mrs. E. M. Sandford, Mrs. Mary Lewis, Mrs. C. N. Hoagland, Mrs. George Stannard, and Mrs. P. A. Resseguie, 2: 937.

46. Ibid., 937.

47. Indeed, just two years after Pilcher gave his paper on surgery and hospitals to the medical society, he read a paper to the National Conference of Charities and Correction annual conference in Baltimore entitled "The Public Hospitals of Brooklyn," in which he stated the need for investigating the way the city paid private hospitals for the care of poor patients, alleging that many hospitals received payment out of proportion to the number of patients they treated. One can't help but feel that Mary Dixon Jones's hospital was indirectly being indicted here; the Woman's Hospital does appear on his list of institutions receiving funds. *Brooklyn Medical Journal* 4 (August 1890): 531–543.

48. Monkkonen, *America Becomes Urban*, 118.

49. Syrett, *City of Brooklyn*, 70–87.

50. Ibid., 91.

51. Gerald W. McFarland, *Mugwumps, Morals, and Politics, 1884–1920* (Amherst: Univ. of Mass. Press, 1975), 50.

52. Schroth, *The Eagle and Brooklyn*, 79–83; Syrett, *City of Brooklyn*, 92–106.

53. Syrett, *City of Brooklyn*, 103.

54. *Eagle*, April 4, 1877, quoted in ibid., 103, 107; see also Schroth, *The Eagle and Brooklyn*, 82.

55. Syrett, *City of Brooklyn*, 106.

56. Quoted in ibid., 134.

57. Ibid., 120–137, esp. 133–134.

58. Ibid., 157–158; Stiles, *History of the County of Kings*, 2, 517.

59. Syrett, *City of Brooklyn*, 113.

60. Ibid., 161–162.

61. Edwin Emery, *The Press and America* (Englewood Cliffs, N.J.: Prentice Hall, 1962), 345.

62. See Timothy Gleason, *The Watchdog Concept: The Press and the Courts in Nineteenth-Century America* (Ames: Iowa State Univ. Press, 1990), 64; Michael Schudson, *Discovering the News: A Social History of American Newspaper* (New York: Basic Books, 1978), passim.

63. Schudson, *Discovering the News*, 97. Gunther Barth, *City People: The Rise of Modern City Culture in Nineteenth-Century America* (New York: Oxford Univ. Press, 1980), 48–109; Lewis Worth, "Urbanism as a Way of Life," in Wirth, *On Cities and Social Life* (Chicago: Univ. of Chicago Press, 1964), 60–83; Alan Trachtenberg, *The Incorporation of America* (New York: Hill and Wang, 1982), 122–126.

64. Trachtenberg, *Incorporation of America*, 124, 125. The remark on village gossip is the sociologist Robert Park's, quoted by Trachtenberg.

65. John B. Thompson, *The Media and Modernity: A Social Theory of the Media* (Cambridge: Polity Press, 1995), 202.

66. Schudson, *Discovering the News*, 18–30; Gaye Tuchman, *Making News: A Study in the Construction of Reality* (New York: Free Press, 1978), 158–161; Frank Luther Mott, *American Journalism: A History of Newspapers in the United States: 1690–1950* (New York: Macmillan, 1950), 232–233.

67. Ibid., 442.

68. Dan Schiller, *Objectivity and the News: The Public and the Rise of Commercial Journalism* (Philadelphia: Univ. of Pennsylvania Press, 1981), 65, 184. Schiller analyzes the reportage of the notorious Richard Robinson–Helen Jewett murder case of 1836, in which a beautiful prostitute was hatcheted to death by a young, respectable, handsome, middle-class clerk who was eventually acquitted, to demonstrate the way the penny press played on class antagonisms. See esp. 57–65. Emery, *The Press and America*, 345.

69. Sidney Kobre, *Development of American Journalism* (Dubuque, Iowa: William C. Brown, 1969), 358, 360, 384; Mott, *American Journalism*, 447.

70. Mott, *American Journalism*, 436, 438; Emery, *The Press and America*, 379; Helen MacGill Hughes, *News and the Human Interest Story* (Chicago: Univ. of Chicago Press, 1940), 18–19. It is interesting to note that by 1887, with New York at its feet, the *World* began to tone down some of its sensationalism.

71. Mott, *American Journalism*, 436.

72. Ibid.

73. Ibid., 436, 438.

74. Bernard A. Weisberger, *American Newspaperman* (Chicago: Univ. of Chicago Press, 1961), 135.

75. Hughes, *News and the Human Interest Story*, 18; Kobre, *Development of American Journalism*, 382.

76. Indeed, the contradiction between public responsibility and corporate and capitalist enterprise was one of the central tensions embodied in late nineteenth-century journalism. See Timothy W. Gleason, *The Watchdog Concept: The Press and Courts in Nineteenth-Century America* (Ames: Iowa State Univ. Press, 1990), 52. Still very useful on libel is Morris L. Ernst and Alexander Lindey, *Hold Your Tongue! Adventures in Libel and Slander* (London: Methuen & Co., 1936).

77. Gleason, *Watchdog Concept*, 52, 54, 63–65, 76; Mott, *American Journalism*, 509.

78. Schudson, *Discovering the News*, 71.

79. Ibid., 77; Tuchman, *Making News*, 158–159.

80. Schudson, *Discovering the News*, 118–119.

81. Ibid., 118.

82. Ibid., 110–117.

83. Quoted in ibid., 116.

84. This is Schudson's argument, ibid., 116–117.

85. Quoted in Hughes, *News and the Human Interest Story*, 18, from Don Seitz, *Joseph Pulitzer: His Life and Letters* (New York: Simon & Schuster, 1924), 422. See also Fred Inglis, *Media Theory: An Introduction* (London: Basil Blackwell, 1990), 28–29. Gunther Barth has argued that the newspapers eroded narrow prejudices and fostered a tolerant cosmopolitanism. *City People*, 106–109.

86. The exact figure is 261,700 foreign born out of a total population of 806,343. Schroth, *The Eagle and Brooklyn*, 104.

87. The cities were consolidated into Greater New York in 1898.

88. Schroth, *The Eagle and Brooklyn*, 110.

89. Ibid., 92.

90. Ibid., 97–99. On McElway, see *The Outlook*, 110 (July 28, 1915): 697; Edgar M. Cullen, "St. Clair McKelway, the Citizen," Oswald Garrison Villard, "St. Clair McKelway, the Journalist," and Chester S. Lord, "St. Clair McKelway, the Educator," in University of the State of New York, *Fifty-First Convocation Proceedings*, 1915, Albany, New York, 10–22.

91. Schroth, *The Eagle and Brooklyn*, 140.

92. See Martin Weyrauch, ed., *The Pictorial History of Brooklyn Issued by the Brooklyn Daily Eagle* (New York: Brooklyn Daily Eagle, 1916), 45–46.

93. Schroth, *The Eagle and Brooklyn*, 95.

94. Ibid., 132. Quotes from *Eagle* special issue, *How a Modern Newspaper Is Made* (Brooklyn, N.Y.: Brooklyn Eagle Press, 1911).

95. Schroth, *The Eagle and Brooklyn*, 446.

96. Another interesting piece of evidence suggesting that for the *Eagle*, as well as for the lawyers involved, the Dixon Jones libel trial was a significant event, is a beautifully bound leather scrapbook now residing in the Brooklyn Historical Society Archives. The scrapbook is gilt-edged, and on each page, perfectly symmetrical, neatly applied, and encased in a bold black border, is the entire collection of *Eagle* newspaper clippings on the libel trial. The inscription reads "A. D. Lamb, a well deserved souvenir. With kind regards of Jesse Johnson." Jesse Johnson was Lamb's law partner and a former U.S. District Attorney.

97. Howard, ed., *The Eagle and Brooklyn*, 99–100.

98. Rosner, *A Once Charitable Enterprise*, 22–23.

99. Kasson, *Rudeness and Civility*, 99. On the figure of the confidence man, see Karen Halttunen, *Confidence Men and Painted Women: A Study of Middle-Class Culture in America, 1830–1870* (New Haven; Yale Univ. Press, 1982), 1–33. Angus Mclaren argues that in the new, commercializing world of the late nineteenth century, concern for reputation increased prodigiously. He believes the stark increase in the incidence of the crime of blackmail indirectly points to this need to defend one's reputation. See *A Prescription for Murder: The Notorious Serial Killings of Dr. Thomas Neill Cream* (Chicago: Univ. of Chicago Press, 1993), 91.

NOTES TO CHAPTER THREE

1. See *Delaware Index Cards of Marriages, 1680–1850*. Salt Lake City: Church of Jesus Christ of Latter Day Saints. n.d. Microfilm SL #6417, for record of the marriage of Noah Dixon and Sally Turner, her parents, on December 22, 1807. It is interesting to note that the household of Noah Dixon, her father, contained five female slaves, one adult, two young women, and two children (Bureau of the Census, *Fifth Census of the United States, 1830: Population Schedules, Maryland*, vol. 4, Dorchester County, 8th Election District, sheet 265).

2. The rest of the biographical information on Dixon Jones was gleaned from the following sources: trial testimony printed in the *Eagle*, February 4, 5, 1892; biographical sketches in Howard A. Kelly and Walter L. Burrage, eds., *Dictionary of American Medical Biography* (New York: D. Appleton, 1928, 677, and Irving A. Watson, ed., *Physicians and Surgeons of America* (Concord, N.H.: Republican Press Association, 1896), 808–810. The Watson sketch was, according to its editor, provided by the subject, and it is in this sketch that we hear about Dixon Jones's grandfather. Perhaps this information is a case of self-aggrandizement, because it appears the Dixons were from Delaware, and there is no record of a James Dixon who could have been her grandfather. On the Reverend James Dixon, see Leslie Stephen and Sidney Lee, eds., *The Dictionary of National Biography* (London: Oxford Univ. Press, 1937), vol. 5: 1029. See also for the Dixon Family, Elias Jones, *New Revised History of Dorchester County, Maryland* (1902; rpt. Cambridge, Md.: Tidewater Publishers, 1966), 62, 106, 143. On Dixon Jones's student and teaching career, see *Catalogue of the Officers and Students of the Wesleyan Female Collegiate Institute, of Wilmingon, Del. 1838–1848* (Wilmington: Evans and Vernon, 1848), 1, 13, 17, 23, 26, 40–41.

3. For information on Bond and Askew, see Howard Kelly and Walter Burrage, eds., *American Medical Biographies* (Baltimore: Norman, Remington, 1920), 122, 43–44, and Eugene Fauntleroy Cordell, *The Medical Annals of Maryland, 1799–1899*, Baltimore, 1903, 326.

4. A biographical sketch in the *Woman's Medical Journal* 4 (November 1895): 307–309, claims that she met her husband at a school musical reception while principal of the Young Ladies' Seminary of southern Maryland. He was a graduate of Jefferson College.

5. On John Quincy Adams Jones, see *Seventh Census of the United States, 1850. Population Schedules, Maryland, Somerset County Dames Quarter District, Sheet 446*, and James Wingate, *Wingate's Maryland Register for 1874–75–76: A Legal, Political and Business Manual* (Baltimore, 1875), 7.

6. Politicians often left families at home during the congressional season, and, by the end of the century, two-career couples were occasionally living apart as well.

7. Testimony of Dixon Jones's son, the Reverend Henry Jones, Brooklyn *Citizen*, February 28, 1892; on Dixon Jones's appearance, see *Citizen*, February 1, 1892. The

Hygeio-Therapeutic Medical College was founded in 1857 by a regular physician named Russell B. Trall, who had strong reformist leanings. Trall edited the *Water-Cure Journal,* an important health reform publication, and trained dozens of hydropathic physicians every year.

8. For accounts of other women physicians, see Regina Morantz-Sanchez, *Sympathy and Science: Women Physicians in American Medicine* (New York: Oxford Univ. Press, 1985), 90–183. The term "sectarian" refers not to religious affiliation, but to competing groups of medical practitioners vying with the orthodox medical profession for public patronage in the middle third of the nineteenth century. Each of these groups had its own distinct theory of disease causation and treatment modality. Thomsonians rejected the harsh mineral drugs of the regulars in favor of botanical treatment. Homeopaths, followers of a system invented in the late eighteenth century by German physician Samuel Hahnemann, administered infinitesimal doses of drugs that would imitate disease symptoms. Hydropathic, or water-cure physicians, used water internally and externally as a mainstay of treatment. With the exception of the Thomsonians, who were anti-elitist and adopted the motto "Every man his own physician," sectarian practitioners founded their own medical schools and associations. These were particularly congenial to women students, who helped to swell their ranks. For information on Dixon Jones, see *The Revolution* 4 (28 October 1869): 270; and ibid., "Dr. Mary Dixon Jones," 267–268. On her income, see *Eagle,* February 2, 1892. On the income of male physicians, see Charles Rosenberg, "The Practice of Medicine in New York a Century Ago," in Judith Leavitt and Ronald Numbers, *Sickness and Health in America* (Madison: Univ. of Wisconsin Press, 1978), 57.

9. "The Status of Gynecology in 1876 and 1900," American Gynecological Society, *Transactions* 25 (1900): 425–426.

10. In her medical articles she mentions having witnessed well-known practitioners operate quite often.

11. See Morantz-Sanchez, *Sympathy and Science,* 66–68. Like Dixon Jones, Lucy Waite, a surgeon who became chief of staff at the Mary Thompson Hospital for Women and Children in 1895, began her medical career as a homeopath.

12. Gulielma Fell Alsop, *History of the Woman's Medical College of Pennsylvania* (Philadelphia: Lippincott, 1950), 109.

13. See her fond reminiscences of Wilson in "College Memories," *Transactions of the Alumnae Association of the Woman's Medical College of Pennsylvania* (1897), 60–63.

14. On Hunt's career, see Kelly and Burrage, eds., *American Medical Biographies,* 579–580.

15. Considerably younger than Dixon Jones, Putnam Jacobi had returned only in 1871 from her medical studies in Paris where she became the second woman to graduate from the École de Medicine. Although not a surgeon, Putnam Jacobi was a prodigious figure among women physicians and much admired among the male medical community in New York, Boston, and Philadelphia. See Morantz-Sanchez, *Sympathy and Science,* 184–202.

16. See Morantz-Sanchez, *Sympathy and Science,* 122–123; *Transactions of the Alumnae Association of the Woman's Medical College of Pennsylvania* (1900), 98.

17. "College Memories," 60–61.

18. For the offer of a position, see Caroline Pease to Clara Marshall, January 18, 1892, Marshall MSS, Archives and Special Collections on Women in Medicine, Medical College of Pennsylvania, Philadelphia.

19. Dixon Jones did not entirely shun female physicians' networks. She was an

associate editor of the *Woman's Medical Journal* briefly in the early 1890s. She occasionally published papers there as well, but they were always reprinted from mainstream medical journals. Putnam Jacobi, by comparison, was more loyal to her female associates, serving on the faculty of the Woman's Medical College of the New York Infirmary, maintaining an active relationship with women's medical institutions, alumnae associations, and medical societies, working constantly on behalf of opening up medical opportunities for women, and publicly supporting women's suffrage.

20. The *Citizen*, June 8, 1889, quotes the entire letter. A biographical sketch in the *Woman's Medical Journal* claims that "The Dean of the College, Prof. R. D. Bodley, wrote as a record of Dr. Jones's examinations: 'White 70. Black 0.' and said 'It was the most perfect record in the twenty-five years history of the College.' Prof. Bodley also wrote: 'The record of the faculty-vote entitles her to rank in her class as distinguished' " (4 (December 1895): 309).

21. Charles Rosenberg, "Making It in Urban Medicine: A Career in the Age of Scientific Medicine," *Bulletin of the History of Medicine* 64 (Summer 1990): 163–183.

22. For this changing context of professional socialization, see the following: John Harley Warner, *The Therapeutic Perspective* (Cambridge, Mass.: Harvard Univ. Press, 1986); Charles Rosenberg, *The Care of Strangers* (New York: Basic Books, 1987); Kenneth Ludmerer, *Learning to Heal* (New York: Basic Books, 1985); George Rosen, *The Structure of American Medical Practice, 1875–1911* (Philadelphia: Univ. of Pennsylvania Press, 1985); Rosemary Stevens, *American Medicine and the Public Interest* (New Haven: Yale Univ. Press, 1971).

23. For the importance of training abroad for many American women physicians, see Thomas Neville Bonner, *To The Ends of the Earth: Women's Search for Education in Medicine* (Cambridge: Harvard Univ. Press, 1992).

24. See Audrey D. Stevens, *America's Pioneers in Abdominal Surgery* (Melrose, Mass.: American Society of Abdominal Surgeons, 1968), 12. See information on the following: In Howard Kelly, ed., *A Cyclopedia of American Medical Biography* (Philadelphia: W. B. Saunders, 1912), sketches of Emily Blackwell, 89–90, Emmeline Cleveland, 187, Marie Mergler (misprinted in this edition as Meigler), 188–189, Sarah Hackett Stevenson, 408–409, Mary Harris Thompson, 442–443; in Kelly and Burrage, *Dictionary of American Medical Biography*, see sketch on Mary Almira Smith, 1132. For Waite, who was married to her mentor, F. Byron Robinson, see William K. Beatty, "Lucy Waite: Surgeon and Free Thinker," Medical Institute of Chicago *Proceedings*, 45 (1992): 52–58; on Broomall, see Morantz-Sanchez, *Sympathy and Science*, 78–79, 169–70; on Keller, ibid., 8–9, 221; Cleveland, who took training in Paris, was performing ovariotomy as early as 1875. See Emmeline Cleveland ["reported by one of her lady pupils"], "Successful Ovariotomy at the Woman's Hospital of Philadelphia," *The Clinic* (Cincinnati) 9 (1875): 100–102. Cleveland wrote "There have been seven cases of ovariotomy in all, at the Woman's Hospital, four of which have recovered, which is certainly a fair proportion for a hospital. . . . The rapid advances that will be made in this direction in the next few years, will go far towards dispelling the doubts of those who consider the point still unsettled, as to whether or not women can make good surgeons." See also Emmeline Cleveland, "Complicated Case of Vesico-Vaginal Fistula," in Philadelphia Obstetrical Society *Transactions* 5 (1877): 62–64.

25. I draw this conclusion after reading extensively in the published articles of other women surgeons, and I offer the following representative samples: Elizabeth C. Keller, "Case of Hemato-Salpynx," Alumnae Association of the Women's College of Pennsylvania *Proceedings* (1889): 79–81; Anna Broomall, "A Case of Rupture of an Ovarian Cyst into the Intestines," *American Journal of Obstetrics and Gynecology* 7

(1884): 1019–1021; Elizabeth Cushier, "Sarcoma of the Ovary," *Medical Record* 28 (1885): 498; Anna Fullerton, "Studies in Gynecology from the Service of the Woman's Hospital of Philadelphia,"*Journal of the American Medical Association* 29 (December 25, 1897): 1298–1301; Marie Mergler, "What Are the Indications for the Removal of the Uterine Appendages?," *Medical and Surgical Reporter* 69 (July 1893): 117–120, and "Fibroid Tumors of the Uterus—Their Complications," *Woman's Medical Journal* 3 (November 1894): 113–118; Lucy Waite, "Removal of the Uterus in Bilateral Diseases of the Appendages: Report of Cases," *Chicago Medical Recorder* 10 (June 1896): 383–387. See also Metta M. Loomis, "The Contributions Which Women Have Made to Medical Literature," *New York Medical Journal* 100 (September 1914): 522–524, which confirms that Dixon Jones was probably one of the most prolific of women physicians, in her generation. 523.

26. See Virginia Drachman, "Gynecological Instruments and Surgical Decisions at a Hospital in Late-Nineteenth Century America," in Edith Mayo, ed., *American Material Culture: The Shape of Things Around Us* (Bowling Green, Ohio: Bowling Green State Univ. Press, 1984), 66–78; Morantz-Sanchez, *Sympathy and Science*, 180–182.

27. On women in surgery, Earle remarked in 1891, "Many who have admitted that a woman might, perhaps, find a place in medicine, have denied her ability to be a surgeon. The facts which we have observed in every day practice deny this assertion." See his Doctorate Address to the Chicago Women's Medical College Graduates, "Progress in the Study and Practice of Medicine by Women," *North American Practitioner* 11 (September 1891): 1–11, 9. I thank Tom Bonner for this cite.

28. See Morantz-Sanchez, *Sympathy and Science*, chs. 4–6. For the Jacobi-Blackwell exchange, see Jacobi to Blackwell, December 25, 1888, Blackwell MSS., Library of Congress.

29. See Morantz-Sanchez, *Sympathy and Science*, 90–183.

30. See Gert Brieger, "Surgery," in Ronald Numbers, ed., *The Education of American Physicians* (Berkeley: Univ. of California Press, 1980), 175–204.

31. John B. Wheeler, *Memoirs of a Small-Town Surgeon* (New York: Stokes, 1935), 43; Arthur E. Hertzler, *The Horse and Buggy Doctor* (New York: Harper & Bros., 1938), 51.

32. John A. Wyeth, *With Sabre and Scalpel: The Autobiography of a Soldier and Surgeon* (New York: Harper Bros., 1914), 347–351.

33. Franklin H. Martin, *Fifty Years of Medicine and Surgery: An Autobiographical Sketch* (Chicago: Surgical Publishing, 1934), 71–84. E. C. Dudley noted that Mercy was the only hospital in Chicago at the time that gave valuable clinical experience. Internships were less formally structured than later, however, and most medical graduates could not get them. E. C. Dudley, *The Medicine Man, Being the Memoirs of Fifty Years of Medical Progress* (New York: J. H. Sears, 1927), 197.

34. Dudley, *The Medicine Man*, 203.

35. Ibid., 209–210.

36. Women physicians actually founded hospitals in this period to gain clinical experience and provide it for their students, but women's hospitals run by women were few, and available clinical appointments even more scarce. Occasionally, as in Chicago and Philadelphia in the 1880s, some of the large city hospitals began to let women stand for their competitive examinations, but in New York City, no hospital other than the New York Infirmary for Women and Children, a female-run institution, admitted women until Emily Dunning Barringer challenged the policy and won an appointment at Bellevue in 1907. See Morantz-Sanchez, *Sympathy and Science*, passim, and Virginia Drachman, *Hospital with a Heart* (Ithaca: Cornell Univ. Press, 1984).

37. This tension and rivalry was particularly acute in England, because the profession was differently organized, with obstetricians being considered physicians, not surgeons. See Ornella Moscucci, *The Science of Woman* (Cambridge: Cambridge Univ. Press, 1990).

38. Martin, *Fifty Years*, 105; Dudley, *Medicine Man*, 198; Audrey Davis, *Dr. Kelly of Hopkins Surgeon, Scientist, Christian* (Baltimore: Johns Hopkins Univ. Press, 1959), 37–38.

39. Martin, *Fifty Years*, 105, 118–119.

40. Ibid., 118–119, 166–167.

41. See, for example, her interesting self-portrait at the beginning of "Personal Experiences in Laparotomy," *Medical Record* 52 (August 1897): 182–192.

42. See Howard A. Kelly, "History of Gynecology in America," in Howard A. Kelly, ed., *A Cyclopedia of American Medical Biography* I:xxxix–liv.

43. Laparotomies were radical and dangerous because they involved surgical incision through the abdominal wall, which increased the possibility of both infection and hemorrhage.

44. Mary McKibben Harper, "Anna E. Broomall, M.D.," *Medical Review of Reviews* 39 (March 1933): 132–139, 137.

45. Morantz-Sanchez, *Sympathy and Science*, 180–182.

46. On Heitzman, sometimes listed as Carl, see W. B. Atkinson, *Physicians and Surgeons of the United States* (Philadelphia: Charles Robson, 1878), 714.

47. See mention of this trip in Dixon Jones, "Two Cases of Removal of Uterine Myoma: One, Suprapubic Hysterectomy; the Other, Complete Hysterectomy. A New Method of Disposing of the Stump. Microscopical Examination of the Appendages. Remarks on the Treatment of Uterine Myoma by Electricity," *New York Medical Journal* 49 (August 25, 1888): 198–205, 199.

48. On the Post-Graduate School in the context of other polyclinics organized around the same time, see Steven J. Peitzman, " 'Thoroughly Practical': America's Polyclinic Medical Schools," *Bulletin of the History of Medicine* 54 (Summer 1980): 166–187, and John A. Wyeth, *With Sabre and Scalpel*, 461–466. Lawson Tait was quite favorably impressed with the school when he visited it in 1884, commenting that "there is nothing of this kind in Great Britain, and I never saw anything on the Continent with which I could compare it." W. J. Stewart McKay, *Lawson Tait: His Life and Work* (New York: William Wood, 1922), 257.

49. For information on Dawson, see Kelly and Burrage, eds., *American Medical Biographies*, 296.

50. See testimony of the following witnesses at the trial, printed in the Brooklyn *Eagle*: James Tanner, February 6; George G. Reynolds, Paul Gruening, February 9; Mrs. Cornelia Plummer, Dr. Annie Brown, and Elizabeth Meachem, February 5, 6, 9, 1892. Plummer quote is from February 6. See also the report of the Committee on Ethics of the New York Pathological Society, May 23, 1889, Pathological Society Mss., New York Academy of Medicine. For a sketch of the rise of community and proprietary hospitals and the increasing tension between surgeons and lady managers, with surgeons caring less about the "worthiness" of charitable patients and surgeons more concerned with getting enough clinical material by admitting interesting cases, see Edward Atwater, "Women, Surgeons, and a Worthy Enterprise: The General Hospital Comes to Upper New York State," in Diana Long and Janet Golden, eds., *The American General Hospital: Communities and Social Contexts* (Ithaca: Cornell Univ. Press, 1989), 40–66.

51. For the distinct personality of women's hospitals, see Morantz-Sanchez, *Sympathy and Science*, 110, 168, 170, 174, 203–221; Drachman, *Hospital with a Heart.*

52. See the sketch of Dixon Jones in Irving A. Watson, ed., *Physicians and Surgeons of America: A Collection of Biographical Sketches of the Medical Profession* (Concord, N. H.: Republican Press Association, 1896), 868–870. See also "Manual of the Medical Society of the County of Kings," *Brooklyn Medical Journal* 2 (October 1888): 317–352. For information on Rockwell see the sketch and obituary in the *Brooklyn Medical Journal* 3 (May 1889): 614–622, 498–500, and the obituary in the Brooklyn *Eagle*, May 1, 1889. Burge was a prominent local surgeon who graduated from the medical school of New York University and taught surgery on the wards of the Long Island College Hospital. See Dale Smith, "A Historical Overview of the Recognition of Appendicitis—Part I," *New York State Journal of Medicine* 86 (November 1986): 577. Charles Dixon Jones was his mother's colleague and surgical assistant throughout her career. When she died in 1908, he continued to practice medicine in New York City. He published a couple of clinical papers that were spin-offs of his mother's surgical interests. He also had a strong interest in pediatric orthopedics, and some of the patient testimony indicates that parents brought their children to him. Dixon Jones also had a unmarried daughter, an accomplished singer who died in her twenties, and a son who graduated from Harvard and became a minister.

53. She testified at the libel trial to 300 operations, but her published case records, which are not necessarily complete, suggest the lower number. See *Eagle*, February 4, 5, 1892. See also Mary Dixon Jones, "Personal Experiences in Laparotomy," *Medical Record* 52 (August 1897): 182–192.

54. See "Removal of the Uterine Appendages—Nine Consecutive Cases," *Medical Record* 30 (August 1886): 198–208, 206 n. On Jacobus see typescript memorial in the New York Academy of Medicine Archives. Morris was a pioneer in ovarian transplants. See Robert T. Morris, *Fifty Years a Surgeon* (New York: E. P. Dutton, 1935). On Wylie see Kelly and Burrage, *Dictionary of American Medical Biography* (1920), 1340–1341; On Coe, *Album of the Fellows of the American Gynecological Society* (1901), 60; on Lee, see Kelly, ed., *Cyclopedia of American Medical Biography* II: 91–92. On King, see Thomas Herrinshaw, ed., *American Physician and Surgeon Blue Book* (Chicago: American Blue Book Publishers, 1919), 266. Tait was a supporter of medical education for women, and during his trip to the United States in 1884, he visited both Jefferson Medical College and the Woman's Medical College of Pennsylvania in Philadelphia. He was very impressed with the latter, especially the fact that the majority of the members of the faculty were "ladies." He met Anna E. Broomall for the second time, having welcomed her on a visit to Birmingham the previous year. He felt the physical plant, operating theater, lying-in wards, and general hospital to be exemplary and left feeling "quite satisfied that the lady graduates of Philadelphia are quite as carefully trained as those in any other medical school." Although he admitted it was still rough going for the women occasionally in the United States, he felt American physicians had traveled much further along the path of acceptance than his British compeers. See Lawson Tait, "American Notes," *Birmingham Medical Review* (December 1884): 20–24, 21.

55. Hertzler, *Horse and Buggy Doctor*, 199.

56. Dixon Jones was an associate editor of the *Philadelphia Times and Register, A Weekly Journal of Medicine and Surgery* from May 21, 1892, to December 16, 1893. Her name appears on the editorial staff of the *Woman's Medical Journal* from January 1894 to December 1896. She guest-edited the *American Journal of Surgery and Gynecology* in January 1899. Besides those journals, her articles were published in mainstream periodicals, including the *Medical Record*, the *New York Medical Journal*, the *American Journal of Obstetrics and Diseases of Women and Children*, the *Buffalo Medical and Surgical Journal*, and the *Annals of Gynecology and*

Pediatry. Abroad, she published several articles in the *British Gynaecological Journal.*

57. See W. F. Bynum and Janice C. Wilson, "Periodical Knowledge: Medical Journals and Their Editors in Nineteenth-Century Britain," in W. F. Bynum, Stephen Lock, and Roy Porter, eds., *Medical Journals and Medical Knowledge: Historical Essays* (New York: Routledge, 1992), 41. See Ella Marble, "Woman's Contribution to Medical Literature," *Woman's Medical Journal* 5 (March 1896): 59–63, for a brief attempt to track women physicians' publications. Marble acknowledges Putnam Jacobi as the most-published, but says of Jones that she "has probably written more of abdominal surgery than any other woman" (62).

58. Mortality from surgery was reduced markedly in the 1880s, so that surgeons and patients alike seemed more willing to resort to the knife at the earliest signs of disease. Tait even advised exploratory operations for diagnostic purposes. Those who fell into the "conservative" camp were generally less willing to operate unless signs of disease were absolutely apparent, and often advised partial rather than total removal of the organs. "Radical" surgeons believed in early operations and total excision. See Chapter 3, and Gert Brieger, "From Conservative to Radical Surgery in Late Nineteenth-Century America," in Christopher Lawrence, ed., *Medical Theory, Surgical Practice: Studies in the History of Surgery* (New York: Routledge, 1992), 216–231. Tait and Dixon Jones both identified with the radicals.

59. Dixon Jones could have chosen the American ovariotomist Robert Battey as her role model, but I believe, though I cannot prove, that she admired Tait's flamboyance. On Tait and his world, see Jane Eliot Sewall, "Bountiful Bodies: Spencer Wells, Lawson Tait, and the Birth of British Gynaecology," Ph.D. dissertation, Johns Hopkins University, 1991. See Fred Byron Robinson, "A Sketch of Mr. Lawson Tait and His Work," *Journal of the American Medical Association* 18 (January 1892): 77–79, 99–103, 129–132, for a serious assessment of Tait's work by an American admirer.

60. See Chapter 5.

61. Mary Dixon Jones, "A Case of Tait's Operation," *American Journal of Obstetrics* 17 (November 1884): 1155–1161.

62. See abstract of the Obstetrical Society meeting, May 15, 1883, reprinted in *American Journal of Obstetrics* 16 (December 1883): 1191–1192.

63. If Dixon Jones was referring to general practitioners, then her remarks are an example of tension between the two groups over specialization. She might also be indicting gynecologists who disapproved of radical surgical techniques. See, for example, this statement: "One young physician said to me a short time since, 'What is the use of studying these intangible subjects? What we want to know is, when and how to operate.' Do we not know when and how best to operate, when we know the momentousness of the disease, and can weigh all the solemn responsibilities? I studied because I wanted to know, and wanted to learn the best thing to be done to help these suffering young women. I believe many young women have been lost from a lack of recognition of all the seriousness of their disease, and the necessity of giving immediate relief. Many more have perished in this way than by having the ovaries removed when some may have imagined there was no necessity, or there was no immediate danger, or there was possibly some other way of relief. As I said in 1886, 'the fault is not with the surgeons who are trying to help the sick women, but with those who have gone before.' " See "The Fourth Hitherto Undescribed Disease of the Ovary; Colloid Degeneration," *Medical Record* 56 (November 1899): 657–667, 666.

64. Mary Dixon Jones, "Removal of the Uterine Appendages—Recovery," *Medical Record* 27 (April 1885): 1155–1161.

65. Ibid., 402.

66. For an example of her subjective diagnosis, see "Removal of the Uterine Appendages: Five Cases," *American Journal of Obstetrics* 21 (February 1888): 169.

67. In a survey of the publications of Dixon Jones's female contemporaries who performed surgery, using the Index Medicus from 1882–1905, I found that of the sixteen women identified, the most active was Sarah E. Post, who published twenty-four articles in this period, although only a few were on surgical topics. Of the women who specialized only in gynecology and surgery, Anna Fullerton published eighteen articles, though six of them were on nonsurgical topics. Elizabeth Cushier published thirteen articles, all in surgery or obstetrics, and Lucy Waite published ten, most of them on surgical and gynecological subjects. Dixon Jones published a total of fifty-seven articles, letters to the editor, and case reports.

68. Lawson Tait, "A Discussion of the General Principles Involved in the Operation of Removal of the Uterine Appendages," *New York Medical Journal* 44 (November 1886): 561–567.

69. "Laparotomy for Diseases of Women from 1879 to 1889," *American Journal of Obstetrics* 26 (July 1897): 74–91.

70. Mary A. Dixon Jones, "A Consideration of Some Criticisms," *Woman's Medical Journal* 2 (April 1894): 80–82, 81.

71. See Robert Frank, "American Physiologists in German Laboratories, 1865–1914," in Gerald Geison, ed., *Physiology in the American Context, 1850–1940* (Bethesda, Md.: American Physiological Society, 1987), 11–46, 38.

72. H. MacNaughton Jones, "Presidential Address: The Position of Gynecology Today," *British Gynaecological Journal* 14 (May 1898): 8–30. It is worth noting that Emory Lanphear, editor of the *American Journal of Surgery and Gynecology*, took pains to point out MacNaughton Jones's remarks about Dixon Jones in his own editorial praise for her. See that Journal 12 (January 1899): 148. For an enormously self-referential account of the 1886 visit, published a decade after the fact, see Dixon Jones, "Reminiscences of Travels in Europe in 1886, Nos. 1, 2, 3," in *Woman's Medical Journal* 4 (December 1895): 299–304, 332–337; ibid. 5 (January 1896): 11–14. Dixon Jones was eventually admitted to the British Gynaecological Society in 1903. See Membership Rolls, Royal College of Physicians and Surgeons, London.

73. See *Citizen*, June 14, 1889. She allegedly saw the following people: Dr. Alexander, of the Woman's Hospital of Liverpool, Dr. Wallace of the Royal Infirmary, Sir Spencer Wells, Dr. James Paget, Granville Bantock, Dr. Mary Garrett Anderson, Lawson Tait, Dr. Thomas Savage, Mendes de Leon (the great Dutch surgeon), Schroeder of Berlin (surgeon to the Frauenklinik), and August Martin. She stayed seven weeks in Germany, visiting Leopold, Billroth, John Van Rennsalaer Haff, Winckel, and Hegar, and she also saw Paen and Charcot in Paris.

74. "Two Cases of Removal of Uterine Myoma: One, Suprapubic Hysterectomy; The Other, Complete Hysterectomy. A New Method of Disposing of the Stump. Microscopical Examination of the Appendages. Remarks on the Treatment of Uterine Myoma by Electricity," *New York Medical Journal* 49 (August 1888): 198–205. For examples of her vigilant insistence that she be given credit for this achievement, see Mary Dixon Jones, "Suppurating Endothelioma—Myofibroma in a Condition of Necrobiosis—Remarks on the Treatment of the Pedicle, etc.," *Medical Record* 38 (September 1890): 262–269; Charles Dixon Jones's letter to the editor of the *American Journal of Obstetrics*, "Removal of Uterine Myoma by Combined Abdominal and Vaginal Hysterectomy," 21 (June 1888): 604–605; and her own long correspondence, "The First Total Removal of the Fibroid Uterus," *American Journal of Obstetrics* 23 (June 1896): 405–414, and "The So-Called 'Total Hysterectomy' of Dr. R. E. Haughton, of Richmond, Indiana," *Amer-*

ican Journal of Surgery and Gynecology 12 (January 1899): 133–135. For recognition by other leading surgeons for her work in hysterectomy, see H. J. Boldt, "The Operative Treatment of Myo-Fibroma of the Uterus," *American Journal of Obstetrics* 27 (January-June 1893): 837–838; E. C. Dudley, "Pressure Forceps versus the Ligature and the Suture in Vaginal Hysterectomy," American Gynecological Society, *Transactions* 13 (1888): 191–208, 201 n.; Ernest W. Cushing, "The Evolution in America of Abdominal Hysterectomy and Total Extirpation of the Uterus," *Annals of Gynaecology and Paediatry* 8 (June 1895): 573–598, 578–579; "Transactions of the New York Academy of Medicine, Section on Obstetrics and Gynecology, May 28, 1895," *American Journal of Obstetrics* 32 (June 1895): 113; Joseph Eastman, "Uterine Fibroids," Cincinnati *Lancet-Clinic* 33 (December 1894): 599–602; Charles P. Noble, "Development and Present Status of Hysterectomy for Fibromyomata," *British Gynaecological Journal* 13 (May 1897): 48–90, 52.

75. The phrase is John Harley Warner's. See Warner, "History of Science and History of Medicine," in Arnold Thackray, ed., *Constructing Knowledge in the History of Science. Osiris* 10 (1995), 164–193. MacNaughton Jones was not the only one to call attention to Jones's work in pathology. See Henry C. Coe, "Endothelioma of the Ovary," *American Journal of the Medical Sciences* 104 (July 1892): 119.

76. This discussion is indebted to Russell Maulitz's work in the history of pathology, especially his articles " 'Physician versus Bacteriologist': The Ideology of Science in Clinical Medicine," in Charles Rosenberg and Morris Vogel, eds., *The Therapeutic Revolution* (Philadelphia: Univ. of Pennsylvania Press, 1979), 91–108, and " 'The Whole Company of Pathology'—Pathology as Idea and as Work in American Medical Life," in Teizo Ogawa, ed., *History of Pathology, Proceedings of the 8th International Symposium on the Comparative History of Medicine—East and West* (Shizuoka, Japan: Susono-shi, 1983), 139–161. I am also grateful to Dr. Maulitz for his generous willingness to talk to me about these issues, and his help in enlightening me with regard to the historical context in which Dixon Jones worked.

77. Even Simon Flexner, then at Pennsylvania, sent her a specimen of fibrocystic tumors. See "The Origin and Formation of Fibroid Tumors of the Uterus," *Medical Record* 60 (September 1901): 401–406; "Fibrocystic Tumors of the Uterus: Their Etiology," *Medical Record* 64 (October 1903): 561–572.

78. JoAnne Brown, *The Definition of a Profession* (Princeton: Princeton Univ. Press, 1992), 21.

79. See Maulitz, " 'Physician versus Bacteriologist.' "

80. Kelly and Burrage, *Dictionary of American Medical Biography*, 677.

81. *Eagle*, March 9, 1892.

82. We can sympathize better with these difficulties when we note that similar disagreements rage today over the indications for hysterectomy or diagnosing fibrocystic disease of the breast.

83. See Joel Howell, *Technology in the Hospital* (Baltimore: Johns Hopkins Univ. Press, 1995), for a discussion of the complex factors involved in such transitions to new technology.

NOTES TO CHAPTER FOUR

1. Thomas Laqueur, *Making Sex: Body and Gender from the Greeks to Freud* (Cambridge, Mass.: Harvard Univ. Press, 1990), 6; Londa Scheibinger has shown that the new sex differences were represented even in anatomists' renderings of skeletons, which deliberately played up masculine and feminine features, in *The Mind Has No Sex?*

Women in the Origins of Modern Science (Cambridge, Mass.: Harvard Univ. Press, 1989), 189–201.

2. For an interesting account of the relationship between emerging social, economic, and political institutions and gender ideology, see Mary Poovey, *Making a Social Body: British Cultural Formation, 1830–1864* (Chicago: Univ. of Chicago Press, 1995). For changes in science itself, see Caroline Merchant, *The Death of Nature: Women, Ecology, and the Scientific Revolution* (New York: Harper and Row, 1976); Schiebinger, *The Mind Has No Sex*, 119–188, 265–277; and Cynthia Russett, *Sexual Science: The Victorian Construction of Womanhood* (Cambridge, Mass.: Harvard University Press, 1989).

3. See Christopher Lawrence, "Democratic, Divine, and Heroic: The History and Historiography of Surgery," in Lawrence, ed., *Medical Theory, Surgical Practice: Studies in the History of Surgery* (London: Routledge, 1992), 1–47, 23. See also John Harley Warner, *The Therapeutic Perspective: Medical Practice, Knowledge and Identity in America, 1820–1885* (Cambridge, Mass.: Harvard Univ. Press, 1986), 235–243, "Remembering Paris: Memory and the American Disciples of French Medicine in the 19th Century," *Bulletin of the History of Medicine* 65 (Fall 1991): 301–325; Charles Rosenberg, "The Therapeutic Revolution: Medicine, Meaning and Social Change in Nineteenth-Century America," in C. Rosenberg and M. Vogel, eds., *The Therapeutic Revolution: Essays on the Social History of American Medicine* (Philadelphia: Univ. of Pennsylvania Press, 1979), 3–26; Erwin Ackerknecht, *Medicine at the Paris Hospital, 1794–1848* (Baltimore: Johns Hopkins Univ. Press, 1967); and Russell Maulitz, " 'Physician versus Bateriologist': The Ideology of Science in Clinical Medicine," in Rosenberg and Vigel, eds., *Therapeutic Revolution*, 91–107; and Maulitz, *Morbid Appearances: The Anatomy of Pathology in the Early Nineteenth Century* (New York: Cambridge Univ. Press, 1987).

4. For the importance of placing medical innovation within the larger history of technology and its attendant intellectual problems, see Joel Howell, *Technology in the Hospital: Transforming Patient Care in the Early Twentieth Century* (Baltimore: Johns Hopkins Univ. Press, 1995), 30–68.

5. Lawson Tait, *Diseases of Women and Abdominal Surgery* (Philadelphia: Lea Brown, 1889), 1–5, 3.

6. Ornella Moscucci, *The Science of Woman: Gynecology and Gender in England, 1800–1929* (Cambridge: Cambridge Univ. Press, 1990), 5–6. See also Toby Gelfand, *Professionalizing Modern Medicine* (Westport, Conn.: Greenwood Press, 1980).

7. On Sims's experience in New York, see James V. Ricci, *One Hundred Years of Gynaecology, 1800–1900* (Philadelphia: Blakeston, 1945), 130; Seale Harris, *Woman's Surgeon: The Life Story of J. Marion Sims* (New York: Macmillan, 1950); J. Marion Sims, *The Story of My Life*, ed. H. Marion Sims (New York: D. Appleton, 1886); Deborah Kuhn McGregor, *Sexual Surgery and the Origins of Gynecology: J. Marion Sims, His Hospital, and His Patients* (New York: Garland, 1989); see also Henry O. Marcy, "Some Special Reasons Why the Laparotomist Should Consider the Medico-Legal Aspects of Abdominal Surgery," *Journal of the American Medical Association* 15 (August 2, 1890): 174–77, 175.

8. The quote regarding cutting "like an executioner" is from Jeffrey Berlant, *Profession and Monopoly*, quoted in Martin Pernick, *A Calculus of Suffering: Pain, Practitioners and Anesthesia in Nineteenth Century America* (New York: Columbia Univ. Press, 1985), 86.

9. See Lawrence, "Democratic, Divine, and Heroic," 29–31.

10. Thomas S. Cullen, "The Evolution of Gynecology," *Ohio State Medical Jour-*

nal 20 (1924): 484–95. Pernick's book is still the most sophisticated analysis of the introduction of anesthesia into the American medical world.

11. Harvey Graham, *Eternal Eve* (London: Hutchinson, 1960), 226–227; Ricci, *One Hundred Years*, ch. 1; Washington L. Atlee, *A Table of All the Known Operations of Ovariotomy, from 1701 to 1851: Including Their Synoptical History, and Analysis* (Philadelphia: T. K. and P. G. Collins, 1851).

12. Christopher Lawrence makes a cogent case for not viewing surgery as solely stimulated by the discovery of anesthesia and antisepsis. He points out, for example, that surgeons operated without anesthesia before 1850 in various instances, and that its acceptance was selective and not instantaneous. Similar was the case with antisepsis. Indeed, he points out, "the making of these two innovations into historical landmarks was itself an historical process," which surgeons themselves validated only in retrospect. It took time for both innovations to be used by the majority of practitioners, and, in the case of Listerism, the technology of cleanliness was not uniform. Some, including Lawson Tait, rejected Listerism altogether in favor of their own unique and idiosyncratic procedures. An occasional contemporary saw the origin of antisepsis not in Listerism, but in obstetrics. John Erichsen argued in 1881 that surgery was "most indebted to obstetricians . . . for it is to them we owe the great precautions which independently of antiseptic or Listerian method, tended to lower the morality of ordinary surgical cases." See Lawrence, "Democratic, Divine, and Heroic," 25–26.

13. Henry J. Bigelow, *Introductory Lecture to the Course on Surgery Delivered at the Massachusetts Medical College in Boston* (Boston: David Clapp, 1850), 10. On images of the surgery and the surgeon, see Lawrence, "Democratic, Divine, and Heroic," 5–6.

14. See Jane Eliot Sewell, "Bountiful Bodies: Spencer Wells, Lawson Tait, and the Birth of British Gynecology," Ph.D. dissertation, Johns Hopkins University, 1991, pp. 112–114.

15. Lawrence's synthesis is invaluable here. See "Democratic, Divine, and Heroic," 14–15. Harold Speert, *Obstetrics and Gynecology in America: A History* (Baltimore: Waverly Press, 1980), 177; see also Oswei Temkin, "The Role of Surgery in the Rise of Modern Medical Thought," in Temkin, *The Double Face of Janus and Other Essays in the History of Medicine* (Baltimore: Johns Hopkins Univ. Press, 1977), 487–496.

16. Speert, *Obstetrics and Gynecology in America*, 177.

17. Ibid., for discussion of the condition and the Dieffenbach quote, translated from the German.

18. McGregor, *Sexual Surgery and the Origins of Gynecology*, 36–81, offers a cogent discussion on medicine and slavery and the racial and gender implications of Sims's work. Her book on Sims has been helpful in the following discussion. See also Todd Savitt, *Medicine and Slavery* (Urbana: Univ. of Illinois Press, 1978). On the resistance of white patients, see Seale Harris, *Woman's Surgeon*, 108–109. On theories of differential experience of pain, see Pernick, *A Calculus of Suffering*, 148–167.

19. Sims, *The Story of My Life*, 240.

20. Ibid., 243; J. Marion Sims, *Silver Sutures in Surgery* (New York: Samuel and William Wood, 1857), 60.

21. "On the Treatment of Vesico-Vaginal Fistula," *American Journal of Medical Sciences* 23 (January 1852): 59–82.

22. "Normal Ovariotomy—Case," *Atlanta Medical & Surgical Journal* 10 (September 1872/73): 321–329, and *Richmond & Louisville Medical Journal* 14 (January 1873): 711–729. Lawrence D. Longo's "The Rise and Fall of Battey's Operation: A

Fashion in Surgery," *Bulletin of the History of Medicine* 53 (Summer 1979): 244–267, is still the most informative discussion of this procedure and has been useful in framing the ensuing discussion.

23. W. F. Westmoreland, "Report on Battey's Operation," *Atlanta Medical & Surgical Journal* 9 (1872/73): 231.

24. R. Battey, "Extirpation of the Functionally Active Ovaries for the Remedy of Otherwise Incurable Diseases," American Gynecological Society *Transactions* 1 (1876): 102. Battey's thinking reflected the assumptions of physicians that after menopause women's problems with their reproductive systems often lessened.

25. Ibid., 113.

26. R. Battey, "Is There a Proper Field for Battey's Operation?," American Gynecological Society *Transactions* (1877): 279–305.

27. See, for example, Sims's admission of ignorance and his qualified support of Battey's work in J. Marion Sims, "Remarks on Battey's Operation," *British Medical Journal* 2 (December 29, 1877): 916–918. See also Ann Dally, *Women Under the Knife* (New York: Routledge, 1992), passim, for examples of unclear indications for surgery that was not gynecological. On appendicitis, see Dale Smith, "A Historical Overview of the Recognition of Appendicitis," *New York State Journal of Medicine* 86 (Fall 1986): 571–583, 639–647.

28. Spencer Wells, Alfred Hegar, and Robert Battey, "Castration in Mental and Nervous Diseases: A Symposium," *American Journal of the Medical Sciences* 9 (October 1886): 484.

29. Fibroids are located in the uterus, but Tait's willingness to perform ovariotomy to cure them lends credence to the view that there was a great deal of ignorance still about how these various organs functioned.

30. International professional discussions of the operation often linked Tait's, Hegar's, and Battey's names, despite sharp differences in their approach to indications for surgery. Such disagreements led to confusion over the meaning of terms like ovariotomy, oöphorectomy, and ovariectomy, which became rife on both sides of the Atlantic in this decade. The term "ovariotomy" was first used by Sir James Young Simpson in correspondence with his colleague Charles Clay. Although the American E. R. Peaslee deplored the word as a "barbarous compound of Latin and Greek" that inaccurately described the actual procedure, preferring to speak of oophorotomy or oöphorectomy, no uniform language was ever adopted and authors often had to offer definitions in published articles in the interests of clarity. For evidence of this confusion, see Ricci, *One Hundred Years*, 72; J. Clarence Webster, "Removal of the Uterine Appendages," in Howard A. Kelly and Charles P. Noble, eds., *Gynecology and Abdominal Surgery* (Philadelphia: W. B. Saunders, 1907), 608; and Fred Byron Robinson, "A Sketch of Mr. Lawson Tait and His Work," Pt. 1, *Journal of the American Medical Association* 18 (January 16, 1892): 79.

31. For Wells's use of antisepsis, see John A. Shepherd, *Spencer Wells: The Life and Work of a Victorian Surgeon* (Edinburgh and London: E. and S. Livingstone, 1965), 97. For statistics, see Sewell, "Bountiful Bodies," 122–124. Sewell's discussion of the mortality trend in general in these early years is excellent; see 114–127.

32. Sims's letter was published in *British Gynaecological Journal* 1 (January-June 1886): 202. For a general account of the importance of the hospital setting to a variety of new techniques see Howell, *Technology in the Hospital*, 1–29, and Charles Rosenberg, "Community and Communities: The Evolution of the American Hospital," in Diana Long and Janet Golden, eds., *The American General Hospital* (Ithaca: Cornell Univ. Press, 1989), 12.

33. "How Gynecology Is Taught," *Journal of the American Medical Association* 11 (August 1888): 181–185.

34. See this emphatic stance in the speeches of leading surgeons, for example, T. Galliard Thomas, "The Gynecology of the Future and Its Relation to Surgery," Presidential Address before the American Gynecological Society, *Transactions* 4 (1879): 41; W. Kennedy, "In Memoriam: Joseph Price," *American Journal of Obstetrics* 65 (January 1912): 96; T. Gaillard Thomas, "An Address in Obstetrics and Gynecology," *New York Medical Journal* 40 (November 22, 1884): 563. Howard Kelly, "History of Gynecology in America," in Howard Kelly, ed., *A Cyclopedia of American Medical Biography* (Philadelphia: W. B. Saunders, 1912), 1: xlviiii–liv, xlviiii.

35. Here it is worth recalling Christopher Lawrence's insight that solutions to technical problems in medicine often arise out of "conflict between different communities with differing interests." See Lawrence, "Democratic, Divine, and Heroic," n. 20.

36. Commented W. Kennedy in a biographical sketch of Joseph Price, a well-respected gynecological surgeon from Philadelphia, "During these years the older surgeons, who occupied positions of authority, as teachers and hospital surgeons, either rejected *in toto* the new surgery, or accepted it as an experiment only" ("In Memoriam: Joseph Price," 96).

37. Jane Sewell and Ornella Moscucci have made an excellent case for the central role desires for upward mobility played in motivating gynecological surgeons in Great Britain. Sewall, "Bountiful Bodies," and Moscucci, *Science of Woman*, passim.

38. Lawrence points out that American surgeons boasted of being practical and empirical. It might also be prudent to observe that in England and on the continent, medicine was organized differently than in the United States, with physicians enjoying much status and prestige, while surgeons, until the late nineteenth century, were viewed as craftsmen, devoid of a gentlemanly education, and thus subservient. Though surgeons rapidly gained prestige in England by the end of the century, my comparisons between the two countries are cautiously aware of different social context, and my focus is primarily on the United States ("Democratic, Divine, and Heroic," 14). The issue of malpractice and its specific relationship to the Dixon Jones case will be taken up in the last two chapters.

39. Kennedy, "In Memoriam: Joseph Price," 96. In keeping with surgeons' identification with progressive science, critics attacked not only new operative procedures but the "new pathology," which utilized the microscope to help diagnose infections, ectopic gestation, and appendicitis.

40. See John Harley Warner, *The Therapeutic Perspective: Medical Practice, Knowledge, and Identity in America, 1820–1885* (Cambridge, Mass.: Harvard Univ. Press, 1986), 225–228; Maulitz, " 'Physician versus Bacteriologist,' " and Toby Appel, "Biological and Medical Societies and the Founding of the American Physiological Society," 155–176, in Gerald Geison, ed., *Physiology in the American Context* (Bethesda, Md.: American Physiological Society, 1987). There is a mature and sophisticated literature on the social construction of science, which for reasons of space cannot be cited here. John Harley Warner's work has been especially helpful to me on changing meanings of science in medicine, as have been the publications of Joel Howell, Robert Kohler, Gerald Geisen, Charles Rosenberg and Morris Vogel, Charles Rosenberg and Janet Golden, and Keith Wailoo.

41. Alfred Stillé, "An Address Delivered to the Medical Classes of the University of Pennsylvania on Withdrawing from His Chair, April 10, 1884," *Medical News* 44 (1884): 433–438, quoted in John Harley Warner, "Ideals of Science and Their Discontents in Late Nineteenth-Century American Medicine," *Isis* (1991): 462–463. Warner

points out that the split was not categorically generational, and there were a few younger physicians who displayed a more traditional mind-set.

42. Warner, "Ideals of Science," 461–463.

43. Warner has given us a detailed account of one fault line around which such difficulties coalesced: the debate in the 1870s and 1880s over revision of the consultation clause of the AMA Code of Ethics, when many younger members rebelled against prohibitions barring the seeking of counsel from homeopathic and other alternative practitioners. There were other sites of contention as well, including the suspicion of specialization as elitist and dehumanizing. Warner, "Ideals of Science," 464–477.

44. See Barbara Rosencrantz, "The Search for Professional Order in Nineteenth-Century American Medicine," in Judith Leavitt and Ronald Numbers, eds. *Sickness and Health in America* (Madison: Univ. of Wisconsin Press, 1985), 219–232.

45. Regina Morantz-Sanchez, "The Gendering of Empathic Expertise: How Women Physicians Became More Empathic than Men," in Maureen A. Milligan and Ellen Singer More, eds., *The Empathic Practitioner* (New Brunswick: Rutgers Univ. Press, 1994), 40–58. See also Morantz-Sanchez, "Feminist Theory and Historical Practice: Rereading Elizabeth Blackwell," *History and Theory* 31 (1992) 51–69.

46. Kelly, "History of Gynecology in America," xxxviiii-xl. Kelly's view that freedom from the pain of surgery was a first step in a series of events that allowed surgeons to fabricate and perfect operating room technique was widely shared. "The most brilliant manipulator alive," observed Henry McNaughton-Jones, president-elect of the British Gynecological Society in 1898, "must feel that he can never repay the anesthetist for his coolness and skill, qualities which in many of the prolonged operations in abdominal surgery are tested to the utmost." "The Position of Gynecology Today," *British Gynaecological Journal* 14 (May 1898): 20–21. But recent historians are less comfortable with the notion of "a moment of discovery," because it implies a kind of technological determinism that discredits the possibility that anesthesia and antisepsis were discovered largely because surgery became the therapy of choice. Lawrence, "Democratic, Divine, and Heroic," 24. Given the cultural construction of white middle-class women as unable to endure sustained physical pain, however, one is tempted to conclude that anesthesia was essential to the willingness of surgeons to perform ovariotomy on that class of patients. One very instructive aspect of the story of Sims's experiments with slave women is the way in which it exposes prevailing assumptions that black women were less sensitive to pain than their white sisters. Martin Pernick's work on the introduction of anesthesia shows that it was used differentially when first introduced, and most often on white middle-class women. His findings imply that the discovery of anesthesia *was* possibly crucial to further developments in the field. See Martin Pernick, *A Calculus of Suffering: Pain, Professionalism and Anesthesia in Nineteenth-Century America* (New York: Columbia Univ. Press, 1985), 148–167.

47. Thomas, "An Address in Obstetrics and Gynaecology," 584.

48. T. Galliard Thomas, "The Gynecology of the Future and Its Relation to Surgery," American Gynecological Society *Transactions* 4 (1879): 36.

49. "Letter from I. L. Watkins, M.D.," *Alabama Medical & Surgical Age* 2 (1889–90): 188–190.

50. See, for example, Ricci, *One Hundred Years*, 344–345, for the use of pessaries. On debates regarding trachelorrhaphy, the surgical repair of the torn cervix developed by Thomas Addis Emmet of the New York Woman's Hospital, see Speert, *Obstetrics and Gynecology in America*, 51; Willis E. Ford, "The Ultimate Results of Trachelorrhaphy," *American Gynecological and Obstetrical Journal* 6 (June 1895): 783–793, and

discussion, 921–927; Henry Garrigues, "Fashions in Gynecology," *Yale Medical Journal* 4 (December 1897): 170–174. Tait opposed trachelorrhaphy. See Fred Byron Robinson, "A Sketch of Mr. Lawson Tait and His Work, Pt. 3," *Journal of the American Medical Association* 18 (January 30, 1892): 129–132, 130.

51. He did do so, however, especially in his early career when he was establishing himself as a skilled and experienced ovariotomist, and before he began to emphasize diseased tubes as the seat of the problem. See Lawson Tait, "Note on Oophorectomy," *British Medical Journal* 2 (July 10, 1880): chart on 49.

52. See Fred Byron Robinson, "A Sketch of Mr. Lawson Tait and His Work, Pt. 2," *Journal of the American Medical Association* 18 (January 23, 1892): 101; Lawson Tait, "Indications for Abdominal Section and the Details for Its Performance," *Medical Press and Circular* 100 (April 9, 1890): 369. "Tait's Law," as his injunction to exploratory surgery was labeled, was as follows: "I venture to lay down a surgical law that in every case of disease in the abdomen or pelvis, in which the health is destroyed or life threatened, and in which the condition is not evidently due to malignant disease, an exploration of the cavity should be made." Quoted in Harvey Graham, *Eternal Eve* (London: Hutchinson, 1960), 269–270. There were those who disapproved of exploratory surgery as not necessary if a better knowledge of the pathology of the female reproductive system were acquired, and critics characterized "Tait's Law" crudely as "When in doubt, open the belly and find out!" See Henry Clarke Coe, "The Old and the New Gynecology," reprinted from the *Dominion Medical Monthly* (August 1910): 4, mss. in the New York Academy of Medicine Archives. See also Coe's criticism of Tait's operation and Tait's response, Henry Clarke Coe, "Is Disease of the Uterine Appendages as Frequent as It Has Been Represented," *American Journal of Obstetrics and Disease of Women and Children (Am. J. Obst.)* 19 (June 1886): 570; (September 1886): 947–950. Dixon Jones favored exploratory surgery but, unlike Tait, accepted the germ theory of disease and followed careful antiseptic procedures.

53. Lawson Tait, "A Contribution to the Debate on the Present Position of Abdominal Surgery," *Medical Press and Circular* 100 (April 23, 1890): 419.

54. Mary Dixon Jones, "Removal of the Uterine Appendages—Five Cases," *Am. J. Obst.* 21 (February 1888): 169. Mundé believed it was important to be very clear about his terms. He referred to "ovariotomy" chiefly as the removal of tumors of the ovaries without involvement of the tubes. Tait's operation, which included the removal of diseased tubes and ovaries, he labeled "salpingo-oophorectomy." The term "oophorectomy" was reserved for "the removal of the ovaries and tubes which *macroscopically* do not appear diseased, the operation being performed for the purpose of bringing on the menopause either for the relief of reflex neuroses, menstrual, psychic or physical (Battey's operation), or to check the growth and symptoms of uterine fibroids (Hegar's operation)." Paul F. Mundé, "A Year's Work in Laparotomy," *Am. J. Obst.* 21 (January 1888): 16–18.

55. Howell, *Technology in the Hospital,* passim, is especially good on this. See Regina Morantz-Sanchez, "Entering Male Professional Terrain: Dr. Mary Dixon Jones and the Emergence of Gynecological Surgery in the Nineteenth-Century United States," *Gender and History* 7 (August 1995): 212.

56. See Ricci, *One Hundred Years,* 42, 56.

57. See C. C. Stockard, "Fibro-Cyst of Uterus Weighing One Hundred and Thirty-Five Pounds," *Medical Record* 26 (August 16, 1884): 177–178.

58. Walter Coles, "A Large Fibro-Cyst of the Uterus and Ovarian Cystoma, Co-Existing with Pregnancy; Operation; Recovery," *St. Louis Courier of Medicine* 8 (December 1882): 490–505, esp. 502 on hemorrhage.

59. Developed by Professor Apostoli of France and adopted briefly by a number of practitioners, this procedure consisted of a galvanic kit with two electrodes that were passed through the uterus, applying current to the offending tumors as a means of cauterization. Supporters believed electricity to be less dangerous than laparotomy, claiming that it cured or greatly relieved the symptoms of fibroids. Some practitioners also used it in the treatment of cancer. For the use of electricity, pro and con, see John Byrne, "On the Relative Merits of Total or Partial Hysterectomy for Cancer of the Cervix by Ordinary Methods, and Supravaginal Excision by Galvano-Cautery," *American Gynecological and Obstetrical Journal* 9 (July 1896): 32–44. See discussion at the end, especially Coe's remarks.

60. Joseph Price, "The Past, Present and Future of Abdominal and Pelvic Surgery," *Journal of the American Medical Association* 15 (January 25, 1890): 110.

61. See discussion at the Fifth Annual Meeting of the American Gynecological Society, Speert, *Obstetrics and Gynecology in America,* 54. See also 65, 69. Also William Goodell, "A Case of Spaying for Fibroid Tumor of the Womb," *American Journal of the Medical Sciences* 76 (July 1878): 36–50.

62. See Lawson Tait, "A Contribution to the Debate on the Present Position of Abdominal Surgery," *Medical Press and Circular* 50 (April 23, 1890): 420, for a discussion of various techniques to control bleeding and an acknowledgment by Tait of the extreme difficulties encountered in these operations.

63. Howard A. Kelly, "Pre-History of Gynecology in Maryland, Pt. 1," *Medical Annals of Maryland, 1899–1925, Maryland State Medical Journal* 29 (March 1980): 82. For various debates over hysterectomy, its technique, indications, and effectiveness, see Charles P. Noble, "Development and Present Status on Hysterectomy for Fibromyomata," *British Gynaecological Journal* 13 (1897): 48–90, and "The History of Early Operations for Fibroid Tumors," *Am. J. Obst.* 40 (July 1899): 171–202; A. Reeves Jackson, "Vaginal Hysterectomy for Cancer," *Journal of the American Medical Association* 5 (August 15, 1885): 169–171; Ernest W. Cushing, "Choice of Methods in Hysterectomy," American Gynecological Society *Transactions* 23 (1898): 209–220; William M. Polk, "Extirpation of the Entire Uterus by the Suprapubic Method," *Am. J. Obst.* 26 (November 1892): 727–742; Joseph Price, "Abdominal Hysterectomy," *Am. J. Obst.* (November 1892): 743–751. Tait preferred the removal of the ovaries and appendages to hysterectomy. See discussion on Electricity in Gynecology at British Gynecological Society meetings published in *Medical Record* 36 (September 21, 1889), 328.

64. LeRoy Broun, "A Review of the Evolution of the Modern Surgical Treatment of Fibroid Tumors of the Uterus," *Medical Record* 70 (July 1906): 136. Broun's article is also a good review of the various approaches to fibroids from the late 1870s through 1906. See also Mary Dixon Jones's presentation in the minutes of the New York Pathological Society meeting for December 1888, published in *Medical Record* 36 (February 1889): 189 in which she describes "Subrapubic hysterectomy, the Stump Removed per Vaginam, as in Kolpo-Hysterectomy." See also Mary Dixon-Jones, "Two Cases of Uterine Myoma: One Suprapubic Hysterectomy, the Other Complete Hysterectomy," *New York Medical Journal* 48 (August 25 and September 1, 1888): 198–205, 226–232. For references to her work in hysterectomy, see Kelly, "History of Gynecology in America," xlvi; Charles P. Noble, "The Development and the Present Status of Hysterectomy for Fibro-Myomata and for Inflammation of the Uterine Appendages in America," *British Gynecological Journal* 13 (May 1897): 52, and "Abdominal Hysteromyomectomy and Myomectomy," in Howard Kelly and Charles P. Noble, eds., *Gynecology and Abdominal Surgery* (Philadelphia: W. B. Saunders, 1907), 661; Ernest W. Cushing, "The Evolution in America of Abdominal Hysterectomy and Total Extirpation of the Uterus," *Annals of*

Gynaecology and Paediatry 8 (June 1895): 579; Albert Mathieu, "The History of Hysterectomy," *Western Journal of Surgery, Obstetrics and Gynecology* 42 (January 1934): 9. Hysterectomy because the treatment of choice even for diseased tubes and ovaries.

65. My discussion is indebted to Maulitz's work in the history of pathology, especially his articles " 'Physician versus Bacteriologist' " and " 'The Whole Company of Pathology': Pathology as Idea and as Work in American Medical Life," in Teizo Ogawa, ed., *History of Pathology, Proceedings of the 8th International Symposium on the Comparative History of Medicine—East and West* (Shizuoka, Japan: Sosono-shi, 1983), 139–161. Quote is from ibid., 142.

66. Thomas Savage, "Diseases of the Fallopian Tubes," *Birmingham Medical Review* 13 (1883): 28.

67. See Maulitz, " 'Physician versus Bacteriologist' "; Warner, *Therapeutic Perspective*, esp. 239–250; "Ideals of Science and Their Discontents in Late Nineteenth-Century American Medicine," *Isis* 82 (1991): 454–478; and "The History of Science and the Sciences of Medicine," *Osiris* 10 (1995): 164–193.

68. This discussion relies heavily on Warner, "Ideals of Science and Their Discontents," 456–458; quote is from Warner, *Therapeutic Perspective*, 258. For another version of these worries about professional identity, see Howell, *Technology in the Hospital*, 207–221. Howell recounts some very public concerns voiced by an old-style surgeon about the meaning and utility of blood tests for appendicitis, espressing many of the same doubts about laboratory medicine recounted here, doubts that were apparently carried well into the twentieth century, according to Howell, and often repeated as new technologies became available.

69. Warner, "Ideals of Science and Their Discontents," 456.

70. Ibid. 464.

71. Quoted in Maulitz, " 'Physician versus Bacteriologist,' " 97.

72. Kennedy, "In Memoriam: Joseph Price," 96.

73. "The Wave of Surgical Progress" (Editorial), *Journal of the American Medical Association* 6 (July 1888): 21.

74. John Burdon-Sanderson, "An Address on the Relation of Science to Experience in Medicine," *British Medical Journal* 2 (1899): 133–135. Quoted in Howell, *Technology in the Hospital*, 62.

75. David W. Cheever, "The Future of Surgery Without Limit," *Medical Record* 36 (May 1889): 579. See also Phineas S. Conner, "Address on Surgery," *Journal of the American Medical Association* 6 (June 1889): 15, 18; L. S. McMurtry, "The Present Position of Pelvic Surgery," *Amer. Jour. Obs* 28 (October 1893): 451.

76. Douglas, "Responsibilities of the Abdominal Surgeon," *Journal of the American Medical Association* 22 (May 12, 1894): 692.

77. Quoted in Lawrence, "Democratic, Divine, and Heroic," 9.

78. Henry Clarke Coe, "Is Disease of the Uterine Appendages as Frequent?" 562–563: "The aid of the microscope is invoked only incidentally by the laparotomist. A piece of a tumor is examined by the pathologist who pronounces it to be malignant, whereupon the surgeon extirpates it; a mass of tissue removed from the uterine cavity presents the microscopical appearances of sarcoma—the gynecologist determines upon a radical operation. These are the natural sequences. But the same gynecologist will remove the ovaries and tubes, and will afterward call upon the pathologist to justify the wisdom of the operation, which, to tell the truth, it is often extremely difficult to do."

79. Dixon Jones, "Ovariotomy and Disease of the Fallopian Tubes" (Letter to the Editor), *Medical Record* 30 (August 1886): 252.

80. Dixon-Jones, "Colpo-Hysterectomy for Malignant Disease—Some Consider-

ations in Regard to the Operation, Technique, etc., with a Report of My First Five Cases," *Am. J. Obst.* 27 (May 1893): 663.

81. JoAnne Brown, *The Definition of a Profession* (Princeton: Princeton Univ. Press, 1992), 21.

82. Coe, "Is Disease of the Uterine Appendages as Frequent?," 561–575. For information on Coe, see Floyd Elwood Keene, *Album of the Fellows of the American Gynecological Society, 1876–1930* (Philadelphia: Wm. J. Dornan, 1930), 134.

83. Dixon Jones often cited Coe in her own publications, and he was aware of her pathological work as well. See a notice he penned on "Endothelioma of the Ovary," published in the *American Journal of the Medical Sciences* (for which he was editor of the monthly section on Gynecology) 104 (July 1892): 119.

84. Coe, "Is Disease of the Uterine Appendages as Frequent?," 562–563.

85. See the admission of David W. Cheever, president of American Surgical Association, that "the older physiology is obsolete and discarded; but in the newer physiology the functions of some of the large and important organs are still undetermined. . . . An ignorance of their functions renders the surgeon unable to predict the consequences of their removal" (*Medical Record* 36 (May 1889): 579).

86. Helen Clapesattle, *The Doctors Mayo* (Minneapolis: The University of Minnesota Press, 1941), 301. For use of the term "furor operandi," see Henry Clarke Coe, *The Old and the New Gynecology*, 3: "Then came the *furor operandi*, which swept over the United States and Canada, until he who could not report a series of laparotomies (with a mortality of 25 per cent!) could not lay claim to be even a local gynecologist."

87. S. C. Gordon, "A Review of the Surgery of the Female Pelvic Organs," American Gynecological Society *Transactions* 31 (1906): 177.

88. "Complications During and Following Abdominal Operations," *Journal of the American Medical Association* 17 (December 19, 1891): 946. For a reference to "Western gynecologists" catching "the infection" of too much operating, see New York correspondent of the *Indiana Medical Journal*, notice "The Craze for Spaying Women" *Medical Record* 36 (March 1889): 327.

89. Clifton E. Wing of Boston argued that "unscrupulous practitioners can much increase their incomes by doing as many 'surgical operations' as possible." See "Unnecessary Surgical Operations in the Treatment of the Diseases of Women," *Boston Medical and Surgical Journal* 104 (April 1881): 389.

90. "Conservatism in Gynecology and Obstetrics," *Medical Record* 35 (December 1889): 676. See Dr. W. H. Link's remarks at the Philadelphia Obstetrical Society, January 1, 1891, in *Annals of Gynecology and Psychiatry* 4 (February 1891): 802. He disagreed with Joseph Price's complaint that young practitioners were being mercenary and blamed the situation on the improper guidance of leading surgeons. There is no end to this kind of offhand self-criticism in the medical journals during this period, though obviously no commentator believed that he himself was guilty of the behavior he was describing.

91. D. MacLean, "Sexual Mutilation of Women," *California Medical Journal* 15 (1894): 382. Marie Zakrzewska, who founded and ran the New England Hospital for Women and Children, was unsympathetic to women's desires for operations, and suspected many married women requested ovariotomies as a means of birth control. "Material comfort, indulgence in luxurious living, dislike to work & self abnegation," she remarked, "are the motives which prompt women to seek operations." Marie Zakrzewska to Elizabeth Blackwell, March 21, 1891. Blackwell MSS, Schlesinger Library.

92. Albert Brinkman, "A Case of Ovariotomy," *Brooklyn Medical Journal* 3 (1889): 458.

93. See Skene's testimony in the *Eagle*, February 19, 1892.

94. See Nancy Theriot, "Women's Voices in Nineteenth-Century Medical Discourse: A Step Toward Deconstructing Science," *Signs* 19 (Autumn 1993): 23.

95. Gert Brieger has done an excellent job sketching out the meaning to surgeons of the terms radical, conservative, and heroic in the last two-thirds of the century. The terms changed meaning, and even among gynecological surgeons, as we shall see later in this chapter, the terms radical and conservative, certainly by the 1890s, became somewhat blurred. See Brieger, "From Conservative to Radical Surgery in Late-Nineteenth Century America," in Lawrence, ed., *Medical Theory, Surgical Practice*, 216–230.

96. Edwin A. Lewis, "Influence of Public Opinion on Surgical Practice," *Brooklyn Medical Journal* 5 (1891): 257, 258, 259.

97. The literature on this subject is vast and diverse; Representative examples would include the work of Cynthia Russett, Nancy Stepan, Sander Gilman, Anne McClintock, Ann Stoler, Mary Poovey, Louise Newman, Marianna Torgovnick, Robert Rydell, Vron Ware, Charles Rosenberg, Jean and John Comaroff, and many others.

98. For example, George W. Kaan, "A Plea for Conservatism in Gynecology," *Boston Medical and Surgical Journal* 156 (April 25, 1907): 539; "To Limit the Castration of Women" (Editorial), *Journal of the American Medical Association* 13 (December 21, 1889): 887; Letter from Henry Savage to the *British Medical Journal* 5 (June 24, 1885): 966; on vivisection, see letter to the editor by Keith, *British Medical Journal* 3 (January 22, 1881): 133; Spencer Wells, "Recent Advances in the Surgical Treatment of Intraperitoneal Tumours," *British Medical Journal* 4 (August 27, 1881): 358.

99. See letter published as an appendage to Howard Kelly's "Conservatism in Ovariotomy," *Journal of the American Medical Association* 26 (February 8, 1886): 250; and Howard Kelly "The Ethical Side of the Operation of Oophorectomy," *Am. J. Obst.* 27 (1893): 207–208.

100. Quoted in Speert, *Obstetrics and Mynecalagy in America*, 69. For Emmet's early opposition to the operation for cancer, see 57. Henry Garrigues, also a gynecologist working in the field for over 25 years, voiced his suspicions of indiscriminate hysterectomy. See "Fashions in Gynecology," 173.

101. "The Fetich of the Ovary," *Am. J. Obst.* 54 (July 1906): 371.

102. See Mary Putnam Jacobi's interesting letter to Blackwell, December 25, 1888, in the Blackwell MSS. Library of Congress, in which she rejects Blackwell's views, retorting that "there is not such special sanctity about the ovary!"

103. "Woman in Medicine," *Women's Medical Journal 3* (July 1894): 15–16.

104. Many Dixon Jones, "Misplacements of the Uterus," *Pittsburgh Medical Review* 3 (October 1889): 305, and "Suppurating Endothelioma—Myofibroma in a Condition of Necrobiosis," *Medical Record* 38 (September 6, 1890): 263, and a quotation from William Byford, n. 1.

105. See John Farley, *Gametes and Spores: Ideas about Sexual Reproduction, 1750–1914* (Baltimore: Johns Hopkins Univ. Press, 1982), 160. On ovulation, see Janet Farrell, *Contraception and Abortion in 19th-Century America* (Ithaca: Cornell University Press, 1994), 80–84.

106. See Coe, "Is Disease of the Uterine Appendages as Frequent?" 564, 567, 568–569; Tait's snide reponse to Coe's cautionary remarks can be found in the Correspondence Section, *Am. J. Obst.* 19 (Sept 1886): 947–951. See also "The Ultimate Results of Laparotomy for the Removal of Diseased Appendages," *Medical Record* 23 (April 19, 1890): 440–443; and Coe's observation that his position in the beginning was "exceedingly unpopular," in Henry Clarke Coe, "Another view of Conservative Surgery of the Tubes and Ovaries," American Gynecological Society *Transactions* 23 (1898): 382.

107. This is a long and detailed article. C. H. F Routh, "On Castration in Females:

Its Frequent Inexpediency and the Signal Advantages of Conservative Surgery in These Cases,'' *Medical Press and Circular* 108 (April-May 1894): 435, 457.

108. *Medical News* 57 (November 29, 1890): 561. See also A. W. Johnstone, ''Clinical Importance of the Menstrual Wave,'' *American Gynecological and Obstetrical Journal* 9 (July 1896): 62–71. Especially interesting, perhaps, because of Skene's cautious acceptance of the use of technology like the microscope, is the discussion after the presentation of Johnstone's paper, in which Skene remarks that surgeons are rethinking their understanding of the relation of the sexual organs to women's general organization. In 1900, when Skene penned a retrospective of the accomplishments of the last quarter-century, he admitted how little was really known of this topic: ''The breath of scientists had blown away the mystical fog that had for ages hung around the function of menstruation. Now it was known to be conducted upon the same principles as all other physical phenomena, and more rational ideas were entertained regarding its utility in the economy. Still, the histology of the structures concerned, its advent at puberty, the physical necessity for it, the inducing conditions, the laws governing and the beneficial results obtained by menstruation were being evolved, but not definitely settled.'' ''The Status of Gynecology in 1876 and 1900,'' American Gynecological Society *Transactions* 25 (1900): 427.

109. S. C. Gordon, ''A Review of the Surgery of the Female Pelvic Organs,'' American Gynecological Society *Transactions* 31 (1906): 178.

110. See Joseph Price, ''The Past, Present and Future of Abdominal and Pelvic Surgery,'' *Journal of the American Medical Association* 14 (January 25, 1890): 109 for a radical view; Thomas Addis Emmet, ''A Protest Against the Removal of the Uterine Appendages,'' *Medical Record* 36 (December 1889): 711–712; and Malcolm McLean, ''Conservatism in Gynecology and Obstetrics,'' read at a November meeting of the Medical Society of the County of New York, including discussion and remarks by Emmet, Coe, H. J. Boldt, A. P. Dudley, and others, all of whom seem sympathetic to McLean's carefully reasoned position. *Medical Record*, ibid.

111. For condemnation of inexperience of general practitioners, see Rufus B. Hall, ''Complications During and Following Abdominal Operations,'' *Journal of the American Medical Association* 17 (December 1891): 946–948. For a helpful discussion of the emerging hierarchy among surgeons, see Dale Smith, ''Appendicitis, Appendectomy, and the Surgeon,'' *Bulletin of the History of Medicine* 70 (Fall 1996): 418–19.

112. As an example of this trend, see Howard A. Kelly, ''Abdominal Myomectomy,'' American Gynecological Society *Transactions* 23 (1898): 221–239, and ''The Conservative Treatment of Myomatous Uteri,'' *Journal of the American Medical Association* 29 (October 2, 1897): 668–669.

113. See Breiger, ''From Conservative to Radical Surgery,'' 222. For quote, see Charles P. Noble, ''True Conservatism in Gynecology,'' *Pennsylvania Medical Journal* 2 (1899): 463, 466, 467, and ''The Question of Operation in Cases of Chronic Oophoritis,'' American Gynecological Society *Transactions* 18 (1893): 398–410. See also Henry Clarke Coe's thoughtful article ''Another View of Conservative Surgery of the Tubes and the Ovaries,'' American Gynecological Society *Transactions* 23 (1898): 381–395, and G. Granville Bantock, ''A Plea for Conservative Gynecology,'' *British Medical Journal* (August 12, 1899): 454–458. This article is especially interesting because it reverses his earlier position. See Bantock, *A Plea for Early Ovariotomy* (London, H. K. Lewis, 1881).

114. For examples see Mordecai Price, ''A Plea for Early Operation in Ovariotomy and Abdominal Work,'' *Medical and Surgical Reporter* 61 (July 13, 1889): 31–34; H. J. Boldt, ''Salpingo-Oophorectomy and its Results,'' *Medical Record* 37 (May 17, 1890):

545–551; Joseph Price, "A Plea for Early Hysterectomy and Puerperal Hysterectomy," *American Association of Obstetricians and Gynecologists Transactions* 4 (1891): 251–269; S. C. Gordon, "A Review of the Surgery of the Female Pelvic Organs," American *Gynecological Society Transactions* 31 (1906): 175–186; Mary Dixon Jones, "Early Operations," Editorial, *Woman's Medical Journal* 2 (May 1894): 110–111.

115. See Skene's remarks during discussion at end of W. J. Corcoran's case report, *Brooklyn Medical Journal* 5 (1891): 453. Skene himself was sympathetic to the conservatives and confessed in 1882 that "I have long entertained the opinion that ovariotomy is the most difficult operation in the whole field of surgery." See "The Essentials of Success in Ovariotomy," *Medical Society of the County of Kings Proceedings* 7 (1882–83): 222.

116. "A Plea for Conservatism in the Treatment of Diseased Uterine Appendages," American Association of Obstetricians and Gynecologists *Transactions* 3 (1890): 309.

117. "On Hysterectomy," *American Gynecological and Obstetrical Journal* 10 (March 1897): 301–317, 303.

118. "The Status of Gynecology in 1876 and 1900," American Gynecological Society *Transactions* 25 (1900): 427.

119. R. C. Wright, "Hysterectomy: Past, Present and Future," *Obstetrics and Gynecology* 33 (1969): 560–563. Quoted in Sue V. Rosser, *Women's Health—Missing from U.S. Medicine* (Bloomington: Indiana Univ. Press, 1994), 59. Although Wright's comment is dated 1969, Rosser's book is very helpful in laying out the ways in which medical research and practice still exploit women. For a more recent example of this same attitude, see Sue Fisher, *In the Patient's Best Interest: Women and the Politics of Medical Decisions* (New Brunswick: Rutgers Univ. Press, 1986), 2–3. It is interesting to point out that physicians' thinking does not take place in a vacuum and always draws from the surrounding culture. Since R. C. Wright complained about too many hysterectomies, the intervention of the feminist movement in health care more generally and the rise in the number of women physicians have created a more complex situation. Women are making themselves heard both as patients and practitioners. For example, there is a very small movement among women with strong histories of breast cancer in their families to undergo preventive mastectomy, but so far doctors resist such operations and are reluctant to comply. Ironically, the argument patients give for wanting such procedures are not very different from gynecologists' justifications for hysterectomy in women who have already had a few children: the organs aren't essential and better to take them out rather than live with the risk of cancer.

An intriguing example of some fascinating parallels with the nineteenth century is the case of a modern-day Dixon Jones, Dr. Vicki Georges Hufnagel, the author of the book *No More Hysterectomies* (New York: New American Library, 1988). Dr. Hufnagel's career was encased in controversy in 1989 when her license to practice was revoked after a two-year investigation and a lengthy hearing by the California Board of Medical Quality Assurance. While some feminist groups hailed her as a "savior of women's reproductive organs"—for example, she lobbied to introduce a bill requiring physicians to obtain written consent from patients before performing a hysterectomy—others, like Dr. Judy Norsigian, accused her of being "into self-aggrandizement in a way that is extremely incompatible with the women's health movement." See *Ms.* magazine (November 1989): 69–71, and Los Angeles *Times*, October 5, 1989.

NOTES TO CHAPTER FIVE

1. See, for example, Ann Douglas (Wood), " 'The Fashionable Diseases': Women's Complaints and Their Treatment in Nineteenth-Century America," *Journal of*

Interdisciplinary History 4 (Summer 1973): 25–52; Barbara Ehrenreich and Dierdre English, *Complaints and Disorders: The Sexual Politics of Sickness* (Old Westbury: Feminist Press, 1973); and *For Her Own Good: 150 Years of Experts' Advice to Women* (New York: Anchor Books, 1979); Virginia Drachman, "Women Doctors and the Women's Medical Movement: Feminism and Medicine, 1850–1895," Ph.D. Thesis, SUNY Buffalo, 1976; Charles Rosenberg and Carroll Smith-Rosenberg, "The Female Animal: Medical and Biological Views of Woman and Her Role in Nineteenth-Century America," *Journal of American History* 60 (September 1973): 332–56; Carroll Smith-Rosenberg, "The Cycle of Femininity: Puberty and Menopause in 19th-Century America," *Feminist Studies* 1 (Winter 1973): 58–72; and "The Hysterical Woman: Sex Roles and Role Conflict in 19th-Century America," *Social Research* 39 (Winter 1972): 652–78; G. J. Barker-Benfield, *The Horrors of the Half-Known Life: Male Attitudes Toward Women and Sexuality in Nineteenth-Century America* (New York: Harper & Row, 1976); Sarah Stage, *Female Complaints: Lydia Pinckham and the Business of Women's Medicine* (New York: W. W. Norton, 1979); John S. and Robin Haller, *The Physician and Sexuality in Victorian America* (Urbana: Univ. of Illinois Press, 1974); Ann Dally, *Women under the Knife: A History of Surgery* (New York: Routledge, 1991); Mary Poovey, " 'Scenes of an Indelicate Character': The Medical 'Treatment' of Victorian Women," *Representations* 14 (Spring 1986): 137–168; Ornella Moscucci, *The Science of Woman: Gynecology and Gender in England, 1800–1929* (New York: Cambridge Univ. Press, 1990); Wendy Mitchinson, *The Nature of Their Bodies: Women and Their Doctors in Victorian Canada* (Toronto: Univ. of Toronto Press, 1991); Elaine Showalter, *The Female Malady* (New York: Penguin Books, 1985); Ludmilla Jordanova, *Sexual Visions* (Madison: Univ. of Wisconsin Press, 1988); Patricia A. Vertinsky, *The Eternally Wounded Woman: Women, Doctors, and Exercise in the Late Nineteenth Century* (Urbana: Univ. of Illinois Press, 1994); Cynthia Russett, *Sexual Science* (Cambridge, Mass.: Harvard Univ. Press, 1989). Also of interest, Alexandra Dundas Todd, *Intimate Adversaries: Cultural Conflict Between Doctors and Women Patients* (Philadelphia: Univ. of Pennsylvania Press, 1989); Athena Vrettos, *Somatic Fictions: Imagining Illness in Victorian Culture* (Stanford, Calif.: Stanford Univ. Press, 1995); Emily Martin, *The Woman in the Body* (Baltimore: Johns Hopkins Univ. Press, 1987); Sue Fisher, *In the Patient's Best Interest* (New Brunswick, N.J.: Rutgers Univ. Press, 1986); Sue V. Rosser, *Women's Health—Missing from U.S. Medicine* (Bloomington: Indiana Univ. Press, 1994); Alice E. Adams, *Reproducing the Womb* (Ithaca: Cornell Univ. Press, 1994). There is an equally abundant literature on the medicalization of childbirth, which I will not cite here.

2. For the increased faith in medical science among women, see Regina Morantz, "Making Women Modern: Middle-Class Women and Health Reform in the 19th Century," *Journal of Social History* 10 (June 1977): 490–507.

3. Moscucci, *Science of Woman*, 102.

4. Mitchinson, *Nature of Their Bodies*, 47.

5. W. T. Smith, "Lectures on Parturition, and the Principles and Practice of Obstetricy," *Lancet* 2 (1848): 119; Arthur Edis, *Diseases of Women: A Manual for Students and Practitioners* (Philadelphia: 1882), 20; Robert Barnes, "Women, diseases of," in R. Quain, ed., *A Dictionary of Medicine: Including General Pathology, General Therapeutics, Hygiene, and the Diseases Peculiar to Women and Children*, 2 vols. (London, 1882), 2:1790. Quotes from Barnes and Smith are cited in Moscucci, *Science of Woman*, 102.

6. Sally Shuttleworth has shown that ads for female pills assumed a "direct continuity between the operation of the menstrual cycle and mental health." Shuttleworth, "Female Circulation: Medical Discourse and Popular Advertising in the Mid-Victorian Era," in Mary Jacobus, Evelyn Fox Keller, and Sally Shuttleworth, eds., *Body/Politics:*

Women and the Discourses of Science (New York: Routledge, 1990), 47–68. Andrew Scull and Diane Fabreau make this point as well in " 'A Chance to Cut Is a Chance to Cure': Sexual Surgery for Psychosis in Three Nineteenth-Century Societies," *Research in Law, Deviance, and Social Control* 8 (1986): 17. See also Nancy Theriot, "Women's Voice in Nineteenth-Century Medical Discourse: A Step Toward Deconstructiing Science," *Signs* 19 (Autumn 1993): 1–31; Regina Morantz-Sanchez, *Sympathy and Science: Women Physicians in American Medicine* (New York: Oxford Univ. Press, 1985), 215–216. Also interesting in terms of patient attitudes is Edward Shorter, *From Paralysis to Fatigue: A History of Psychosomatic Illness in the Modern Era* (New York: Free Press, 1992), chs. 2 and 3. See also Mitchinson, *Nature of Their Bodies*, who suggests that the medical perception of female ill-health gained credibility at least partly because it reinforced what people already believed (50). Of course medical ideas both reflected as well as helped shape ideas about women.

7. George H. Rohé, "The Relation of Pelvic Disease and Psychical Disturbance in Women," *Transactions* of the American Association of Obstetricians and Gynecologists 5 (1892) 321.

8. For a clear exposition of the reflex theory and its origins, see Shorter, *From Paralysis to Fatigue*, 40–94. Ruth Harris's *Murders and Madness: Medicine, Law, and Society in the fin de siècle* (Oxford: Clarendon Press, 1989) offers an excellent chapter on the medical approach to neurological and physiological problems in general which contributes intelligently to our understanding of the way physicians approached mind-body issues in the period. See 24–64.

9. On Clarke, his theories and influence, see Morantz-Sanchez, *Sympathy and Science*, 54–55; Rosalind Rosenberg, *Beyond Separate Spheres: Intellectual Roots of Modern Feminism* (New Haven: Yale Univ. Press, 1982), 1–27; and Sue Zschoche, "Dr. Clarke Revisited: Science, True Womanhood, and Female Collegiate Education," *History of Education Quarterly* 29 (Winter 1989): 545–569. On thermodynamics and its application to theories of human energy, see Russett, *Sexual Science*, 104–129. See E. C. Dudley, "Infancy; Puberty; Maturity; Menopause; Senility," *American Gynecological and Obstetrical Journal* 6 (January 1895): 125. Dudley felt the jury was still out regarding higher education for women, but he acknowledged the social power of these beliefs.

10. See Theriot, "Women's Voice in Nineteenth-Century Medical Discourse," passim, for tensions between specialties. Scull and Fabreau also flag disagreements between alienists, neurologists, and surgeons over such operations. For some women physicians' opposition to surgery, see Morantz-Sanchez *Sympathy and Science*, 195–196. Contemporary articles on hysteria and surgery are abundant, and I cite here only a few representative examples: Augustus P. Clarke, "A Consideration of Some of the Operative Measures Employed in Gynecology," *Journal of the American Medical Association* (February 1893): 141; Thomas More Madden, "Constitutional Treatment of Chronic Diseases Peculiar to Women," *Medical Press and Circular* (May 1890): 497–500, and "The Relation of Hysteria to Structural Changes in the Uterus and Its Adnexa," *Transactions* of the American Association of Obstetricians and Gynecologists 7 (1894): 435–441; Spencer Wells, Alfred Hegar, and Robert Battey, "Castration in Mental and Nervous Diseases: A Symposium," *American Journal of the Medical Sciences* 92 (October 1886): 455–490; Henry MacNaughton-Jones, "The Correlation of Sexual Function with Insanity and Crime," *British Gynaecological Journal* 15 (February 1900): 524–552; E. W. Cushing, "Melancholia; Masturbation; Cured By Removal of Both Ovaries," *Journal of the American Medical Association* 8 (April 1887): 441–442; William Goodell, "Two Successive Cases of Laparotomy, For Ovarian Cyst and For Ovarian Insanity," *The Medical News*

56 (May 1890): 521–22; Robert T. Edes, "Ovariotomy for Nervous Disease," *Boston Medical and Surgical Journal*, 130 (January 1894): 105–110; A. J. C. Skene, "Gynecology as Related to Insanity in Women," reprint from *Archives of Medicine*, (New York: G. P. Putnam, 1880). Skene mentions the differences between gynecologists and alienists, who were skeptical about the direct relationship of insanity to diseases of the reproductive organs, p. 2. For representative examples of women physicians who operated, some of them cautiously, for mental disturbances, see Elizabeth Keller's response to E. W. Cushing on Oophorectomy at a meeting of the Gynecological Society of Boston, 1887 in *Journal of the American Medical Association* 8 (April 1887): 441; Anne H. McFarland, "The Relations of Operative Gynecology to Insanity," *Woman's Medical Journal* 2 (February 1894): 40–42. H. A. Tomlinson and Mary E. Bassett, in "Association of Pelvic Diseases and Insanity in Women, and the Influence of Treatment of the Local Disease upon the Mental Condition," *Journal of the American Medical Association* 33 (September 1899): 827–831 were two alienists, one a woman, who did not believe surgery cured insanity.

11. Poovey, *Uneven Developments: The Ideological Work of Gender in Mid-Victorian England* (Chicago: Univ. of Chicago Press, 1988) 1–23, quote on 10. See also Ruth Bloch, "American Feminine Ideals in Transition: The Rise of Moral Motherhood, 1785–1815," *Feminist Studies* 4 (June 1978): 101–126. Also helpful in charting the redefinition of female sexuality in the eighteenth and nineteenth centuries is Nancy Cott, "Passionlessness: An Interpretation of Victorian Sexual Ideology," *Signs* 4 (Winter 1978): 219–236.

12. In a somewhat problematic, but interesting reading of the debates over the uses of chloroform in childbirth, Mary Poovey sees these two representations coming into conflict as professionalizing physicians attempted to assert their authority over this increasingly culturally loaded event. Although doctors believed that women were chaste, they feared that under the influence of anesthesia they would regress to a state of nature in which they would be sexually uncontrollable. Poovey, *Uneven Developments*, 24–51.

13. Carol Groneman, "Nymphomania: The Historical Construction of Female Sexuality," *Signs* 19 (Winter 1994): 337–367.

14. See Barker-Benfield, *Horrors of the Half-Known Life*; Showalter, *Female Malady*; Poovey, " 'Scenes of an Indelicate Character' "; Jane E. Sewell, "Bountiful Bodies: Spencer Wells, Lawson Tait, and the Birth of British Gynaecology," Ph.D. dissertation, Johns Hopkins University, 1991, p. 290. The word "transgressive" is Sewell's, but she is much more careful than other authors to explain internal developments within medical practice other than the desire to keep women in their place that might have motivated physicians to try such procedures. Her work is complex and rewarding.

15. See Morantz-Sanchez, *Sympathy and Science*.

16. Nancy Theriot, "Women's Voices in Nineteenth-Century Medical Discourse: A Step Toward Deconstructing Science," *Signs* 19 (Autumn 1993): 2.

17. See Kelly's assessment of his work in Howard A. Kelly and Walter Burrage, eds., *Dictionary of American Medical Biography* (Baltimore: Norman, Remington, 1928), 383.

18. Emmet, *The Principles and Practice of Gynecology* (Philadelphia: Henry C. Lea's Son, 1879). A second edition was published in 1880 and a third in 1884. For Kelly's remarks, see Kelly and Burrage, eds., *Dictionary of American Medical Biography*, 383.

19. Note, for example, this recognition of the importance of pathology to diagnosis: "By studying the physical, chemical and microscopical characters it is almost always possible to diagnosticate ovarian cysts, *even without knowing anything about the patient*, and, of course, still more so when the result is combined with the other features of the case" (emphasis mine). On the next page, however, he continues to put his faith in

bedside diagnosis and clinical judgment, demonstrating that his faith in the laboratory is tentative: "We have certainly not yet reached a stage where the operator can afford to throw aside his own judgment, if based on a fair experiment in physical examinations. In two instances of doubt it has occurred to me to operate and remove ovarian tumors after experts were unable from an examination of the fluid, to give me the slightest information in regard to the character of the tumor." *The Principles and Practice of Gynaecology*, 3rd ed. (Philadelphia: Henry C. Lea's Son, 1884), 681–682.

20. See the works cited above, as well as Tom Laqueur, *Making Sex* (Cambridge, Mass.: Harvard Univ. Press, 1990); Russett, *Sexual Science*; Mary Poovey, *Making a Social Body: British Cultural Formation, 1830–1864* (Chicago: Univ. of Chicago Press, 1995); Judith Walkowitz, *City of Dreadful Delight* (Chicago: Univ. of Chicago Press, 1992).

21. *The Principles and Practice of Gynecology* (1879), 18.

22. Ibid., 20.

23. E. H. Clarke, *Sex in Education: A Fair Chance for Girls* (Boston, 1873), 41. On the significance of Clarke see note 9 above.

24. *The Principles and Practice of Gynecology* (1879), 22.

25. Ibid., 21–22.

26. Ibid., 654.

27. On Austin Flint's views and his role in the AMA Code of Ethics controversy, see Warner, "Ideals of Science and their Discontents in Late Nineteenth-century America," *Isis* 82 (1991): 454–478, 463, 467–468.

28. See Robert Latou Dickinson's obituary in American Gynecological Society *Transactions* 26 (1901): 393–396, which was reprinted in Kelly and Burrage, eds., *American Medical Biographies* (Baltimore: Norman, Remington Co., 1920), 1058–1059. Skene's name is still known by medical students because of Skene's glands, the paraurethral glands named and described by him in 1880.

29. See A. J. C. Skene, *Education and Culture as Related to the Health and Diseases of Women* (Detroit: George S. Davis, 1889).

30. A. J. C. Skene, *Medical Gynecology: A Treatise on the Diseases of Women from the Standpoint of the Physician* (New York: D. Appleton, 1895), 32–33, 64. *Education and Culture* was incorporated verbatim as the first six chapters of *Medical Gynecology* (1895), so the page citations will be from the latter work.

31. Ibid., 79–80, 224–225.

32. Ibid., 320.

33. Ibid., 45–48, 83.

34. See Regina Morantz-Sanchez, "Rereading Elizabeth Blackwell," *History and Theory* 31 (December 1992): 51–69, and *Sympathy and Science*, 47–63, 209–213; Ella Ridgeway, "The Causes of Uterine Diseases," M.D. thesis, Woman's Medical College of Pennsylvania, 1873; Anna Longshore-Potts, *Discourses to Women on Medical Subjects* (San Diego, 1897), 122.

35. As early as 1874, a group of women in Boston urged Dr. Mary Putnam Jacobi to enter an essay in Harvard Medical School's celebrated Boylston Essay competition, of which the topic chosen that year was the effect of menstruation on women. Jacobi did submit an essay, anonymously, entitled "The Question of Rest for Women During Menstruation," which actually won the prize, to the chagrin of supporters of the Clarke thesis. The study challenged conservative medical opinion on the subject with state-of-the-art statistical analyses and case studies, concluding that there was "nothing in the nature of menstruation to imply the necessity, or even the desirability, of rest for women whose nutrition is really normal." See Mary Putnam Jacobi, *The Question of Rest for*

Women During Menstruation (New York, 1877), 227. See C. Alice Baker's letter to Jacobi, urging her to submit an entry in the Schlesinger Library, Radcliffe College, Baker to Putnam Jacobi, 7 November 1874, Jacobi MSS. Examples of other studies that made important contributions to rethinking the issue of women's health include Elizabeth C. Underhill, "The Effect of College Life on the Health of Women Students," *Woman's Medical Journal* 22 (Febrary 1912): 31–33; Mary E. B. Ritter, "Health of University Girls," *California State Medical Journal* 1 (1902–3): 259–264; Clelia Mosher, "Normal Menstruation and Some Factors Modifying It," *Johns Hopkins Hospital Bulletin* 12 (1901): 178–179; Elizabeth R. Thelburg, "College Education a Factor in the Physical Life of Women," *WMCP Alumnae Transactions* (1899), 73–87. For a good study of changing attitudes toward physical exercise for women and its larger implications regarding the female body see Martha H. Verbrugge, *Able Bodied Womanhood: Personal Health and Social Change in Nineteenth-Century Boston* (New York: Oxford Univ. Press, 1988).

36. For an extensive discussion of this point, and how women physicians balanced their womanhood, professional aspirations, and dominant medical theory, see Morantz-Sanchez, *Sympathy and Science*, 203–231.

37. Margaret Colby, "Presidential Address," *Woman's Medical Journal* 12 (July 1902): 154.

38. M. Carey Thomas, "Present Tendencies in Women's College and University Education," *Education Review* 25 (1908): 58.

39. Charles A. L. Reed, ed., *A Text-book of Gynecology* (New York: D. Appleton, 1901), 7–8.

40. Emmet, *Principles and Practice of Gynaecology* (1884), 24.

41. Anna Fullerton, "Studies in Gynecology from the Service of the Woman's Hospital of Philadelphia," *Journal of the American Medical Association* 29 (December 25, 1897): 1301. On gynecology's contribution to monitoring female health, see also A. J. C. Skene, *Medical Gynecology* (1895), 22: "Physicians ought to be at all times ready to give advice to and prescribe for those who are undergoing physical culture and development, for here they can do more for the human race than at any other time of life . . . it is wiser to employ a physician to superintend the physical education of girls than to employ him to cure their ill health during womanhood." On the bicycle see Robert Latou Dickinson, "Bicycling for Women from the Standpoint of the Gynecologist," *American Journal of Obstetrics and Gynecology* 31 (October 1895): 25–35; James F. Prendergast, "The Bicycle for Women," ibid. 34 (November 1896): 247–253; and Thomas R. Evans, "Harmful Effects of the Bicycle upon the Girl's Pelvis," ibid. 33 (May 1896): 554; Editorial, "Bicycling for Women," *Atlanta Medical and Surgical Journal* 12 (1895–96): 421.

42. See Charlotte Blake Brown, "The Health of Our Girls," California State Medical Society *Transactions* 26 (1896): 193–202.

43. Fullerton, "Abdominal Surgery at the Woman's Hospital of Philadelphia," Philadelphia County Medical Society *Proceedings* 28 (1892): 177–180, and *Philadelphia Times & Register* 24 (June 1892): 626. It is likely that this exchange was catalyzed by an article Fullerton published in the *Annals of Gynaecology and Pediatry* 4 (November 1890): 76–81, titled "Surgery or Electricity in Gynaecology?," in which she took a dim view of electrical treatment. The issue also published a written response from Massey and an answer by Fullerton. See Ibid., 151–154 and 216–220.

44. For representative examples, see Charlotte Blake Brown, "Report of the Surgical Work of the Children's Hospital from March 1, 1886 to October 1, 1887— A Period of 19 Months," *Pacific Medical and Surgical Journal and Western Lancet* 30

(December 1887): 688–689; Helene Kuhlmann, "A Few Cases of Interest in Gynecology in Relation to Insanity," *State Hospital Bulletin*, Utica, New York, 1 (1896): 172–179.

45. Mary Dixon Jones, "Sterility in Woman—Causes, Treatment, and Illustrative Cases," *Medical Record* 40 (September 19, 1891): 321–323; Mary Fullerton, "Abdominal Surgery in the Woman's Hospital of Philadelphia," *Philadelphia Times and Register* 24 (June 1893): 619–625.

46. "Reminiscences of Travels in Europe in 1886, No. 3," *Woman's Medical Journal* 5 (January 1896): 12.

47. Mary Dixon Jones, "Insanity, Its Causes: Is There in Woman a Correlation of the Sexual Function with Insanity and Crime?" *Medical Record* 58 (December 1900): 931.

48. "Reminiscences of Travels, No. 3," 13.

49. "Removal of the Uterine Appendages: Nine Consecutive Cases," *Medical Record* 30 (August 21, 1886): 207; see also "A Hitherto Undescribed Disease of the Ovary: Endothelioma Changing to Angeioma and Haematoma," *New York Medical Journal* 50 (September 28, 1889): 338: "This patient had long complained of tenderness and soreness in the pelvis, and that the marital relations were not only painful but repulsive and unendurable. After the operation her emphatic statement to me, as well as similar statements of many other patients, disprove the assertion that the removal of the ovaries destroys sexual desires. So far from it, this patient assured me to the contrary, and similar statements have been made to me by other patients." See also this statement about menstruation, which is clearly addressed to more conservative male physicians: "We regard menstruation as a physiological function, and not necessarily attended with pain. If the genital organs are healthy, and the system in a proper condition, there will be no special trouble or distress . . ." ("Removal of the Uterine Appendages—Recovery," *Medical Record* 27 (April 1885): 399). When she felt justifiably beleaguered, Dixon Jones seems to have deliberately taken stands publicly that would vindicate her from some of the *Eagle*'s more heartless representations. I have already mentioned that it was during this time that she published an article against abortion, not necessarily surprising since she was accused by the *Eagle* of performing one. In a couple of other articles she waxed rather eloquent on the subject of motherhood, writing, for example, in 1894 that she published the piece on abortion because "I was impelled to write that paper from my great love and admiration of children; it was written partly in defense of the unborn babe, and for its protection. To me nothing in life is so beautiful as a child, nothing so interesting, whether we consider its opening and growing intelligence, or the perfection of its physical structure, the Adonis like beauty of its form; the beauty of every baby of every land, showing that God has formed of one blood all nations of the earth, and all in His likeness and image." Though I do not deny Dixon Jones may have been sincere in the expression of these feelings, I believe self-promotion was also at work, especially at the end of the piece, when she publishes several letters praising her work from male members of the profession. There is not a trace of this kind of sentimentality to be found in her articles published before the trial. See Mary Dixon Jones, "An Open Letter—The Summing Up," *Woman's Medical Journal* 3 (December 1894): 145–149. See also "Criminal Abortion—Its Evils and Its Sad Consequences," *Woman's Medical Journal* (August 1894): 28–31, 60–70. Also published in *Medical Record* a few months earlier, "Shall Mothers Nurse Their Babies?" *Philadelphia Times and Register* 25 (August 20, 1892): 220–221.

50. "A Case of Tait's Operation," *American Journal of Obstetrics and Diseases of Women and Children* 17 (November 1884): 1191–1193. See also "Removal of the

Uterine Appendages—Recovery,'' ''Removal of the Uterine Appendages: Nine Consecutive Cases.''

51. For evidence of her knowledge, see Dixon Jones, ''Removal of the Uterine Appendages—Five Cases,'' *American Journal of Obstetrics* 21 (February 1888): 162, n. 1. For evidence of her trip coinciding with this event, see Dixon Jones, ''Oophorectomy in Diseases of the Nervous System,'' *Medical and Surgical Reporter* 68 (May 1893): 800, n. 17) and ''Letters of Travel in Europe in 1886,'' *Woman's Medical Journal* 4 (December 1895): 299–304.

52. See Dixon Jones, ''Letters of Travel in Europe,'' 304.

53. Dixon Jones, ''Removal of the Uterine Appendages—Five Cases.'' In a similar vein, she wrote, ''I wish to emphasize that however alarming the nervous and mental symptoms may be, or however serious the general constitutional condition, yet the operation of oöphorectomy should not for a moment be considered, unless there is unmistakable proof that the ovaries are themselves seriously and irreparably diseased, and in such a state as to destroy the health, comfort, and comparative usefulness of the individual. This I have stated several times . . .'' ''Diagnosis and Some of the Clinical Aspects of Gyroma and Endothelioma of the Ovary,'' *Buffalo Medical and Surgical Journal* 32 (November 1892): 212.

54. Page 171.

55. Ibid.

56. Dixon Jones, ''Oophorectomy in Diseases of the Nervous System,'' *Medical and Surgical Reporter* 68 (May 1893): 804; emphasis mine. It is not necessarily disingenuous for a physician to argue in this manner about diagnosis; in part it can mean simply that she was doing the best she could with all the ways of knowing that were available to her.

57. ''A Plea for Conservatism in Gynecology,'' *Boston Medical and Surgical Journal* 156 (April 1907): 539–541.

58. *Treatise on the Diseases of Women*, 3rd ed. (New York: D. Appleton, 1899), 444.

59. See Skene, *Education and Culture*, 9, 38, 26–27. See also Horatio Bigelow's reference to ''a human life mutilated, *deprived of its distinctive characteristics*, and rendered miserable!'' (emphasis mine) in ''Conservative Gynecology,'' *Annals of Gynecology* 1 (November 1887): 67–74. For other remarks on ''castration,'' ''unsexing,'' ''spaying,'' ''mutilation,'' and race suicide, see Howard Kelly, ''The Ethical Side of the Operation of Oöphorectomy,'' *American Journal of Obstetrics and Diseases of Women and Children* 27 (1893): 206–207, and ''Conservatism in Ovariotomy,'' *Journal of the American Medical Association* 26 (February 8, 1896): 249–252; Ely Van de Warker, ''The Fetch of the Ovary,'' *American Journal of Obstetrics and Diseases of Women and Children* 54 (July–December 1906): 366–373; Editorial, ''To Limit the Castration of Women,'' *Journal of the American Medical Association* 8 (December 21, 1889): 887–888.

60. Gert Brieger, ''Surgery,'' in Ronald Numbers, ed., *The Education of American Physicians* (Berkeley: Univ. of California Press, 1980), 175–204; Oswei Temkin, ''The Role of Surgery in the Rise of Modern Medical Thought,'' in Temkin, *The Double Face of Janus and Other Essays in the History of Medicine* (Baltimore: Johns Hopkins Univ. Press, 1977), 487–96; ''Rudolph Virchow, Julius Cohnheim and the Program of Pathology,'' *Bulletin of the History of Medicine* 52 (Summer 1978): 162–182.

61. See L. J. Rather, *The Genesis of Cancer* (Baltimore: Johns Hopkins Univ. Press, 1978), 169–174.

62. Dixon Jones, ''The Opinions of Different Surgeons and Pathologists as to the

Origins and Cause of Fibroid Tumors," *Medical Record* 62 (August 30, 1902): 324, 325.

63. Page 325.

64. Ibid.

65. Ibid., 325, 327.

66. See Howard Kelly and Charles P. Noble, eds., *Gynecology and Abdominal Surgery* (Philadelphia: W. B. Saunders, 1907). The women physicians who were asked to write for the volume were Anna Fullerton, who was a surgeon at the Woman's Hospital in Philadelphia for part of her career, and Elizabeth Hurdon, a Johns Hopkins M.D. and a protégée of Howard Kelly's.

67. Henry Parker Newman, "Woman and Her Diseases vs. Gynaecology," *American Gynaecological and Obstetrical Journal* 9 (October 1896): 416–417.

68. It may also be true that, by the end of the century, such discussions were no longer necessary in some venues—gender ideology had become socially inscribed in powerful ways. This is not to say that twentieth-century medicine did not continue to play a crucial role in determining images and treatment of women's bodies. The work of Emily Martin on misogyny in contemporary medical textbooks cautions us to note that language may have changed more than attitudes. See Emily Martin, *The Woman in the Body: A Cultural Analysis of Reproduction* (Boston: Beacon Press, 1987). Nancy Stepan and Sander Gilman have found that, by the early decades of the twentieth century, the metaphors of scientific language, which once were "open, varied, metaphorically porous," in literary form, eventually became "more tightly controlled." "The modern scientific text," they argue, "had replaced the expansive scientific book, and the possibilities of multivalent meanings being created out of scientific language were thereby curtailed." Stepan and Gilman, "Appropriating the Idioms of Science: The Rejection of Scientific Racism," in Dominick La Capra, ed., *The Bounds of Race* (Ithaca: Cornell Univ. Press, 1991), 62. For changing scientific language, see also Londa Schiebinger, *The Mind Has No Sex?* (Cambridge, Mass.: Harvard Univ. Press), 150–159.

69. Quoted in Moscucci, *Science of Woman*, 134.

70. Ironically, this gradual shift to a "one body" model of disease, devoid of the consideration of social context, has also proved problematic for women, as Sue Rosser has recently pointed out. It has allowed twentieth century researchers on major life-threatening illnesses to ignore sex differences when they should have been taken into account. See Rosser, *Women's Health: Missing from U.S. Medicine* (Bloomington: Indiana Univ. Press, 1994).

71. Stepan and Gilman, "Appropriating the Idioms of Science," 62. For Jewish responses to race science, see John Efron, *Defenders of the Race: Jewish Doctors and Race Science in Fin-De-Siecle Europe* (New Haven: Yale Univ. Press, 1994). It would take half a century or more for minority groups and women to begin to understand the way the concept of scientific objectivity itself could be used to oppress marginal groups. There is a vast literature on this subject, but a good place to begin would be Evelyn Fox Keller, *Reflections on Gender and Science* (New Haven: Yale Univ. Press, 1985), and Ruth Bleier, *Feminist Approaches to Science* (New York: Pergamon Press, 1986).

72. Female educators paid particular attention to women doctors' findings, and many colleges and universities hired women physicians to monitor their female students' health. Women reformers of all stripes also took seriously women physicians' alternative notions of the female body. See Morantz-Sanchez, *Sympathy and Science*, 203–231, 266–311.

73. See Lawson Tait, "A Discussion of the General Principles Involved in the Operation of Removal of the Uterine Appendages," *New York Medical Journal* 44 (November 1886): 561–567; Henry MacNaughton-Jones, "Presidential Address: The Posi-

tion of Gynaecology Today," *British Gynaecological Journal* 14 (May 1898): 8–30. Tait was known to be supportive of women physicians, and occasionally hired a female assistant, but he also believed that, except for a few, women were intellectually inferior to men and most should stay at home. On the other hand, he was also beloved by most of his patients, and fondly remembered for the courses in physiology he gave to young women. See Letter to Fausett Welsh from Miss Kathleen Haseler, November 7, 1944; Louisa Annie Harbarge to Fausett Welsh, January 2, 1945; February 17, 1945; Sarah J. Young to Welsh, March 8, 1945, on his encouragement regarding nursing. Also "Nurse Bayley" to Welsh, December 29, 1944. Lawson Tait Centenary Collection, Birmingham Medical Institute, Birmingham, England.

74. Four works making this argument are Vrettos, *Somatic Fictions*; Poovey, *The Making of a Social Body*; Anne McClintock, *Imperial Leather: Race, Gender and Sexuality in the Colonial Contest* (New York: Routledge, 1995); Elaine Showalter's *Sexual Anarchy: Gender and Culture at the Fin de Siècle* (New York: Viking, 1990), although in a less careful way.

NOTES TO CHAPTER SIX

1. "The Hysterical Woman: Sex Roles and Role Conflict in Nineteenth-Century America," *Social Research* 39 (Winter 1972): 258; Joan Brumberg, *Fasting Girls: The Emergence of Anorexia Nervosa as a Modern Disease* (Cambridge, Mass.: Harvard Univ. Press, 1988); Mary Poovey, " 'Scenes of an Indelicate Character': The Medical 'Treatment' of Victorian Women," *Representations* 14 (Spring 1986): 148, 152, 153.

2. This is not to say that husbands and fathers are totally absent, but their presence is decidedly less pervasive than past histories would have us believe. For participation of husbands and fathers and parents, see Mary Dixon Jones, "Personal Experiences in Laparotomy," *Medical Record* 52 (August 7, 1897): 182–191, esp. cases 1, 69, 4, 55; and "Diagnosis and Some of the Clinical Aspects of Gyroma and Endothelioma of the Ovary," *Buffalo Medical and Surgical Journal* 32 (November 1892): 200, 205, 207, 208.

3. This fact underscores Edward Shorter's argument that, in contrast to the traditional patient, who had a high pain threshold and greater tolerance for chronic illness, the modern patient displays greater sensitivity to the body's vicissitudes, and seeks advice from experts more quickly. See *Bedside Manners: The Troubled History Between Doctors and Patients* (New York: Simon and Schuster, 1985), 61. In addition, knowledge that women moved from doctor to doctor would not surprise modern medical sociologists, who have found that, although women may appear passive in the doctor's office, they take a more active role in managing their health outside the formal clinical setting. Apparently, even today women are more likely to change their doctors more often than men. Some scholars argue that they also turn more readily to "unconventional methods of healing." In short, writes Alexandra Dundas Todd of present-day female attitudes, "Women use medical care more than men, perhaps because of a more help-oriented socialization and their need of health services for reproductive care as well as disease. The literature . . . illustrates that in seeking this care, women report many dissatisfactions. There is no evidence, however, that these dissatisfactions are voiced to doctors. In fact, women's complaints, in general, seem to take the form of silent rebellion, such as noncompliance and changing practitioners, rather than direct confrontation." See Todd, *Intimate Adversaries: Cultural Conflict Between Doctors & Women Patients* (Philadelphia: Univ. of Pennsylvania Press, 1989), 40–41.

4. Dixon Jones's case records abound with reports of other physicians' therapies and diagnoses, and this is just a representative example. Given my reading of the gy-

necological literature, these treatments are perfectly plausible. All were used. See Dixon Jones, "Removal of the Uterine Appendages: Nine Consecutive Cases," *Medical Record* 30 (August, 1886): 200.

5. *Eagle*, May 11, 14, 1889; *Citizen*, June 20, 1889.

6. Mary Dixon Jones, "Another Hitherto Undescribed Disease of the Ovaries. Anomalous Menstrual Bodies," *New York Medical Journal* 51 (May 10, 1890): 511–551; "Diagnosis and Some of the Clinical Aspects of Gyroma and Endothelioma of the Ovary," *Buffalo Medical and Surgical Journal* 32 (November 1892): 209.

7. *Eagle*, February 13, 1892. Though parts of Scholtz's story are contradictory, her incessant search for the perfect doctor is not.

8. *Citizen*, February 24, 1892.

9. *Eagle*, February 26, 1892.

10. *Eagle*, February 9, 1892.

11. *Eagle*, February 25, 1892. See also the following cases: Mrs. Bruggeman, *Eagle*, May 7, 1889, *Citizen*, February 12, 1892; Mrs. Hulten, *Eagle*, May 11, 1889; Mrs. Fisher, *Eagle*, May 14, 1889; February 10, 1892; *Citizen*, February 10, 1892; Mrs. Nash, *Eagle*, May 17, 1889, February 12, 1892; Miss Olsen, *Eagle*, June 14, 1889; Ida Hunt, *Eagle*, May 31, 1889, February 17, 1892; Mrs. Rettinger, *Eagle*, February 13, 15, 1892; Mrs. Clara Hartisch, *Citizen*, June 10, 1889; Margaret Walsh, *Citizen*, June 10, 1889; Miss Hattie Coulson, *Citizen*, June 20, 1889; Mrs. Maggy Laklbreunar, *Eagle*, February 24, 1892; Charlotte Mason, *Eagle*, February 25, 1892. Dixon Jones's case records tell exactly the same story.

12. The question of the trial's female audience and its meaning will be taken up in the last chapter. For comments on the larger numbers of women who attended the libel trial see *Eagle*, February 12, 1892.

13. *Eagle*, May 7, 1889, February 12, 1892.

14. *Eagle*, May 10, 1889.

15. *Eagle*, February 20, 1890, February 17, 1892.

16. *Eagle*, May 6, 1889.

17. *Eagle*, May 2, 1889. So apparently did Mrs. Bruggeman, who had been seeing the Misses McNutt in New York. These two physicians were sisters who had graduated from the New York Infirmary Medical School and were treating Bruggeman with electricity. *Eagle*, May 7, 1889.

18. *Eagle*, February 11, 1892.

19. Male physicians worried constantly that women physicians would be an economic threat, not only by glutting the market with practitioners but by charging lower fees. See Regina Morantz-Sanchez, *Sympathy and Science: Women Physicians in American Medicine* (New York: Oxford Univ. Press, 1985), 53.

20. Dixon Jones, "Another Hitherto Undescribed Disease," 515.

21. Ibid., 543.

22. *Eagle*, May 19, 1889.

23. *Citizen*, June 10, 1889; *Eagle*, February 24, 1892.

24. *Citizen*, June 7, 1889.

25. *Eagle*, February 20, 1890; *Citizen*, February 20, 1890. See also Dixon Jones, "Another Hitherto Undescribed Disease of the Ovaries," where she reports that a particular patient and her husband "both" insisted on an operation being performed, 515.

26. Nancy Theriot, "Women's Voice in Nineteenth-Century Medical Discourse: A Step Toward Deconstructing Science," *Signs* 19 (Autumn 1993): 1–31.

27. Mary Dixon Jones, "A Hitherto Undescribed Disease of the Ovary: Endothelioma Changing to Angeioma and Haematoma," *New York Medical Journal* 50 (Septem-

ber 28, 1889): 339, 340, 341, and "A Case of Tait's Operation," *American Journal of Obstetrics* 17 (November 1884): 1156; and "Misplacements of the Uterus: History of Cases Showing How in Many Instances They Are Produced; The Accompanying Condition; Microcopical Examinations," *Pittsburgh Medical Review: A Monthly Journal of Medicine and Surgery* 3 (October 1897): 302, 303; "Removal of the Uterine Appendages—Recovery," *Medical Record* 27 (April 1885): 401; "Removal of the Uterine Appendages: Nine Consecutive Cases," *Medical Record* 30 (August 1886): 202, 204.

28. Dixon Jones, "Removal of the Uterine Appendages: Nine Consecutive Cases," 201.

29. Dixon Jones, "The Fourth Hitherto Undescribed Disease of the Ovary; Colloid Degeneration," *Medical Record* 56 (November 1899): 661; "Removal of the Uterine Appendages: Nine Consecutive Cases," 206.

30. For example, see Dixon Jones, "Fibroid Tumors of the Uterus, Their Relation to Diseased Adnexae. Origin of Fibroid Tumors, When Is the Proper Time for Their Removal?," *Annals of Gynecology and Pediatry* 14 (April 1901): 469, for mention of a patient, Mrs. E, who, from the case record description is Mina Emerich. According to Dixon Jones's report, the patient begged for an operation. Emerich corroborated this characterization of her behavior in the *Citizen*, June 10, 1889.

31. "Removal of the Uterine Appendages: Nine Consecutive Cases," 200.

32. "A Case of Tait's Operation," 1156–1157; "Removal of the Uterine Appendages: Nine Consecutive Cases," 204.

33. Mary Dixon Jones, "Diagnosis and Some of the Clinical Aspects of Gyroma and Endothelioma of the Ovary," *Buffalo Medical and Surgical Journal* 32 (November 1892): 206. This is especially interesting testimony in view of Carroll Smith-Rosenberg's argument that doctors were in collusion with husbands in the hostility they felt toward hysterical patients. The fact that Dixon Jones was a woman, and that clearly in these cases the wife was perhaps even more eager than the husband to alleviate symptoms, qualifies some of her otherwise acute insights. See Smith-Rosenberg, "The Hysterical Woman."

34. Dixon Jones, "Diagnosis and Some of the Clinical Aspects of Gyroma and Endothelioma of the Ovary," *Buffalo Medical and Surgical Journal* 32 (November 1892): 205, 211.

35. See Dixon Jones, "Sterility in Woman—Causes, Treatment, and Illustrative Cases," *Medical Record* 40 (September 19, 1891): 317–326.

36. Two important works on infertility in America are Margaret Marsh and Wanda Ronner, *The Empty Cradle: Infertility in America from Colonial Times to the Present* (Baltimore: Johns Hopkins Univ. Press, 1996), esp. 41–74, and Elaine Tyler May, *Barren in the Promised Land: Childless Americans and the Pursuit of Happiness* (New York: Basic Books, 1995).

37. "A Hitherto Undescribed Disease of the Ovary," 338. Dixon Jones sided with the surgeons who denied that removal of the ovaries diminished desire. See Chapter 3.

38. Ibid., 340.

39. Ibid., 309.

40. Ibid., 305, 306, 307.

41. "Diagnosis and Some of the Clinical Aspects of Gyroma and Endothelioma," 207, 208.

42. Nancy Theriot's insights into the revelations of the case study have been very important in guiding my analysis in this section. See "The Case Within the Case Study: Uncovering the Voices of Nineteenth-Century Women Patients," paper given at the History of Science Society Meetings, New Orleans, October 1994.

43. *Eagle*, February 15, 1892; *Citizen*, June 8, 12, 17, 1889; *Eagle*, February 23, 24, 1892; *Citizen*, June 10, 1889.

44. *Citizen*, June 10, 1889.

45. *Citizen*, June 20, 1889.

46. "Reminiscences of Travels in Europe in 1886, No. 2," *Woman's Medical Journal* 4 (December 1895): 335.

47. Dixon Jones, "Diagnosis and Some of the Clinical Aspects of Gyroma and Endothelioma of the Ovary," 201, 204; "Removal of the Uterine Appendages: Nine Consecutive Cases," 202; "A Report of Five Laparotomies," 67.

48. *Eagle*, February 11, 1892.

49. *Eagle*, February 12, 1892.

50. *Eagle*, February 19, 1892, May 10, 1889, February 13, 24, 1892. It may be significant to note that all these women lived and were healthy enough to testify in court.

51. *Eagle*, February 10, March 1, February 13, 1892.

52. *Eagle*, February 18, 1892.

53. *Eagle*, February 10, March 1, 1892.

54. *Citizen*, February 11, 1892; *Eagle*, February 23, 1892.

55. Kunigunde Rettinger, *Eagle*, February 11, 1892, May 2, 10, 1889.

56. See testimony of the hospital's nurses, Mrs. Caroline Corey and Nurse Olsen, *Eagle*, February 26, 27, March 1, 1892. None of this testimony deviates from standard hospital practice. For the custom of having hospital patients help with the Nursing, see Charles Rosenberg, *The Care of Strangers* (New York: Basic Books, 1987), 212–217; Susan M. Reverby, *Ordered to Care: The Dilemma of American Nursing, 1850–1945* (New York: Cambridge Univ. Press, 1987), 26–27.

57. *Eagle*, February 13, 19, 1892.

58. *Eagle*, February 13, 1892; Dixon Jones, "Carcinoma on the Floor of the Pelvis," *Medical Record* 43 (March 1893): 292.

59. *Eagle*, February 12, 13, 1892.

60. See testimony of Julia Shute, *Eagle*, February 18, 1892; Sophia Sass, June 4, 1889; Kate Thompson, February 12, 1892.

61. See Dudley's comments made at a meeting of the New York Academy of Medicine's Section in Obstetrics and Gynecology on January 24, 1889, *Medical Record* 36 (March 1889): 245–247.

62. Charles P. Noble, "The Question of Operation in Cases of Chronic Oophoritis," American Gynecological Society *Transactions* 18 (1893): 409; Lawson Tait, like Dixon Jones, favored early operations for everybody. See his comments regarding patients' class in a letter to the editors of *The Lancet* 2 (September 21, 1895): 755. See also Donnell Hughes, "The Treatment of Fibroid Tumors of the Womb," American Association of Obstetricians and Gynecologists *Transactions* 3 (1891): 313–331.

63. Information on the class composition of various Brooklyn neighborhoods during this period was gleaned from the following sources: Henry W. B. Howard, ed., *The Eagle and Brooklyn* (Brooklyn Daily Eagle Publication, 1893); Clay Lancaster, *Old Brooklyn Heights* (Rutland, VT: Charles E. Tuttle, 1961); Alter F. Landesman, *A History of New Lots, Brooklyn* (Port Washington, N.Y.: Kennikat Press, 1977); Julian Ralph, "The City of Brooklyn," *Harper's New Monthly Magazine* (April 1893), reprinted in Mary Ellen and Mark Murphy and Ralph Foster Weld, *A Treasury of Brooklyn* (New York: William Sloan Associates, 1949); Harold C. Syrett, *The City of Brooklyn, 1865–1898: A Political History* (New York: Columbia Univ. Press, 1944); and Altina A. Waller, *Reverend Beecher and Mrs. Tilton* (Amherst: Univ. of Massachusetts Press, 1982).

64. *Eagle*, February 10, 1892, May 10, 1889, February 10, 16, 1892.

65. See Nurse Bayley to Fausett Welsh, December 29, 1944: "He made the rich pay for the poor." Lawson Tait Centenary Collection, Birmingham Medical Institute.

66. *Eagle*, February 10, 16, 19, March 4, 1892.

67. See, for example, "Medical Compliance as an Ideology," *Social Science and Medicine* 27 (1988): 1299–1316.

68. In a recent paper, Kathy Powderly has found the same variation of approach to patients in the medical practice of A. J. C. Skene. In an examination of his relations with patients, she learned that Skene sometimes privileged the patient's wishes and judgment, and sometimes behaved paternalistically, with the doctor being the final decision-making authority. See "Patient Consent and Negotiation in the Brooklyn Gynecological Practice of Alexander J. C. Skene: 1863–1900," Paper presented to the New York Consortium on the History of Medicine, Fall, 1998.

69. For a thorough discussion of these issues, see Brian Turner, *Regulating Bodies: Essays in Medical Sociology* (London: Routledge, 1992), esp. the introduction.

70. Smith-Rosenberg first offered a version of this argument in her article on "The Hysterical Woman." In addition, Nancy Theriot's work on generational changes in women's attitudes toward their bodies suggests that daughters coming of age in the 1880s were not as passive as their mothers were in accepting debility and disease as a normal aspect of the female life-cycle. See *Mothers and Daughters in Nineteenth-Century America: A Biosocial Construction of Femininity*, rev. ed. (Lexington: Univ. of Kentucky Press, 1996), 80–81. For a particularly interesting contemporary example of this phenomenon, see Emily K. Abel and Nancy Reifel, "Interactions Between Public Health Nurses and Clients on American Indian Reservations During the 1930's," *Social History of Medicine* 9 (April 1996): 89–108.

71. The argument in this paragraph as well as the quote is drawn from Gregory Pappas's helpful article, "Some Implications for the Study of the Doctor-Patient Interactions: Power, Structure, and Agency in the Works of Howard Waitzkin and Arthur Kleinman," *Social Science and Medicine* 30 (1990): 200.

72. For more on this point, see Morantz-Sanchez, *Sympathy and Science*, esp. chs. 7–10.

NOTES TO CHAPTER SEVEN

1. See *Eagle*, December 19, 21, 1889.

2. *Citizen*, February 18, 1890. The *Eagle* claimed in 1889 that its case against Dixon Jones was not inspired by animus against women physicians. The *Eagle* was a "friend of women in medicine and surgery." Dixon Jones, however, was not representative and "should not be classed with her sex in medicine." She was a "non professional monstrosity." *Eagle*, May 31, 1889.

3. *Eagle*, February 17, 1890. For Ridgway's willingness to drop the Bates case if the Hunt case was lost, see *Eagle*, December 21, 1889, "Moving for Trial: The Jones Family May Be Brought up in February."

4. *Eagle*, February 18, 1890. *Citizen*, February 18, 1890.

5. Ibid.

6. Ibid. On Butler, see Henry W. B. Howard, *The Eagle and Brooklyn* (Brooklyn: Brooklyn Daily *Eagle*, 1893), 700–701, and Howard Kelley and Walter Burrage, eds., *Dictionary of American Medical Biography* (New York: O. Appleton, 1928), 182; on Fowler, see *Dictionary of American Medical Biography*, 430–431, and *The Eagle and Brooklyn*, 676–677.

7. See *Citizen*, February 19, 1890.

8. *Eagle*, February 19, 1890.

9. *Citizen*, February 19, 1890. Note that in the *Eagle*'s report of the Hunt testimony, there is no mention of his infection.

10. *Citizen* and *Eagle*, February 20, 1890. This was the first hint in the *Eagle*'s account that Ida's tumor might have been linked to venereal disease; Reynolds, who did the summation, referred cryptically to that possibility again in his closing remarks. See *Eagle*, February 25, 1890.

11. Nurse Olsen's testimony is found in the *Eagle* and *Citizen*, February 19 and 20; Charles Dixon Jones's, February 20; and Mary Dixon Jones's, February 22, 1889.

12. *Citizen*, February 21, 1890.

13. *Eagle*, February 22, 1890. See also *Citizen*, February 22, 1890. Charles also testified that "he never explained the methods of operations to patients." *Citizen*, February 21, 1890.

14. *Eagle*, February 22, 1890.

15. *Eagle* and *Citizen*, February 20, 1889. The source for this rumor is unclear. This incident was not described in the 1889 *Eagle* articles nor, by my search, in subsequent articles published between then and the manslaughter trial.

16. *Eagle* and *Citizen*, February 21, 1890. On Polk, see Kelly and Burrage, eds., *Dictionary of American Medical Biography*, 1972; Floyd Elwood Keene, ed., *Album of the Fellows of the American Gynecological Society 1876–1930* (Philadelphia: Wm. J. Duncan, 1930), 258.

17. *Eagle*, February 21, 1890. On Coe's career see Thomas Herringshaw, ed., *American Physician & Surgeon Blue Book* (1919), 103; Keene, ed., *Album of the Fellows of the American Gynecological Society*, 134.

18. Keene, ed., *Album of the Fellows of the American Gynecological Society*, 134. See also *Citizen*, February 21, 1890.

19. *Citizen*, February 21, 1890. On Heitzman, see Howard Kelly and Walter Burrage, eds., *American Medical Biographies* (Baltimore: Norman, Remington, 1920), 513.

20. *Citizen*, February 21, 1889. See also *Eagle*, February 21, 1890. For information on Morris, see Hans H. Simmer, "Robert Tuttle Morris (1857–1945): A Pioneer in Ovarian Transplants," *Obstetrics and Gynecology* 35 (February 1970): 314–327; Kelly and Burrage, *Dictionary of American Medical Biography*, 460.

21. *Eagle*, February 21, 1890. On Price, see W. Kennedy, "Joseph Price: In Memoriam," *American Journal of Obstetrics* 65 (1912): 95–98; Kelly and Burrage, *Dictionary of American Medical Biography*, 992–994.

22. *Citizen*, February 21, 1890. For information on Wylie see Kelly and Burrage, eds., *Dictionary of American Medical Biography*, 1340–1341; Keene, ed., *Album of the Fellows of the American Gynecological Society*, 638.

23. *Citizen*, February 24, 1890.

24. *Eagle*, February 24, 1890.

25. *Eagle*, February 25, 1890. See *Citizen*'s editorial, February 23, 1890. For other New York newspapers' coverage of the manslaughter trial, see New York *World*, February 19, 1890; New York *Tribune*, February 19, 20, 22, 25, 1890; New York *Times*, February 20, 22, 23, 25, November 6, 1890.

26. *Citizen*, February 25, 26, 1890.

27. *Eagle*, February 25, 1890.

28. *Citizen*, February 25, 1890.

29. Minutes of the New York Pathological Society, 1888–1902. See Executive Committee Minutes, Minutes of Committee on Admissions and Ethics, and the scrapbook of the Dixon Jones case, New York Academy of Medicine Archives. Dixon Jones's sponsors for admission were George Shrady, editor of the influential New York *Medical*

Record; John A. Wyeth, a distinguished surgeon; and Wesley M. Carpenter, Secretary of the Medical Society of New York. See the society's membership records. Shrady was one of President Grant's consulting physicians. See biographical notes on Shrady in George F. Shrady, *General Grant's Last Days* (New York: privately printed, 1908), 3–5, William B. Atkinson, ed., *Physicians and Surgeons of the United States* (Philadelphia: Charles Robson, 1878), 239; for Wyeth see Kelly and Burrage, eds., *Dictionary of American Medical Biography*, 1928, 1339–1340; and for Carpenter, Daniel Lewis, "Memoir of Dr. Wesley M. Carpenter, Medical Society of the State of New York, *Transactions*, 1888, 568–72.

30. New York *Medical Record* 37 (March 1, 1890): 242–243.

31. This was a legal technicality based on the allegation that the certificates were improperly filed by the attorney at the time of incorporation. But in that sense the *Eagle*'s charges were validated. See *Eagle*, October 9, December 11, 23, 1891.

NOTES TO CHAPTER EIGHT

1. *Eagle*, February 4, 12, 1892. The *Eagle* actually compared the testimony to "a detective novel from a master hand." February 3, 1892.

2. *Eagle*, February 4, March 4, 1892.

3. *Eagle*, March 9, 1892.

4. *Eagle*, February 12, 1892.

5. See *Eagle*, February 2, 1892.

6. *Eagle*, February 1, 1892.

7. *Eagle*, February 2, 1892.

8. Ibid.

9. Dixon Jones increased her income from $100 to $5000 a year in less than a decade. The average earnings of male physicians in New York during this period was between $1500 and $2000 a year. See Charles Rosenberg, "The Practice of Medicine in New York a Century Ago," in Judith Leavitt and Ronald Numbers, eds., *Sickness and Health in America* (Madison: Univ. of Wisconsin Press, 1978), 57. Of course, teachers earned more in the range of $150–$300 a year, while nurse hospital superintendents could earn between $900 and $2000, depending upon the size of the hospital, but the latter were on call twenty-four hours a day, six and a half days a week. Regular nurses earned considerably less. See Polly Welts Kaufman, *Women Teachers on the Frontier* (New Haven: Yale Univ. Press, 1984), 34, and Susan Reverby, *Ordered to Care* (New York: Cambridge Univ. Press, 1987), 106–108.

10. *Eagle*, February 2, 1892.

11. Ibid.

12. Ibid. The phrase "deep mourning" is the *Citizen*'s, February 1, 1892. According to the Brooklyn *Citizen*, Henry Jones testified on February 29, 1892, that his father attended the manslaughter trial but "died a few weeks after it was concluded." See *Citizen* for that date. It is interesting that after two years Dixon Jones was still dressed in mourning, a practice that was not uncommon. But her garb could easily have also been calculated to gain the sympathy of the jury.

13. *Eagle*, February 2, 1892.

14. *Eagle*, February 3, 1892. One of two articles that day, this entitled "Still Reading."

15. *Citizen*, February 3, 1892.

16. Ibid.; *Eagle*, February 3, 1892.

17. *Citizen*, February 3, 1892; *Eagle*, February 3, 1892.

18. *Eagle*, February 4, 1892. Early in the trial Dixon Jones's lawyers took great pains to undermine the credibility of the newspaper. In the cross-examination of George F. Dobson, the *Eagle*'s city editor in 1889 (now in the advertising business), Baldwin inquired several times about the veracity of Sidney Reid, who had apparently published a bogus interview in the *Eagle* between Jim McDermott, a corrupt democratic politico, and Samuel McLean, the editor of the Brooklyn *Citizen*. Apparently Reid had been suspended from the newspaper, but Dobson could not be pinned down on the subject. Ibid. On the figure of the "confidence man" and its resonances in Victorian culture, see Karen Halttunen, *Confidence Men and Painted Women: A Study of Middle-Class Culture in America, 1830–1870* (New Haven: Yale Univ. Press, 1982), ch. 1 and passim.

19. *Eagle*, February 3, 1892.

20. *Citizen*, February 4, 1892. It is worth remembering at this point that the *Eagle* was a hostile reporter of these proceedings throughout the affair, but the corroborative testimony of the *Citizen* leads one to conclude that Dixon Jones's appearances on the stand simply did not help her case.

21. *Eagle*, February 4, 1892. Here Bartlett was referring to the 1890 manslaughter trial regarding the case of Ida Hunt, at which he also presided.

22. Ibid. For the details of Dixon Jones biography, see Chapter 3.

23. *Eagle*, February 3, 1892.

24. Ibid.

25. See Austin Abbott, *Trial Evidence—The Rules of Evidence Applicable on the Trial of Civil Actions (Including Both Causes of Action and Defenses) at Common Law, in Equity, and Under the Codes of Procedure* (New York: Baker and Voorhis, 1881), 670, 672. See also Judge Bartlett's charge to the jury, which included a very clear explication of the concepts of justification and mitigation, which it was imperative for them to understand for their deliberations. *Eagle*, March 11, 1892.

26. Stuart Blumin in *The Emergence of the Middle Class: Social Experience in the American City, 1760–1900* (Cambridge: Cambridge Univ. Press, 1989), finds that memberships on various boards of trustees were "arenas of class-relevant social life" (192). See also Paul Boyer, *Urban Masses and Moral Order in America, 1820–1920* (Cambridge, Mass.: Harvard Univ. Press, 1978); Kathleen D. McCarthy, *Noblesse Oblige: Charity and Cultural Philanthropy in Chicago, 1849–1929* (Chicago: University of Chicago Press, 1982); Stephen Yeo, *Religion and Voluntary Organizations in Crisis* (London: Croom Helm, 1976).

27. *Eagle*, February 4, 1892, morning edition.

28. Perhaps most ironic of all was that Dixon Jones and District Attorney Ridgway had been neighbors for a time, and relations proved cordial enough to prompt him to draw up the articles of incorporation for the second hospital free of charge. Ridgway testified on February 4, 1892. See *Eagle*, evening edition, for that date.

29. *Eagle*, February 4, 1892, evening edition. See also testimony of Judge Augustus Van Wyck, Foster L. Backus *Eagle*, February 4, 1892; James Tanner, Howard N. Smith, *Eagle*, February 6, 1892; Mayor David Boody, George G. Reynolds, and Paul Grening, *Eagle*, February 9, 1892; ex-Mayor Samuel Booth, *Eagle*, February 15, 1892.

30. For Jacobus's testimony, see *Eagle*, February 9, 1892. It is important to note that this comment explains why the New York Pathological Society was so eager to investigate the matter when the *Eagle* articles were first published in 1889, and considered expelling Dixon Jones from the society. Obviously, if its professional integrity and reputation were to be maintained, it needed to make sure that its members were not guilty of unseemly conduct.

31. For information on Garrigues, see Howard Kelly and Walter Burrage, eds., *American Medical Biographies* (Norman, Remington, 1920), 428–429.

32. Testimony of all can be found in *Eagle*, February 23, 1892.

33. Putnam Jacobi, *Eagle*, February 27, 1892. On Jacobi's career see Regina Morantz-Sanchez, *Sympathy and Science: Women Physicians in American Medicine* (New York: Oxford Univ. Press, 1985), 184–202; Kelly and Burrage, eds., *Dictionary of American Medical Biography*, 643–645.

34. Eagle, February 23, 1892. See also similar testimony from John A. Wyatt, February 9, 1892.

35. *Eagle*, February 23, 1892. On Lee see Howard Kelly, *A Cyclopedia of American Medical Biography* (Philadelphia: W. B. Saunders, 1912), 2: 91–92; on Fox, see Syntex Laboratories, *Leaders in Dermatology: George Henry Fox* (Palo Alto, Calif.: Syntex, 1967), 9–20.

36. *Eagle*, February 4, 1892.

37. *Eagle* summary, February 27, 1892. See Chapter 6.

38. On the importance of a reputation for good character and gentility, see Gert H. Brieger, "Classics and Character: Medicine and Gentility," *Bulletin of the History of Medicine* 65 (Spring 1991): 88–109.

39. *Eagle*, February 9, 1892. On Shaw, see Kelly, ed., *Cyclopedia of American Medical Biography*, 2: 364–65; on Richardson, see Henry W. B. Howard, ed., *The Eagle and Brooklyn: The Record of the Progress of the Brooklyn Daily Eagle, Issued in Commemoration of its Semi-Centennial and Occupancy of its New Building: Together with the History of the City of Brooklyn From Its Settlement to the Present Time* (Brooklyn: Brooklyn Daily Eagle, 1893), 695.

40. *Eagle*, February 26, 1892.

41. *Eagle*, February 10, 1892. Other physicians who testified to Dixon Jones's bad reputation were A. W. Shepard, *Eagle*, February 11, 1892; Dr. John Rushmore, Dr. George McNaughton, Eliza Mosher, Lucy Hall Brown, Glentworth Butler, and A. J. C. Skene, *Eagle*, February 19, 1892. For biographical information on Gray, see Henry R. Stiles, ed., *The Civil, Political, Professional and Ecclesiastical History and Commercial and Industrial Record of the County of Kings and the City of Brooklyn, N.Y. from 1683 to 1884* (New York: W. W. Munsell, 1884), 921.

42. Caroline Pease to Clara Marshall, January 18, 1892. Marshall *MSS*, Archives on Women in Medicine, Medical College of Pennsylvania, Philadelphia.

43. *Eagle*, February 9, 1892. See also February 8, 1892, for mention of the Pease testimony in the *Eagle*'s editorial.

44. *Eagle*, February 8, 1892. On Wallace see Kelly, *Cyclopedia of American Medical Biography*, 473.

45. Ibid.

46. See Medical Society of the County of Kings Archives, Council Minutes, 1871–1883, p. 149; April 9, 1884, p. 8; May 14, 1884, p. 11, now located at Downstate Medical Center Library. Note that by 1884 the society had enrolled several female members, including a graduate of Dixon Jones's first medical school, the New York Hydropathic Institute, and a black woman physician, Susan McKinney (Steward) a graduate of the homeopathic New York Medical College for Women. See Warren A. Lapp, "History of the Medical Society of the County of Kings," in Martin Markowitz, ed., *The Sesquicentennial Journal* (Brooklyn: Kings County Medical Society, 1972), 31.

47. *Eagle*, February 9, 1892.

48. Ibid.

49. See "Criminal Abortion—Its Evils and Its Sad Consequences," *Woman's Med-*

ical Journal 3 (August 1894): 28–31, 60–70. The article was also published in the *Medical Record* earlier that year. Americans generally accepted the legitimacy of abortion before quickening until the 1850s, when selected members of the medical profession began a successful public policy campaign against the practice. Many physicians thought abortion to be morally wrong, but they were also quite concerned about enlisting the state to ban alternative practitioners who competed with them for public patronage, and setting precedents for cooperation between government and their own, increasingly status-hungry profession.

50. *Eagle*, February 6, 1892. See also testimony of Elizabeth Meachim, Mary W. Jones (no relation to Dixon Jones), and Dr. Annie Brown, *Eagle*, February 5, 1892. Dixon Jones's version was that she was "put out by one of the foulest conspiracies." See *Eagle*, February 4, March 4, 5, 1892. In a conversation between Bartlett and Jones's lawyer, Robinson, on February 6, the latter explained that he was going into detail to demonstrate defamation of character. In his impatience, the judge made a telling remark: "Some people might think it was a libel to say of a lady that she was skirmishing or that she took the floor and held it against all comers." He was being sarcastic, but the remark resonates nonetheless.

51. *Eagle*, February 11, 1892.

52. Ibid.; the headline on February 12 is worth quoting in full: "More Women Relate the Melancholy Narrative of Their Sufferings After Being on the Operating Table of Mary A. Dixon Jones—Mrs. Kate Thompson Was Not Informed of the Nature of the Ordeal Through which She Had to Pass, and When She Recovered Consciousness in the Night She Had Been Cut Open—Sick Women Left Without Care with the Rain Blowing in Through the Windows and Wetting the Bed Clothes—One Witness Says She Would Gladly Have Taken Poison Rather Than Continue to Endure the Torture to which She Was Subjected. Patients Often Went Hungry and When They Cried Out No Attention Was Paid to Them—How Mrs. Sophia Sass Was Lured to the Operating Table—Startling Array of Facts for the Contemplation of Disinterested Observers."

53. *Eagle*, February 18, 1892. The *Eagle*'s own evidence belies this observation—there were plenty of middle-class patients among Dixon Jones's clientele, and it is clear the newspaper is being caught here in a blatant instance of deliberate self-representation as the champion of the poor.

54. *Eagle*, February 12, 1892. Testimony from former patients appeared in the *Eagle* on February 10–13, 15, 16, 18, and 19, 1892.

55. *Eagle*, February 20, 1892.

56. William Bedford's testimony, *Eagle*, February 9, 1892. See also the statements of Elizabeth Lowden, Kate H. Drillon, and George Lowden, *Eagle*, February 23, 1892, and Mrs. Louise Mckee and Eva Thompson on February 24. Mrs. Carrie Hunt stated that the class size dwindled from fifteen girls to two before Dixon Jones resigned, but provided no explanation or context for this information. See *Eagle*, April 9, 1892.

57. *Eagle*, February 9, 1892.

58. O'Brien and Henry Jones testified on February 29, 1892. For Mary Jones, see *Eagle*, March 1, 1892. Charles testified on March 2, and Mary Dixon Jones on March 4.

59. Ibid. Tenney reported Annie's present status and whereabouts. Dixon Jones and her husband both came from Maryland families that owned a few slaves, which may explain, though not excuse, their cavalier insensitivity to northern protocols for the humane treatment of servants.

60. *Eagle*, February 20, 23, 1892.

61. *Eagle*, February 20, 1892.

62. *Eagle*, February 24, 1892.

63. See testimony of Mrs. Elizabeth Lowden, Mrs. Nellie Dorsey, *Eagle*, February 23, 1892; Clara Schaeckla, Mrs. Mena Emerick, *Eagle*, February 24, 1892. Several of these physicians testified at the trial that Dixon Jones brought cases to them for consultation.

64. See testimony of Mrs. Charlotte Mason and Thomas Robb, *Eagle*, February 25, 1892.

65. Ibid. See also testimony of Norah Kenney, Mrs. Maggie Ellen Dens in *Eagle*, February 26, 1892. Regarding Dixon Jones's behavior, see *Eagle*, February 24, 1892.

66. See, for example, the first time the issue arose on February 9. *Eagle*, February 8, 1892. See also *Eagle*, February 24, 1892.

67. For a description of these procedures see Chapter 4.

68. See *Eagle*, March 8, 1892.

69. *Eagle*, February 11, 1892.

70. *Eagle*, March 3, 8, 1892.

71. *Eagle*, March 5, 1892.

72. Emphasis mine. *Eagle*, March 8, 1892. Chapter 4 deals with these changes from the perspective of long-term developments in the field of gynecology. Dr. George McNaughton, a defense witness, also implied that even five years previously people were not as conservative about operations as they were at present. See *Eagle*, February 19, 1892.

73. See Kelly and Burrage, eds., *American Medical Biographies*, 513.

74. *Eagle*, March 8, 1892.

75. *Eagle*, March 9, 1892. Kelly and Burrage credit her with the discovery of these diseases. See *Dictionary of American Medical Biography*, 677.

76. Kelly and Burrage, eds., *Dictionary of American Medical Biography*, 677.

77. *Eagle*, March 4, 1892.

78. For Buckmaster and King, see *Eagle*, February 11; for Rushmore's testimony, see *Eagle*, February 19. For biographical information on Rushmore see Howard, *The Eagle and Brooklyn*, 694; on Buckmaster see *Brooklyn Medical Journal* 5 (April 1891): 245–257.

79. *Eagle*, February 19, 1892.

80. *Eagle*, March 9, 1892. It might be worth noting here that Wylie was always considered a radical surgeon, and Skene had long thought him beyond the pale in this regard. See *Journal of the American Medical Association* 4 (February 1885): 163–165 for a report of the annual general meeting of the New York Academy of Medicine, where a number of papers were given, including one by Wylie entitled "Diseases of the Fallopian Tubes and Their Relation to the Uterine Displacements and the Use of Pessaries." About this meeting the editor of the journal commented: "It will probably take a smaller mortality than that of one in seven to convince the mass of the profession that this operation is, as a rule, justifiable in the class of cases described by Dr. Wylie, where chronic invalidism is the worst that usually befalls the patient. . . . That Dr. Wylie was inclined to resort too frequently to laparotomy seemed to be the general opinion of the speakers who took part in the discussion of the paper, among whom were such distinguished gynaecologists as Dr. Noeggerath, Dr. A. J. C. Skene, of Brooklyn, and Dr. P. F. Mundé, editor of the *American Journal of Obstetrics*."

81. *Eagle*, March 10, 1892.

82. *Eagle*, March 11, 1892.

83. Bartlett's charge to the jury was printed in full by the *Eagle* on March 11, and in part by the *Citizen* on the same day.

84. *Citizen*, March 12, 1892.

85. During the course of the trial, one juror had developed financial hardships and was excused with the permission of both sides.

86. *Citizen*, March 12, 1892. For the report of a single juror, see *Eagle*, March 12, 1892.

87. *Eagle*, March 13, 1892.

88. Ibid., editorial page. Baldwin did file a motion for a new trial, which Judge Bartlett denied on the ruling that there were no grounds. See *Eagle*, March 14, 1892.

89. *Eagle*, March 17, 20, 1892.

90. For mention of Dixon Jones in the medical literature, see Charles P. Noble, "The Development and the Present Status of Hysterectomy for Fibro-Myomata and for Inflammation of the Uterine Appendages in America," *British Gynecological Journal* 8 (May 1887): 52; Joseph Eastman, "Uterine Fibroids," *The Cincinnati Lancet-Clinic* 33 (December 1894): 599–602; Henry McNaughton-Jones. "Presidential Address," *British Gynecological Journal* 14 (May 1898): 8–30; LeRoy Broun, "A Review of the Evolution of the Modern Surgical Treatment of Fibroid Tumors of the Uterus," *Medical Record* 70 (July 1906): 135–137; Henry C. Coe, "Endothelioma of the Ovary," *American Journal of the Medical Science* 104 (July 1892): 119; H. J. Boldt, "The Operative Treatment for Myo-Fibroma of the Uterus," *American Journal of Obstetrics* 27 (January–June 1893): 832–854; Ernest W. Cushing, "The Evolution in America of Abdominal Hysterectomy and Total Extirpation of the Uterus," *Annals of Gynaecology and Paediatry* 8 (June 1895): 579. For Dixon Jones's last publication, see "Difficulties in Microscopical Work in Smoky Cities," *Medical Record* 67 (April 1905): 667.

NOTES TO CHAPTER NINE

1. Remember the note from the treasurer of the New York Pathological Society to the chairperson of the investigating committee exclaiming that "women doctors are a nuisance."

2. Dixon Jones remained publicly grateful to these men throughout her career. As editor of the Philadelphia *Times and Register, A Weekly Journal of Medicine and Surgery*, she wrote in praise of women physicians ("Like other physicians they work unceasingly for suffering humanity in many instances without accepting the least compensation") as well as the male physicians who came to her aid ("In my troubles, of which I can truly say, 'an enemy hath done this'—it was the great and good men of the profession who stood by and helped me. My debt to them is infinite. I join the whole world in giving the good men of the medical profession their meed of praise"). See editorial, *Times and Register* 26 (December 1893): 1167–1169. For more about these professional controversies, see Chapter 4.

3. On malpractice, see J. R. Weist, "Civil Malpractice Suits," Indiana Medical Society *Transactions* 34 (1884): 132; Dr. Julius Noer, "Suits for Malpractice—Their Cause and Prevention," *Milwaukee Medical Journal* 10 (1902): 66. "In a large proportion of cases the action lies against men prominent, educated and well qualified; the inference from this fact, therefore, is that the mere possession of knowledge and professional skill is not a sufficient safeguard against the misfortune of malpractice litigation." H. B. Favill, "The Avoidance of Malpractice Litigation," State Medical Society of Wisconsin *Transactions* 25 (1892): 378. Bernard Wolff, "Protection Against Fraudulent Malpractice Suits," *Atlanta Journal Record of Medicine* 1 (1899): 82: "In some parts of the country suits against surgeons are almost as common as against railroads and other corporations, and the result has been that the physicians there are disposed to abandon surgery or to entrench themselves behind written contracts before undertaking any op-

eration." See also Kenneth De Ville, *Medical Malpractice in Nineteenth-Century America* (New York: New York Univ. Press, 1990), 221 and passim, and James Mohr, "The Emergence of Medical Malpractice in America," *Transactions & Studies of the College of Physicians of Philadelphia* 14 (1991): 1–21, and *Doctors and the Law* (New York: Oxford Univ. Press, 1993).

4. See Smith W. Bennett, "Malpractice," *Cleveland Medical Journal* 1 (August 1902): 398.

5. For a typical example of such calls to arms, see *Boston Medical and Surgical Journal* 117 (December 1887): 610, for an editorial on a recent case, "Stogdale vs. Baker."

6. A. Vanderveer, "The Medical-Legal Aspect of Abdominal Section," *Journal of the American Medical Association* 15 (July 12, 1890): 41. Vanderveer's article includes a letter he received from Dixon Jones claiming that the laws of New York afford no protection whatsoever to surgeons, who are liable to be sued for malpractice at any time (43–44).

7. William Warren Potter, "What Is the Present Medico-Legal Status of the Abdominal Surgeon?" *Journal of the American Medical Association* 15 (July 5, 1890): 13–17.

8. Ibid. Others worried about the power of newspapers as well. See Bernard Wolff, "Protection Against Fraudulent Malpractice Suits," *Atlanta Journal Record of Medicine* 1 (1899): 80: "The physician is well aware that all will read in the newspapers, with infinite relish, the sensational charges against him, while few will notice his modest rebuttal, for this is the day when the newspaper has notoriously usurped the honorable function of the jury"; Milo Buel Ward, "A Plea for More Surgery in Chronic Disease of Female Pelvic Organs," *Denver Medical Times* 15 (February 1896): 307.

9. *Brooklyn Medical Journal* 5 (1891): 726–727; Edwin A. Lewis, "Influence of Public Opinion on Surgical Practice," ibid., 258, 259.

10. "Malpractice Suits and the Remedy," *Pennsylvania Medical Journal* 1 (1897): 297.

11. Noer, "Suits for Malpractice," 66. See also Lucius Wenschenk, "Malpractice," *Daniel's Texas Medical Journal* 5 (1889–90): 217–218.

12. The ensuring discussion on the expert witness is wholly informed by Mohr, *Doctors & the Law*, esp. 34, 197–199.

13. Ibid., 3.

14. Quoted in ibid., 197.

15. Ibid., 198–199; *Boston Medical and Surgical Journal* quoted on 198.

16. Mohr, 198–199; March 12, 1892.

17. Clark Gapen, "Legal Criticism of Medical Expert Evidence," *Journal of the American Medical Association* 21 (September 23, 1893): 452.

18. See Donald B. Pritchard, "Malpractice Suits. How Best to Protect Ourselves Against Them," *St. Paul Medical Journal* 2 (1900): 444–448; "Malpractice Defense and Its Success," Miscellany Section, *Journal of the American Medical Association* 42 (April 23, 1904): 1092.

19. "The Rights and Duties of Medical Witnesses," *Journal of the American Medical Association* 24 (January 12, 1895): 47–52. See also John A. Sterling, Esq., "The Medical Expert Witness," *Journal of the American Medical Association* 22 (March 17, 1894): 377–382; Morris Fishbein, *A History of the American Medical Association, 1847–1947* (Philadelphia: W. B. Saunders, 1947), 107.

20. See *Brooklyn Medical Journal* 3 (May 1889): 326–333; (June 1889): 435–436; 5 (January 1891): 14–25; editorial, "What Is an Expert?," 7 (February 1893): 375–376;

Landon Carter Gray, "Suggestions for a New Method of Taking Expert Testimony," *New York Medical Journal* 57 (May 20, 1893): 547–550.

21. *Eagle*, February 19, March 9, 1892. We are reminded, of course, of the Imlach affair, discussed in Chapter 4, which pitted followers of Lawson Tait against followers of Spencer Wells. See Ornella Moscucci, *The Science of Woman* (New York: Cambridge Univ. Press, 1990), 160–164.

22. F. J. Groner, "The Causes and the Remedies of Suits for Malpractice," *Medical Record* 39 (August 1890): 144. David W. Cheever, "Surgical Morals," *Boston Medical and Surgical Journal* 134 (March 12, 1896): 281.

23. Joseph Price, "Analysis of Fifteen Months' Work in the Gynecean Hospital, Philadelphia," *Annals of Gynecology* 31 (February 1890): 213–214. Paul Mundé didn't like to say the word "operation" to his patients, arguing that many "shrink from the mere word . . . as they would from a pestilence." He preferred always to qualify the statement that an operation was necessary "by omitting that word, and speaking of 'closing up' or 'sewing a tear,' until the patient has become accustomed to the idea." Many a patient had been frightened away "by incautiously telling her that an 'operation' would have to be performed." See Mundé, *Minor Surgical Gynecology. A Manual of Uterine Diagnosis and the Lesser Technicalities of Gynecological Practice for the Use of the Advanced Student and General Practitioner* (New York: William Wood, 1890), 7. By 1905, Henry J. Garrigues, a prominent New York physician, claimed in his text-book, *Medical and Surgical Outlines for Students and Practitioners* (Philadelphia: J. B. Lippincott, 1905), 326, that "the law requires the operator to obtain the patient's consent to remove her ovaries. Otherwise he is guilty of mayhem and liable to a suit for damages." He did not mean a formal state law, but referred to how malpractice decisions were being decided in court. For clarification of the evolution of these ideas, see Martin Pernick, "The Patient's Role in Medical Decisionmaking: A Social History of Informed Consent in Medical Therapy," President's Commission for the Study of Ethical Problems in Medicine and Biomedical and Behavioral Research, *Making Health Care Decisions: The Ethical and Legal Implications of Informed Consent in the Patient-Practitioner Relationship* (Government Printing Office, 1982) 3: 1–35,

24. *Journal of the American Medical Association* 18 (April 1892): 431–432.

25. *Eagle*, March 15, 1892.

26. Ibid.

27. Ibid.

28. *Eagle*, February 20, 1892. See especially the testimony of Mrs. Elkins.

29. David Rosner, *A Once Charitable Enterprise: Hospitals & Health Care in Brooklyn & New York, 1885–1915* (New York: Cambridge Univ. Press, 1982), 22–23. See also Charles Rosenberg, *The Care of Strangers: The Rise of America's Hospital System* (New York: Basic Books, 1987), 262–286.

30. Ibid. Rosner, *A Once Charitable Enterprise*, 22–23.

31. Athena Vrettos, *Somatic Fictions: Imagining Illness in Victorian Culture* (Stanford: Stanford Univ. Press, 1995), 82–83. There is evidence that women formed a significant portion of the audience during this period at court proceedings with gendered themes. Their attendance at the Dixon Jones trial had other analogues: Women packed the courtroom at the murder trial of Dr. Thomas Neill Cream, the notorious poisoner of prostitutes, for example, and attended faithfully the trial of Madame Cailleux, the wife of a powerful French cabinet minister, who shot and killed the editor of Le Figaro for slandering her husband. See Edward Berenson, *The Trial of Madame Caillaux* (Berkeley: Univ. of California Press, 1992), 15, 122–132, 164–166, 240–244; Angus McLaren, *A Prescription for Murder: The Victorian Serial Killings of Dr. Thomas Neill Cream* (Chi-

cago: Univ. of Chicago Press, 1993), 53. In contrast, though the audience was respectable and the courtroom "tightly packed," only nine women, some of them the defendant's relatives, attended the trial of the assassin Guiteau, a mentally unbalanced misfit who shot president James Garfield in 1881. See Charles Rosenberg, *The Trial of the Assassin Guiteau* (Chicago Univ. of Chicago Press, 1968), 11.

32. Nancy Theriot has cogently argued that the generation of women who came to age in the last two decades of the nineteenth century were less willing than their mothers to accept the physical suffering of their reproductive lives as an uncontested part of the burdens of womanhood. See *Mothers & Daughters in Nineteenth-Century America: The Biosocial Construction of Femininity*, rev. ed. (Lexington: Univ. of Kentucky Press, 1996), 80–81.

33. Quote from David Scobey, "Nymphs and Satyrs: Sex and the Bourgeois Public Sphere in Victorian New York," paper delivered at the Newberry Library, Chicago, November, 1995, 36.

34. *Eagle*, March 10, 1892.

35. Helpful in understanding this process is A. Cheree Carlson, "The Role of Character in Public Moral Argument: Henry Ward Beecher and the Brooklyn Scandal," *Quarterly Journal of Speech* 77 (February 1991): 38–52.

36. *Eagle*, March 14, 1892.

37. For Americans' generally positive views of technology and science, especially in the nineteenth century, see Howard P. Segal, *Technological Utopianism in American Culture* (Chicago: Univ. of Chicago Press, 1985), esp. 19–98, and Segal, *Future Imperfect* (Amherst: Univ. of Massachusetts Press, 1994).

38. Sherlock Holmes novels remained high on American best-sellers lists throughout this period. The Dr. Jekyll and Mr. Hyde metaphor was an available one, and was used by the prosecuting attorney at the Lizzie Borden trial. Indeed, theatrical adaptations of Robert Louis Stevenson's compelling novel, especially one written by T. R. Sullivan and performed by Richard Mansfield, apparently remained popular for a couple of years after the play debuted in May 1887 in Boston. "The Biggest Hits of the Old Days: The Most Popular Plays and Musical Comedies of the American State," Boston *Post*, December 10, 1933. Cara W. Robertson, "Representing 'Miss Lizzie': Cultural Convictions in the Trial of Lizzie Borden," *Yale Journal of Law & Humanities* 8 (Summer 1996): 351–417. For a terrific "medical science gone mad" short story written by a woman doctor, see "The Genius Maker," by Dr. Eleanor M. Hiestand-Moore, Woman's Medical College of Pennsylvania class of 1890, in *Daughters of Aesculapius: Stories Written by Alumnae and Students of the Woman's Medical College of Pennsylvania*, (Philadelphia: George W. Jacobs, 1897). The Brooklyn *Citizen*'s reference to scandalous real-life and literary figures of contemporary French and English culture such as "Madame Chouseuse," "Mere Frochard," and "Jack the Ripper" suggests that Americans were aware of a range of such cultural markers. See *Citizen*, June 8, 1889. Although the *Eagle* did not oppose vivisection and the word does not appear once in its reports of the trial, the antivivisectionist controversy should also be considered a significant cultural referent for some of the negative images of Dixon Jones produced at the trial. Both in the United States and in England the antivivisection movement, which argued that men who tortured animals to advance scientific knowledge were morally corrupt and corrupting, attracted a large percentage of female supporters and was associated as well with opposition to gynecological surgery. Analogies were drawn repeatedly between suffering animals and suffering women.

39. See Mary S. Hartman, *Victorian Murderesses: A True History of Thirteen Respectable French and English Women Accused of Unspeakable Crimes* (New York:

Schocken Books, 1977), 13–42, 215–254, and, on the "crime of passion," 239; Ruth Harris, *Murders and Madness: Medicine, Law, and Society in the Fin de Siècle* (Oxford: Clarendon Press, 1989), 208–242.

40. For a fascinating study of the various negative images of women produced at the end of the nineteenth century from which the *Eagle* drew some of its literary conventions, see Bram Dijkstra, *Idols of Perversity: Fantasies of Feminine Evil in Fin-de-Siècle Culture* (New York: Oxford Univ. Press, 1986), 162, 331–332, passim. I have been able to find only one trial in the United States in this period in which the defense included a version of the crime of passion argument in its English and French incarnation, but I am convinced that these ideas about potential loss of will among females pervaded public notions of femininity in this country as well as in England and France. In studying the Lizzie Borden trial, for example, Cara W. Robertson makes a strong case for the argument that in the American courtroom, a powerful medical-criminological model of womanhood, fashioned by scientists, biologists, criminologists, and physicians in the United States and Europe during this period, argued that "pathological femininity always underlies the norm." Whereas working-class women were inherently depraved, the peculiarities of female biology meant that genteel, middle-class women could also temporarily lose their minds when particular biological and social conditions came into play simultaneously. The crime of passion is just one version of this larger argument. See Robertson, "Lizzie Borden," 415, 375–391. For an unconventional crime of passion, that of a woman killing her female lover because she feared that she would lose her, see Lisa J. Lindquist, "Images of Alice: Gender, Deviancy, and a Love Murder in Memphis," *Journal of the History of Sexuality* 6 (July 1995): 30–61. For a wonderfully suggestive article on lawyers' constructions of male defendants who murdered their wives' lovers in the Victorian period, see Hendrik Hartog, "Lawyering, Husbands' Rights, and 'the Unwritten Law' in Nineteenth-Century America," *Journal of American History* 64 (June 1997): 67–96. Hartog's piece indirectly tells us how little historical work has been done on trials of this sort and how fruitful such research might be. It is also interesting to note that Mark Twain and Charles Dudley Warner savagely critiqued the "crime of passion" defense and the social penchant for sentimentality that tolerated it in their novel, *The Gilded Age: A Tale of Today*, published in 1873. See Laura Hanft Korobkin, "The Maintenance of Mutual Confidence: Sentimental Strategies at the Adultery Trial of Henry Ward Beecher," *Yale Journal of Law & the Humanities* 7 (Winter 1995): 1–48, 41–44.

41. See McLaren, *Prescription for Murder*; Richard Wightman Fox, "Intimacy on Trial: Cultural Meanings of the Beecher-Tilton Affair," in Fox and T. J. Jackson Lears, *The Power of Culture* (Chicago: Univ. of Chicago Press, 1993); Altina Waller, *The Reverend Beecher and Mrs. Tilton* (Amherst: Amherst Univ. Press, 1982). On the Alice Mitchell trial, see Lisa J. Lindquist, "Images of Alice," and Lisa Duggan, "The Trials of Alice Mitchell: Sensationalism, Sexology, and the Lesbian Subject in Turn-of-the-Century America," *Signs* 18 (Summer 1991): 791–814. See also Hartog for three sensational murder-scandals, the Sickles-Key, Cole-Hiscock, and McFarland-Richardson trials, all of which became major media events. George Cooper also covers the McFarland-Richardson affair in *Lost Love: A True Story of Passion, Murder, and Justice in Old New York* (New York: Random House, 1994). For the arrest of Madame Restell, the famous abortionist, see Eric Homberger, *Scenes from the Life of a City: Corruption and Conscience in Old New York* (New Haven: Yale Univ. Press, 1994). For the murder of the robber baron Jim Fiske by Edward Stokes for love and money, see W. A. Swanberg, *Jim Fisk: The Career of an Improbable Rascal* (New York: Scribner's, 1959).

42. See Scobey, "Nymphs and Satyrs," 36, and McClaren, *Prescription for Murder*, 91.

43. The phrase is David Scobey's ("Nymphs and Satyrs," 38).

44. Brooklyn *Eagle*, February 6, 9, March 10, 1892.

45. Leslie Arey, *Northwestern University Medical School, 1859–1959: A Pioneer in Educational Reform* (Evanston and Chicago: Northwestern Univ. Press, 1959), 409–410. I am grateful to Tom Bonner for pointing out the parallels between Dixon Jones and Murphy.

46. See M. M. Ravitch, *A Century of Surgery* (Philadelphia: Lippincott, 1981), 209; Robert Schmitz and Timothy T. Oh, eds., *The Remarkable Surgical Practice of John Benjamin Murphy* (Urbana and Chicago: Univ. of Illinois Press, 1993), 3; Loyal Davis, *J. B. Murphy: Stormy Petrel of Surgery* (New York: Putnam, 1938), 198.

47. Schmitz and Oh, eds., *Remarkable Practice*, 3.

48. See works cited in n. 46, above, plus Sir Berkeley Moynihan, "John B. Murphy—Surgeon," in *Surgery, Genecology and Obstetrics* 31 (December 1920): 549–573.

49. *Eagle*, February 5, 1892.

50. See Deborah Tannenbaum, "Earnestness, Temperance, Industry: The Definition and Uses of Professional Character among Nineteenth-Century American Physicians," *Journal of the History of Medicine and Allied Sciences* 49 (April 1994): 251–283. She argues that the issues for both male and female physicians were also about the changing meaning of "character." See the testimony of Eliza Mosher and Lucy Hall Brown in *Eagle*, February 19, 1892. Mosher to Blackwell, November 3, 1883, Mosher MSS, Bentley Library, University of Michigan, Ann Arbor. The Mosher letter does not specifically mention Dixon Jones by name, but she was the only woman presenting at the Pathological Society at this time, and internal evidence suggests that Mosher is referring to her. For biographical information on Mosher and Lucy Hall Brown, see Regina Morantz-Sanchez, *Sympathy and Science: Women Physicians in American Medicine* (New York: Oxford Univ. Press, 1985), 152, 118–20, 156–158. A sketch of Brown can also be found in Irving Watson, *Physicians and Surgeons of America* (Concord, N.H.: Republican Press, 1896), 74–75, and of Mosher, ibid., 299.

51. For an interesting discussion of the various meanings of the term "sympathy" and the entrance into medical discourse at the end of the nineteenth century of the term "empathy," see Ellen More, "Empathy Enters the Profession of Medicine" and Regina Morantz-Sanchez, "The Gendering of Empathy: Late Nineteenth-Century Concepts of Medical Practice and Ideas of the Good Practitioner," in Ellen More and Maureen Mulligan, eds., *The Empathic Practitioner: Empathy, Gender, and the Therapeutic Relationship* (New Brunswick, N.J.: Rutgers Univ. Press, 1994), and Regina Morantz-Sanchez, "Feminist Theory and Historical Practice: Rereading Elizabeth Blackwell," *History and Theory*, Beiheft 31 (December 1992): 51–69.

52. *Eagle*, May 11, 1889. It might be worth mentioning here that an exploration of late nineteenth-century novels about women doctors yielded only one that represented a woman physician passionate about the pursuit of science. This is the character of Dr. Mary Prance, described in Henry James's *The Bostonians* as "spare, dry, hard, without a curve." Not a surgeon, Dr. Prance is preoccupied by research (*The Bostonians*, ed. Daniel Aaron (London: J. M. Dent, 1886), 37, 314). In all the other novels consulted, the female physicians are quite young and feminine, the plots rather sentimentalized. Most of them are described as intelligent and beautiful, romantically desirable, and often one of the central dilemmas is choosing between profession and love/marriage. The youth and beauty of these characters, the fact that each of them is described as thoroughly ladylike, suggest that there were no positive representations of a figure of Mary Dixon

Jones's age and interests to be found in the popular literature. See Louisa May Alcott, *Jo's Boys and How They Turned Out* (Boston: Little Brown, 1886); William Dean Howells, *Doctor Breen's Practice* (Boston: James R. Osgood, 1882); Graham Travers (Margaret Georgina Todd), *Mona MacLean, Medical Student* (London: William Blackwood, 1892); G. G. Alexander, *Doctor Victoria: A Picture from the Period* (London: Samuel Tinsley, 1880); Elizabeth Stuart Phelps, *Dr. Zay* (Boston: Houghton, Mifflin, 1882); Anonymous (Annie Nathan Meyer), *Helen Brent, M.D.* (New York: Cassell Publishing, 1892); Sarah Orne Jewett, *A Country Doctor* (Boston: Houghton, Mifflin, 1884). For a more general discussion of late-nineteenth-century representations of women physicians, see Lilian R. Furst, "Halfway Up the Hill: Doctresses in Late-Nineteenth-Century American Fiction," in Lilian R. Furst, ed., *Women Healers & Physicians: Climbing a Long Hill* (Lexington: Univ. of Kentucky Press, 1997).

53. Editorial, "Who Was She?" in *Philadelphia Times and Register* 26 (December 16, 1893): 1169. A week earlier in the same publication she wrote, "If by joining the medical profession woman is transformed into a heartless wretch, deaf to the cry of suffering, then let medicine remain in the hands of men," ibid. 26 (December 2, 1893): 1093–1094.

54. See editorial, *Woman's Medical Journal* 2 (January 1894): 10; 4 (October 1895): 278; and "Women Physicians and Surgeons: Biographical Series" 4 (December 1895): 306–309.

55. Laura Hanft Korobkin, "Sentimental Strategies at the Beecher Trial," 10. See also Bernard S. Jackson, "Narrative Theories and Legal Discourse," in Christopher Nash, ed., *Narrative in Culture: The Uses of Storytelling in the Sciences, Philosophy, and Literature* (New York: Routledge, 1990), 23–50; W. Lance Bennett and Martha S. Feldman, *Reconstructing Reality in the Courtroom: Justice and Judgment in American Culture* (New Brunswick: Rutgers Univ. Press, 1981); Nancy Pennington and Reid Hastie, "A Cognitive Theory of Juror Decision Making: The Story Model," *Cardozo Law Review* 13 (November 1991): 519–557; and Janice Schuetz and Kathryn Holmes Snedaker, *Communication and Litigation: Case Studies of Famous Trials* (Carbondale: Southern Illinois Univ. Press, 1988).

56. Korobkin, 11.

57. Ibid., 14–15.

58. It is worth mentioning here how important the trial behavior of key litigants was, even in the nineteenth century. Cara Robertson points out that in the Lizzie Borden trial, Borden's ladylike demeanor and dignified silences worked well in convincing the jury that a young lady of her refinement and self-effacing qualities simply could not have committed such a heinous crime as patricide. See Robertson, "Representing 'Miss Lizzie," 352–353.

59. In her insightful analysis of the Tilton-Beecher trial, Korobkin makes an excellent case for the power of the sentimental narrative in Victorian culture in general and argues persuasively that its ability to move audiences, including juries, was an important factor in that case. There is no reason that her insights about the significance of sentimentality as a familiar cultural trope cannot also be applied to the Dixon Jones affair; indeed, the use of it by both sides is clearly apparent. Korobkin, "Sentimental Strategies," 13–36.

Index

Dixon Jones, Mary: accomplishments/success of, 80, 114–15, 168, 209, 211–12, 213, 214; ambition of, 61, 209; biography of, 9–10, 23, 62, 167–68, 170, 212; death of, 5, 194; early career of, 62–65; education/on the job learning of, 62–69, 167–68; family of, 62; importance of story of, 7–9, 10, 79, 112, 135–36, 195–214; as mother, 30–31, 168, 182, 207; post-trial years of, 4–5, 194, 212; as social counterfeit, 60; uniqueness of career of, 88

Dobson, George, 169, 173

Doctor-patient relationship: and authority of physicians, 153–55; and cultural/social image of women, 143, 145; and female bodies, 153–55; and finding a doctor, 139–42; and libel case, 6, 59, 184; and moral values, 98; motherhood as metaphor in, 98; and patient acquiescence, 153–54; and patients' frustrations with doctors, 142; as power relationship, 115, 145–55; role of choice in, 146, 155; and validation by physicians, 155; women's self-reported symptoms as basis of, 107. *See also* Informed consent; Patients

Domesticity, 7, 98

Donohue, Newcombe and Cardoza, 34

Dorsey, Nellie, 149

Douglas, Richard, 103

Drury, George, 185

Dudley, Augustus P., 150, 184

Dudley, E.C., 68

Dykman, Mr., 166–67, 170–72, 174, 177, 186

The Eagle and Brooklyn (Brooklyn *Daily Eagle*), 39–40, 58–59

Earle, Charles Warrington, 66

Ectopic pregnancy, 92

Edis, Arthur, 116

Education: of Dixon Jones, 62–69, 167–68; on the job learning as, 65–69; nursing, 71; of women, 121, 122, 123, 124, 126–27

Edwards, C.H., 32

Eisenhut, Mrs., 152

Eisenhut, Theodore, 149

Electricity: as therapy, 101, 125

Elites, 14, 39–42, 59–60, 196, 204, 205

Elkins, Horatio B., 28, 33, 183

Emerich, Mina, 32, 142

Emery, Z. Taylor, 25, 176, 178

Emmet, Thomas Addis, 63, 69, 108, 120–22, 124, 125, 126, 129, 133

Empathy, 98

Endothelioma, 78, 79, 186, 187

England: Dixon Jones visit to, 128

Epilepsy, 127

Etheridge, J.H., 199

Europe: Dixon Joneses' tour of, 76–77, 128

Everson, George, 160

Ewing, James, 77

Expert testimony, 174–78, 184–88, 192, 196, 199–202, 203, 206–7

Exploratory surgery, 99–100, 128–29, 187

Fallopian tubes, 116, 127, 133

Fees, 23, 32, 33, 142, 149–50, 152, 153

Female body: and definitions of femininity, 115–19; disease as external to, 145–46; Dixon Jones's views about, 126–30; and doctor-patient relationship, 153–55; gynecological constructs of, 114–37; holistic versus localist views, 134–35; inherent health of, 132–33; and meaning of libel case, 6, 206–7; medical science constructs of, 115–19; as metaphor for Brooklyn, 206–7; new knowledge regarding, 7. *See also* Reproductive system

Female reform community, 8, 63, 64

Female reproductive system. *See* Reproductive system

Femininity: definitions of, 115–19; of Dixon Jones, 80, 187–88, 210–11; and meaning of libel case, 208, 210–11; pathology of, 116; social conceptions of, 112–13; and style, 197

Fibroids/fibroid tumors, 69, 77, 95–96, 100–101, 110, 113, 116, 131–32. *See also* Myomectomy

Fisher, Mrs., 147

Fixing/staining techniques, 109

Flint, Austin, 122

Foote, Edward, 19

Fowler, George R., 140, 142, 158

Fox, George Henry, 175

Fraud, 163, 167, 171, 177. *See also* Mishandling of funds

Frederick, Carlton C., 111

Freeman, Dr., 177–78

French, Mrs., 141

Fullerton, Anna, 124, 125, 126

Galbraith, Anna, 124

Gale, Annie, 18–19, 142, 148, 149, 181

Garrigues, Henry, 174–75

Gearon, Mary, 141, 158, 160

Gedney, Mrs., 184

Gender: and character, 210; definitions of, 119; Dixon Jones's ideology of, 136; ideological work of, 117; and libel case, 6, 188–90, 196, 207–11; and narratives of illness, 142–

22, 96, 196–203; specialization in, 43–46; values in, 42–46. *See also* Brooklyn physicians; Male physicians; Physicians; Professionalism; Women physicians
Medical schools: lack of first-rate, 45. *See also* Medical education; *specific institution*
Medical societies, 203
Meigs, Charles D., 92
Memmem, Emma, 148, 149, 152–53
Menstruation, 106, 113, 116, 144
Mentors, 66, 67, 70
Mergler, Marie, 66
Merritt, John, 72
Microscope, 77–78, 79, 80, 95, 102–3, 104, 109, 128, 130, 185, 187
Middle class: aspirations of, 172–73; birth rates among, 127; in Brooklyn, 39–42, 46–49, 60, 172–73, 196, 205, 213; characteristics of nineteenth century, 7–8; and charity, 172–73, 203–4; concerns about health and illness of, 116; Dixon Jones as role model for women of, 8–9; and Dixon Jones as social counterfeit, 60; and libel case, 172–73, 213; and meaning of libel case, 7–9, 196, 205; policing of, 205; and politics, 46–49; and self-advertisement of Dixon Jones, 152–53; social responsibility of, 196, 203–7
Miller, Charles E., 159
Miller, Mrs. Oliver P., 33–34, 141–42, 181
Miller, Oliver P., 20, 169
Millette, Sarah J., 28, 183
Ministers, 40. *See also specific person*
Mishandling of funds, 27, 167, 179, 191, 204, 211
Mismanagement: of Woman's Hospital of Brooklyn, 27, 166
Misrepresentation, 14–18, 71, 167, 171, 189, 191
Mitchinson, Wendy, 116
Mitigation: and libel case, 171–72, 173, 191
Moffat, Reuben C., 24, 209
Money: Dixon Jones concern about, 152. *See also* Fees; Income
Moore, Alice, 146
Morality, 59, 98, 108–9, 117–18
Morris, Robert T., 33, 72, 161, 185, 186, 196
Mortalities: among Dixon Jones patients, 170; from fibroid tumors, 100; from laparotomies, 160; from myomectomy, 100–101; from ovariotomies, 31, 92, 96; following surgical gynecology, 96; at Woman's Hospital of Brooklyn, 27, 31
Mosher, Eliza, 136, 210, 214
Moss, John C., 28, 33

Motherhood, 115–16, 182–83, 207, 212
Mundé, Paul F., 25, 33, 75, 100, 105
Murphy, James, 135
Murphy, John Benjamin, 209–10
Myoma, 20
Myomectomy, 100–101, 110

Narratives: of illness, 142–44, 181
Nash, Helen, 146
Nash, Mrs. W.R., 26–27
Neighbors, 20–21, 23–24, 26, 172, 173, 182–83, 190
"Neuromimesis," 206
New York Academy of Medicine, 104
New York City: Brooklyn compared with, 36, 38, 41, 42, 206; Brooklyn's rivalry with, 106–7, 204; merger of Brooklyn and, 55–56
New York Infirmary for Women and Children, 64, 66
New York Medical Journal, 75, 187
New York Medical Record, 104, 163–64, 197
New York Obstetrical Society, 71, 74
New York Pathological Society, 68, 73, 77, 101, 104, 163, 173
New York *Times*, 54–55, 58
New York *Tribune*, 4, 33, 58
New York *World*, 4, 13, 33, 52–53, 54, 55, 56, 58
Newcombe, Richard S., 28–29, 34, 158, 159–60
Newman, Henry Parker, 134
News crusades, 53
Newspapers, 49–55, 107. *See also* Press; Reporters; *specific newspaper*
Noble, Charles P., 110, 133–35, 150
Nurses, 71, 160
Nymphomania, 118

O'Brien, William, 182
Obstetricians, 68, 69
Obstetrics and Gynecology (journal), 112
Ochs, Adolph, 54, 55
Offeldt, Augusta, 141, 146
Olsen, Nurse, 149, 159, 160
On the job learning, 65–69
Oöphorectomy, 100
Operations. *See* Surgery; Unnecessary surgery
Otterson, Andrew, 176
Ovarian cysts, 91, 94–95, 116
Ovaries: criteria for performing surgery on, 95; and Dixon Jones's surgery, 127; extirpated, 109; and hysterical symptoms, 125; and reflex theory, 121–22; as site of most disorders, 116; suppurating, 133. *See also* Hysterectomy; Ovarian cysts; Ovariotomies

T., Mrs. (case study), 143
Tait, Lawson: cited in Dixon Jones
  publications, 73–74, 75, 76, 79, 128; as
  consultant for Woman's Hospital of
  Brooklyn, 22, 209; and diagnosis, 99–100,
  109; Dixon Jones's admiration for, 72, 73–
  74, 76, 79, 128; Dixon Jones
  correspondence with, 75, 170; Dixon Jones
  as validation for, 76, 136; and emergence of
  gynecology, 90; and exploratory surgery,
  128–29, 187; and Imlach Affair, 127, 128;
  operation techniques of, 73–94, 96, 100,
  104, 109; and ovariotomies, 95, 99, 100;
  overcharging by, 152; as radical surgeon,
  185, 190; and unnecessary operations, 105;
  U.S. trip of, 72
Taylor, William R., 183
Tenney, A.W., 23–24, 173, 182, 183
Testimonials, 26–27, 32, 33, 146, 152–53, 155,
  160–61, 212
Theriot, Nancy, 145
Thomas, M. Carey, 123
Thomas, T. Gaillard, 12, 92, 99, 105, 140,
  184
Thompson, John B., 50, 51
Thompson, Kate, 148, 150
Thompson, Mary, 66
Trachtenberg, Alan, 50
Trials: as forum for competing stories, 212–13;
  as history, 6; meaning of sensational, 195;
  sensational Victorian, 208; use of specimens
  in, 185, 186–87, 198. See also Expert
  testimony
Trustees: and meaning of libel trial, 204; and
  patient treatment, 205; physician clashes
  with, 40; for Woman's Hospital of
  Brooklyn, 15, 16, 17, 18, 23, 25, 27–28, 71,
  170, 172–73, 189
Tumors: complaints about, 116; fibroid, 69, 77,
  95, 100-101, 131–32; malignant, 19, 20–21;
  origins of, 120; techniques for removal of,
  96
Tweeddale, Euphemia, 20, 22–23, 24, 141,
  149, 152, 192
Tyng, Anita E., 66

Undertakers: and Bates case, 19
University Medical College in New York, 91
Unnecessary surgery: Brooklyn Daily Eagle
  charges of, 3, 14, 18–22, 24–26, 107, 162;
  criticisms about, 105–6; and libel case, 129,
  181, 185, 189, 201, 211; moral concerns
  about, 108–9; and radical versus
  conservative surgeons, 201; and women
  physicians, 72, 76, 108

Unprofessional conduct, 14, 22–26, 176, 177–
  78, 181, 191
Uterus, 76, 91, 96, 100, 109, 116, 132, 142.
  See also Fibroids/fibroid tumors;
  Hysterectomy

Vaginal speculum, 94
Values: in Brooklyn elites, 39–42; in medical
  profession, 42–46; scientific, 196. See also
  Morality
Van Anden, Isaac, 56
Van Benshoten, Harriet, 182
Van Cott, Joshua M., 78–79, 185, 186–87
Van de Warker, Ely, 91, 96, 108, 113, 117,
  129
Van Wyck, Augustus, 17–18
Vanderveer, Albert, 197–98
Venereal disease, 13, 133, 146, 159, 161
Vesico-vaginal fistula, 93–94
Vibert, Mary, 140–41
Virtue, female, 117–18
Vivisection, 21, 107–8
Vrettos, Athena, 206

Waite, Lucy, 66
Walker, Jerome, 176
Wallace, William, 177–78
Walsh, Margaret, 32, 147
Water cure, 63, 64
Weisberger, Bernard, 53
Welch, William, 104
Wells, Spencer, 22, 75, 76, 90, 96, 99, 103,
  104, 127, 128
Westbook, Dr., 140
Westbrook, Dr. B.F., 74, 140, 141
Wheeler, John B., 33–34, 67, 141–42
White, S.V., 15
Williams, Herbert E., 158
Williams, Inspector, 169
Williams, Mrs., 149
Wilson, Benjamin B., 63, 66
Wilson, Janice, 73
Winckel, Franz von, 76
Woman's Homeopathic Hospital of Brooklyn,
  16
Woman's Hospital of Brooklyn: advisory
  board for, 15, 18, 174, 189; Brooklyn Daily
  Eagle exposé about, 11–13; class of patients
  at, 38; Committee of Five report about, 27–
  28, 33; consulting staff for, 22, 25–26, 33,
  46, 170, 173, 175, 176, 189, 209;
  disbanding of, 212; Dixon Jones's prepared
  statement about, 15–16, 17; first (1881), 17,
  23, 32, 46, 71, 168, 176, 179, 183, 184, 204;
  founding of, 23, 46; history of, 17, 18, 27;